CONTRIBUTORS

J. Abraham

C. C. Bartley

Gary C. Chamness

Mark E. Costlow

Wayne E. Criss

Roy O. Greep

John G. Hemington

Russell Hilf

Patricia M. Hinkle

Howard T. Hinshaw

Nobuyuki Kadohama

Kathryn F. Lanoue

Tehming Liang

Shutsung Liao

William L. McGuire

Harold P. Morris

William R. Moyle

Margit M. K. Nass

Robert L. Ney

Tomoko Ohnishi

Roland A. Pattillo

Roger E. Shepherd

Armen H. Tashjian, Jr.

Roger W. Turkington

John R. Williamson

James L. Wittliff

HORMONES AND CANCER

HORMONES AND CANCER

EDITED BY

KENNETH W. McKERNS

Department of Obstetrics and Gynecology
The J. Hillis Miller Health Center
University of Florida
Gainesville, Florida

ACADEMIC PRESS   New York and London   1974
A Subsidiary of Harcourt Brace Jovanovich, Publishers

ACADEMIC PRESS, INC.
111 Fifth Avenue, New York, New York 10003

United Kingdom Edition published by
ACADEMIC PRESS, INC. (LONDON) LTD.
24/28 Oval Road, London NW1

Library of Congress Cataloging in Publication Data

McKerns, Kenneth W
        Hormones and cancer.

        Includes bibliographies.
        1.   Glands, Ductless—Cancer.   2.   Hormones.
3.   Oncology, Experimental.   I.   Title.   [DNLM: 1.   Endocrine glands—Pathology.   2.   Neoplasms—Physiopathology.   QZ200 M159h 1974]
RC280.E55M32   616.9′94′4   74-1634
ISBN 0—12—485350—1

CONTENTS

Chapter VIII   Receptors and Mechanisms of Action of Androgens in Prostates

Shutsung Liao and Tehming Liang

Chapter IX   Structure, Synthesis, and Transcription of Mitochondrial DNA in Normal, Malignant, and Drug-Treated Cells

Margit M. K. Nass

Chapter X   Abnormal Hormonal Control in the Neoplastic Adrenal Cortex

Howard T. Hinshaw and Robert L. Ney

Chapter XI   **Steroid-Secreting Tumors as Models in Endocrinology**
                      William R. Moyle and Roy O. Greep

Chapter XII   **Endocrine and Immunological Factors in Trophoblast Cancers**
                      Roland A. Pattillo

LIST OF CONTRIBUTORS

Numbers in parentheses indicate the pages on which the authors' contributions begin.

S. ABRAHAM (29), Bruce Lyon Memorial Research Laboratory, Children's Hospital Medical Center of Northern California, Oakland, California

J. C. BARTLEY (29), Bruce Lyon Memorial Research Laboratory, Children's Hospital Medical Center of Northern California, Oakland, California

GARY C. CHAMNESS (75), Department of Physiology and Medicine, University of Texas Medical School, San Antonio, Texas

MARK E. COSTLOW (75), Department of Medicine, University of Texas Medical School, San Antonio, Texas

WAYNE E. CRISS (169), Department of Obstetrics and Gynecology, University of Florida College of Medicine, Gainesville, Florida

ROY O. GREEP (329), Laboratory of Human Reproduction and Reproductive Biology, Harvard Medical School, Boston, Massachusetts

JOHN G. HEMINGTON (131), Department of Physiology, Northwestern University Medical School, Chicago, Illinois

RUSSELL HILF (103), Department of Biochemistry, University of Rochester School of Medicine, Rochester, New York

PATRICIA M. HINKLE (203), Laboratory of Pharmacology, Harvard School of Dental Medicine, and Department of Pharmacology, Harvard Medical School, Boston, Massachusetts

HOWARD T. HINSHAW* (309), Department of Medicine, University of North Carolina School of Medicine, Chapel Hill, North Carolina

NOBUYUKI KADOHAMA† (1), Department of Medicine, University of Wisconsin Medical School, Madison, Wisconsin

* Present address: The Nalle Clinic, Charlotte, North Carolina.
† Present address: Department of Clinical Biochemistry, Banting Institute, University of Toronto, Toronto, Ontario, Canada.

KATHRYN F. LANOUE (131), Johnson Research Foundation, University of Pennsylvania, Philadelphia, Pennsylvania

TEHMING LIANG (229), Ben May Laboratory for Cancer Research and the Department of Biochemistry, The University of Chicago, Chicago, Illinois

SHUTSUNG LIAO (229), Ben May Laboratory for Cancer Research and the Department of Biochemistry, The University of Chicago, Chicago, Illinois

WILLIAM L. MCGUIRE (75), Department of Medicine, University of Texas Medical School, San Antonio, Texas

HAROLD P. MORRIS (131), Department of Biochemistry, Cancer Research Unit, College of Medicine, Howard University, Washington, D. C.

WILLIAM R. MOYLE (329), Laboratory of Human Reproduction and Reproductive Biology and Department of Biological Chemistry, Harvard Medical School, Boston, Massachusetts

MARGIT M. K. NASS (261), Department of Therapeutic Research, University of Pennsylvania School of Medicine, Philadelphia, Pennsylvania

ROBERT L. NEY (309), Department of Medicine, University of North Carolina School of Medicine, Chapel Hill, North Carolina

TOMOKO OHNISHI (131), Johnson Research Foundation, University of Pennsylvania, Philadelphia, Pennsylvania

ROLAND A. PATTILLO (363), Cancer Research and Reproductive Endocrinology Laboratories, Department of Gynecology and Obstetrics, Medical College of Wisconsin, Milwaukee, Wisconsin

ROGER E. SHEPHERD (75), Department of Physiology and Medicine, University of Texas Medical School, San Antonio, Texas

ARMEN H. TASHJIAN, JR. (203), Laboratory of Pharmacology, Harvard School of Dental Medicine, and Department of Pharmacology, Harvard Medical School, Boston, Massachusetts

ROGER W. TURKINGTON (1), Department of Medicine, University of Wisconsin Medical School, Madison, Wisconsin

JOHN R. WILLIAMSON (131), Johnson Research Foundation, University of Pennsylvania, Philadelphia, Pennsylvania

JAMES L. WITTLIFF (103), Department of Biochemistry, University of Rochester School of Medicine, Rochester, New York

PREFACE

These twelve selected chapters in the area of hormones and cancer express a diversity of concepts and experimental approaches to the study of regulatory mechanisms in cancer tissues. The tissues studied include those from the breast, liver, pituitary, adrenal cortex, testis, ovary, and trophoblast. Induced, spontaneous, and transplanted tumors are described. The major focus is on a biochemical approach to the study of model systems.

Emphasis is given to hormone receptors in the cytoplasm and nucleus and to receptor levels as a guide to therapy, the regulation of DNA and RNA synthesis in the nucleus and mitochondria, acidic chromatin proteins, enzymatic differences in normal and tumor tissue, anion and electron transport in mitochondria, energy metabolism, immune suppression, and blocking antibodies, as well as to the use of antihormones. The mechanisms of action of hormones such as ACTH, LH, TSH, estrogen, androgen, and glucocorticoids on gene expression and many other processes in the regulation of normal and abnormal tissues are also dealt with in detail.

The description and evaluation of concepts and the future projections in cancer research will be of interest to all investigators concerned with cancer of endocrine tissues.

I wish to thank Mrs. Sally McDonell for general secretarial assistance and for help in the preparation of the Subject Index.

Financial assistance was generously provided by Ayerst Laboratories and The Lilly Research Laboratories.

KENNETH W. McKERNS

CHAPTER I

ACIDIC CHROMATIN PROTEINS: CHANGES IN BREAST CANCER CELLS

NOBUYUKI KADOHAMA AND ROGER W. TURKINGTON

I. Introduction

The chromosomes of eukaryotic cells are generally considered to be comprised of four main classes of macromolecules: DNA; RNA; histones; and the residual, acidic chromosomal proteins. Since their discovery by Miescher in 1874 the histones of the cell nucleus have been extensively characterized in terms of their primary structure and functional properties. Although the non-histone proteins of the nucleus were recognized quite early by Lilienfeld (1893), serious problems in the purification and subfractionation of these proteins prevented their study until very recently. During the past two decades the development of adequate methods for isolation and characterization of the acidic chromatin proteins has made these proteins the subject of intensive investigation. These studies have increasingly implicated this class of proteins as playing an important role in the regulation of gene transcription.

The acidic chromatin proteins are generally assumed to correspond to the residual protein fraction that remains tightly bound to DNA after the removal of saline-soluble acidic proteins (the proteins of the nucleoplasm) and RNA and after the removal of histones by acid extraction or treatment with solutions of high salt concentration (Busch, 1965). These proteins are negatively charged at neutral pH and have a relatively high content of glutamic and aspartic acids. They have a relatively low content of the basic amino acids, and unlike the histones they contain tryptophan. The non-histone, acidic chromosomal proteins are phosphoproteins, as determined by their high content of alkali-labile phosphate groups and by *in vivo* incorporation of ^{32}P by esterification of their serine and threoninine residues (Langan, 1967; Benjamin and Gellhorn, 1968; Patel *et al.*, 1968; Kleinsmith and Allfrey, 1969). Their reported molecular weights range from 5000 to 200,000 (Elgin and Bonner, 1970; Shelton and Allfrey, 1970; Graziano and Huang, 1971; LeStourgeon and Rusch, 1971; Shelton and Neelin, 1971) as estimated by electrophoresis in polyacrylamide gels containing sodium dodecyl sulfate (SDS). Electrophoresis of acidic chromatin proteins in SDS-polyacrylamide gels has revealed extreme heterogeneity in preparations of these proteins derived from a variety of tissues, such as rat brain and kidney (Teng *et al.*, 1971), bovine thymus, kidney, and brain (Platz *et al.*, 1970), mouse mammary gland (Turkington and Kadohama, 1972), chicken erythrocytes (Loeb and Creuzet, 1970), HeLa cells (Stein and Borun, 1972), sea urchin embryos (Hill *et al.*, 1971), and the slime mold *Physarum polycephalum* (LeStourgeon and Rusch, 1971). Despite the existence of a number of common chemical properties among the acidic chromatin proteins, several major difficulties relating to the isolation and characterization of these proteins have been encountered by all investigators. Because of their extreme insolubility in aqueous solutions, it has not been possible to apply classic techniques for their isolation, and consequently a great variety of preparative methods have been devised for the study of these proteins. Because each of these methods has yielded somewhat different results it has been difficult to compare preparations between laboratories, and currently there is no precise agreement among investigators as to the specific composition of chromatin and chromatin acidic proteins.

II.   Isolation and Characterization of Nuclear Acidic Proteins

Three serious problems must be dealt with in the isolation and characterization of acidic chromosomal proteins: (1) potential contamination by nonchromatin proteins from the cell cytoplasm and the nucleoplasm; (2) The extreme insolubility of these proteins and their marked, tendency to aggregate; and (3) proteolysis.

The first of these problems has been minimized by the utilization of procedures by which chromatin is extracted from previously isolated and purified nuclei rather than from whole tissue (Spelsberg and Hnilica, 1971; Wilhelm *et al.*, 1972). However, it has become increasingly more apparent from electron microscopic evidence relating to the ultrastructural characteristics of the nucleus that there may be numerous intranuclear structures which are distinct from chromatin and which remain at present undefined (Bouteille, 1972). Because of the striking tendency of acidic chromatin proteins to bind other proteins, it is likely that many of the preparative procedures currently used yield chromatin contaminated with nucleoplasmic constituents. The additional problem of the tendency of acidic chromatin proteins to aggregate and precipitate during the subsequent steps of purification of chromatin and acidic chromatin proteins has been adequately described by numerous investigators (Gershey and Kleinsmith, 1969; Marushige et al., 1968). A variety of methods have been reported for the dissociation of acidic proteins from chromatin and DNA. The conventional approach involved basically a pretreatment of chromatin with dilute mineral acid and hot trichloroacetic acid for the sequential removal of histones and DNA, respectively, and solubilization of the residual material in alkali (Busch, 1965; Stein and Baserga, 1970). Such procedures expose the proteins to extremes of pH and heat treatment that undoubtedly cause alterations in protein structure. This basic procedure has the additional disadvantage that the full complement of the acidic proteins is generally not recovered. Use of the detergent sodium dodecyl sulfate has been highly successful for the removal of proteins from DNA and maintenance of chromatin proteins in solubilized form (Marushige et al., 1968). However, such detergent treatment has made difficult the interpretation of studies designed to evaluate the functional properties of the isolated proteins. Likewise, use of other agents such as phenol (Teng et al., 1971; Shelton and Neelin, 1971) and high pH (Benjamin and Gellhorn, 1968) also leads to irreversible denaturation of the proteins. Deoxycholate has been reported to act to dissociate and solubilize chromatin proteins in a reversible manner (Wang, 1966; Patel et al., 1968). Salyrgan, an organic mercurial compound, has also been reported to act to solubilize chromatin proteins without leading to irreversible denaturation (Dijkstra and Weide, 1972). In some studies, chromatin preparations have been subjected to shearing forces in order to facilitate the initial solubilization (Marushige et al., 1968; Shaw and Huang, 1970; Hill et al., 1971; Levy et al., 1972; van den Broek et al., 1973), although this procedure may result in the loss of certain proteins (Arnold and Young, 1972).

In recent years preparative methods utilizing mild conditions of extraction have been found for the isolation of acidic chromatin proteins. Most reported procedures involve solubilization of chromatin proteins in high salt–urea buffers (Gilmour and Paul, 1969; Shaw and Huang, 1970; Spelsberg and Hnilica, 1971; Richter and Sekeris, 1972; Yoshida and Shimura, 1972), separation of DNA by ultracentrifugation (Shaw and Huang, 1970; Richter and Sekeris, 1972), gel exclusion chromatography (Graziano and Huang, 1971; van den Broek et al., 1973), or selective precipitation with lanthanum chloride (Yoshida and Shimura, 1972), and separation from histones by ion-exchange chromatography (Gilmour and Paul, 1969; Graziano and Huang, 1970; Richter and Sekeris, 1972; Yoshida and Shimura 1972; van den Broek et al., 1973). Alternatively, the chromatin can be dissociated in guanidinium chloride and subjected to the same separative techniques (Hill et al., 1971; Arnold and Young, 1972; Levy et al., 1972). The availability of such procedures which avoid protein denaturation during extraction should greatly facilitate studies on the functional roles of these proteins.

While the methods described above permit the isolation of non-histone acidic proteins under relatively mild conditions of extraction, fractionation into their individual components on a preparative scale has not yet been achieved. Success in this regard has been limited to fractionation into several large groups of proteins, primarily by ion-exchange chromatography (Wang and Johns, 1968; Levy et al., 1972; Richter and Sekeris, 1972). The great value of these methods is that nucleic acids, histones, and non-histone proteins are separated from one another and quantitatively recovered from a single chromatin sample. The combined use of sodium dodecyl sulfate and electrophoresis in polyacrylamide gels has permitted a high degree of resolution of the individual constituents of acidic chromatin proteins (Graziano and Huang, 1971; Hill et al., 1971; Teng et al., 1971; van den Broek et al., 1973). Although this procedure has been a valuable analytical tool, it has not yet been utilized for purification on a preparative scale. Recently, LeStourgeon and Rusch (1973) have separated the total nuclear proteins of the plasmodial slime mold *Physarum polycephalum* into four distinct solubility classes which exhibit characteristic molecular weight ranges and electrophoretic profiles. Their procedure, as applied to purified nuclei or nucleoli, involves sequential extraction in 0.14 M sodium chloride, extraction in 0.25 N HCl, extraction with 73% phenol at 4°C, and extraction in 5% sodium dodecyl sulfate at 100°C. This procedure has led to the identification of at least 41 electrophoretic bands, indicating that electrophoretic analysis of well-defined subfractions may serve as a more powerful tool for the recognition of individual components than mass electrophoresis of the total extract of acidic chromatin proteins. Their results suggest that both the phenol-soluble acidic proteins and the residual SDS-proteins are firmly associated with DNA, while the saline-soluble proteins and histones are bound to DNA with considerably less ionic strength.

The final major problem in the purification and characterization of acidic chromatin proteins is that of proteolysis (Dounce et al., 1972). Early studies demonstrated contamination of various chromatin preparations with nucleases and proteases which were active even in the presence of 5 M

urea. Elimination of such proteolytic activity was especially desirable in view of the extreme heterogeneity in protein sizes demonstrated by the technique of SDS—polyacrylamide gel electrophoresis. In recent years several techniques have been found to be quite successful in reducing proteolysis to a minimal and highly acceptable level. Proteolysis can be prevented with the use of sodium bisulfite at pH 7.5–8.0 (Panyim *et al.,* 1968) or by the exposure of native chromatin to a low pH (pH 6.0) (Spelsberg *et al.,* 1971; Kadohama and Turkington, 1973a). Other protease inhibitors such as diisopropyl fluorophosphate have also been successful. Le-Stourgeon and Rusch (1973) have reported a surprisingly low proteolytic activity in their method for the preparation of residual acidic proteins from *Physarum* nuclei; homogenates were allowed to stand for periods of nearly four hours at room temperature without affecting quantitative recoveries or electrophoretic profiles of these proteins. Current results indicate that the problem of proteolysis is no longer a formidable barrier to the study of these proteins. Assays providing evidence of acceptably low levels of proteolytic activities within a given preparation should provide sufficient evidence to exclude the factor of proteolysis as a major problem in the interpretation of electrophoretic profiles of acidic chromatin proteins.

III.   Evidence for a Gene Regulatory Function of Acidic Chromatin Proteins

A. *Characteristics of the Isolated Proteins*

Direct evidence which demonstrates a role of the residual acidic nuclear proteins in the regulation of eukaryotic genes is currently lacking. However, a constellation of experimental observations has provided a variety of lines of suggestive evidence which is mutually supportive and which leads to the hypothesis that these proteins play some role in gene regulation. The extreme electrophoretic heterogeneity of these protein preparations is consistent with their proposed role in the recognition of individual polydeoxynucleotide sequences (MacGillivray *et al.,* 1971). Unlike the histones, these proteins display both tissue specificity and species-specific interactions with DNA (Paul and Gilmour, 1968; Teng *et al.,* 1970). Both of these observations are consistent with their proposed role in the determination of cell differentiation and the regulation of transcription by differential binding to specific genes (Stellwagen and Cole, 1969; Baserga and Stein, 1971; Elgin *et al.,* 1971). Kleinsmith and his co-workers (1970) have shown that tissue-specific acidic chromosomal proteins bind only to the DNA of the tissue of origin. A dramatic degree of species specificity of the electrophoretic profiles of acidic chromatin proteins has been demonstrated by all investigators in this field. Tissue and species specificity has also been demonstrated by immunochemical techniques (Chytil and Spelsberg, 1971). All of these observations are thus consistent with the proposed role of the acidic chromatin proteins in the determination of cell differentiation and in the regulation of transcription by differential binding to specific genes. In attempts to obtain more direct evidence for an effect of these proteins on transcription, several workers have demonstrated that histone-inhibited transcription of RNA *in vitro* can be reversed by the addition of acidic protein constituents of the template chromatin (Wang, 1968; Teng and Hamilton, 1969). However, the relevance of these effects is unclear because of the tendency of acidic proteins to form insoluble complexes with histones and DNA. This problem has been reviewed in great detail by MacGillivray *et al.* (1972). Whether such reported effects are fortuitous or not, other experiments have shown that acidic proteins are indeed responsible for directing *in vitro* transcription with a high degree of specificity. Spelsberg *et al.* (1971) demonstrated by the reconstitution of various components of the chromatins of rat liver or rat thymus that patterns of RNA synthesized on each of these templates (as characterized by RNA–DNA hybridization) can be altered specifically by the acidic protein molecules. Similarly, Gilmour and Paul (1970) have fractionated and reconstituted chromatins from various rabbit tissues and have reported that the non-histone, acidic fractions were capable of interacting with DNA and modifying transcription in a manner specific for the tissue from which the acidic proteins were derived. Kostraba and Wang (1972a,b) have reported that non-histone proteins added to condensed chromatin (heterochromatin) stimulated the template activity to almost the level observed with diffuse chromatin (euchromatin), suggesting that acidic proteins may activate previously repressed sites of transcription. These experiments thus provide evidence to indicate that the acidic chromatin proteins can exert both activating and inhibitory effects on the transcription of DNA. Although they lend strong support to the concept that acidic chromatin proteins are important regulators of eukaryotic genes, they are open to the criticism that the reconstituted chromatin may not possess some significant properties of native chromatin. These results are also subject to the limitations inherent currently in the experimental techniques of RNA–DNA hybridization and electron microscopic characterization of the reconstituted chromatin (Bishop, 1972; Paul *et al.*, 1972).

B. Synthesis during Cell Proliferation

Additional evidence for the involvement of acidic chromatin proteins in gene regulation is provided by numerous observations on the activation of synthesis of these proteins in relation to activation of cell proliferation. Unlike the histones, which are synthesized almost exclusively during the DNA-replicative phase of the cell cycle and exhibit little turnover, the acidic chromosomal proteins are synthesized throughout the cell cycle and exhibit relatively high rates of turnover, as demonstrated in such diverse tissues as rat liver (Buck and Shauder, 1970), mouse mammary gland (Turkington and Kadohama, 1972), and HeLa cells (Borun and Stein, 1972). Stein and Baserga (1970) demonstrated that synthesis of these proteins is maximal in the prereplicative phase of the cell cycle in the isoproterenol-stimulated proliferation of salivary cells. These workers also reported that synthesis of the acidic chromatin proteins continues throughout the cell cycle of HeLa cells, with maximal rates of synthesis observed in the G_1 phase just preceding the initiation of DNA synthesis. Synthesis of acidic chromatin proteins has been shown to be one of the earliest responses to activation of lymphocyte proliferation by phytohemagglutinin (Levy *et al.,* 1972; Weisenthal and Ruddon, 1972). An immediate increase in the synthesis of acidic nuclear proteins is observed when density-inhibited cultures of human fibroblasts are stimulated to proliferate by changing the medium (Rovera and Baserga, 1971; Tsuboi and Baserga, 1972), and infection of monkey kidney cells with the oncogenic SV40 virus induces a similar phenomenon (Rovera *et al.,* 1972). Kostraba and Wang (1970) reported stimulation of the synthesis of acidic chromatin proteins in parallel with DNA synthesis during regeneration of rat liver following partial hepatectomy. Because this system represents a relatively low degree of synchronization of cell cycles there was no apparent correlation of activation of acidic chromatin protein synthesis with the presumed G_1 period. In one of the most extensively characterized models for self proliferation, the insulin-induced proliferation of mouse mammary cells in organ culture, Turkington and Kadohama (1972) demonstrated activation of acidic chromatin protein synthesis in mid to late G_1 phase with a peak of acidic chromatin protein synthesis preceding the peak of DNA synthesis. A second peak of synthesis was observed during the post-DNA synthetic phase of culture.

A widely held concept is that multiple genes are activated to direct specific events at specific stages of the cell cycle. It may be anticipated from this hypothesis that changes in rates of synthesis or in nuclear content of specific molecular forms of acidic proteins would occur at discrete time points in the cycle related to activation or inhibition of specific genes. Small, quantitative changes have been observed in the electrophoretic radioactivity profiles of partially synchronized mammary cells induced to divide by insulin (Kadohama and Turkington, 1973a) and in synchronized HeLa cells (Bhorjee and Pederson, 1972; Stein and Borun, 1972) although induction of distinct qualitative changes in acidic protein profiles in relation to the progression of the cell cycle has not yet been reported.

C. Changes during Cell Differentiation

Whereas the tissue and species specificity of the acidic chromatin proteins, their specific interactions with DNA, and activation of synthesis of these proteins during cell proliferation imply a gene regulatory function for these proteins, perhaps more direct evidence concerning their roles in gene regulation is provided by studies on differentiating cells. It is a widely accepted concept that the differentiated state of eukaryotic cells is determined by variable or differential gene expression. Thus, it would be anticipated that transitions in the state of cell differentiation would be marked by the synthesis of new species of nuclear acidic proteins and a change in the electrophoretic profiles of these proteins as the newly differentiated cells appear. LeStourgeon and Rusch (1971, 1973) have presented evidence for dramatic changes in acidic chromatin proteins during cell differentiation in the slime mold, *Physarum polycephalum*. This multinucleate organism is a highly undifferentiated eukaryotic syncytium which can be induced by light to sporulate after a requisite threshold period of starvation. The development of the photosensitive state during differentiation is marked by the appearance of 6 specific protein bands and nearly complete disappearance of 2 other major protein bands. If the photosensitized plasmodia are then fed, vegetative growth returns and the electrophoretic profile characteristic of this state of cell differentiation is reinduced. The acidic chromatin protein profile remains unchanged throughout somatic growth, but during the period of synthesis of the new proteins involved with coalescence, stalk formation, meiosis, and pigment and spore wall formation, specific and reproducible changes occur within the acidic chromatin proteins. Most of these changes have been shown to occur in the chromatin-associated proteins ranging in molecular weight from 32,000 to 160,000. These studies further show that the new proteins which appear during differentiation are newly synthesized, as indicated by incorporation studies with ^{14}C-labeled amino acids, and that protein species that disappear during differentiation do not become radioactively labeled during development of the new cell states. These workers have also extracted 7 specific acidic proteins from nucleoli and have demonstrated that one of these proteins with a molecular weight of 86,500 disappears during differentiation. Thirty-nine easily detectable and highly reproducible polypeptide bands have been found to be of chromosomal origin, and they may thus act to regulate changes in the transcription of specific genes.

Developing sea urchin embryos represent a somewhat more complex system in which definite changes in acidic chromatin proteins have been demonstrated during cell differentiation. Extensive studies in this system have demonstrated the validity of methods for the isolation of nuclei and chromatin from these embryos. Furthermore, studies on transcription in these organisms by Marushige and Ozaki (1967) have demonstrated that the template activity of this chromatin increases between the blastula and pluteus stages. RNA–DNA hybridization studies have also demonstrated that the isolated chromatin retains information for stage-specific patterns of transcription (Chetsanga et al., 1970). While the studies of Hill et al. (1971) demonstrated primarily quantitative changes in the acidic chromatin proteins during development from blastula to pluteus, the studies of Cognetti et al. (1972) implicated qualitative changes in specific electrophoretic bands. Their studies demonstrated that four bands that appear at the bastula stage are no longer present at the pluteus stage and that three bands which emerge during the pluteus stage are not detectable by their methods at the bastula stage. These comparisons were most apparent in comparisons with the 16-cell stage of development. Hnilica and Johnson (1970) have reported similar changes in the acidic nuclear proteins in sea urchin embryos verified not only by electrophoresis but also by changes in amino acid composition.

Changes in acidic chromatin proteins during the differentiation of mammalian cells have also been reported, as demonstrated by studies on mouse mammary cells (Kadohama and Turkington, 1973a). Differentiation of mammary epithelial stem cells into secretory, alveolar cells occurs as a consequence of cell division. The progenitor cells can be induced to divide in vitro by addition of insulin to the chemically defined medium. After the sequential actions of hydrocortisone and prolactin acting in concert with insulin on the newly formed cells, the daughter cells form specific milk proteins which are uniquely characteristic of the mammary secretory alveolar cell (Turkington et al., 1973). Treatment of the cell cultures with various inhibitors of DNA synthesis or mitosis completely prevents the new expression of the genes for milk proteins, indicating that chromosomal replication and cell division are requirements for the new expression of these genes (Turkington, 1971b). Definite and highly reproducible differences in the electrophoretic profiles of acidic chromatin proteins have been observed in comparing the protein populations derived from undifferentiated epithelial cells (from virginal mammary glands) and cell populations containing large numbers of alveolar cells (lactational mammary gland). In particular, a complex of 6 high molecular weight proteins which are not detectable in the undifferentiated cells represents a dominant component of the nuclear acidic proteins derived from lactational tissue. In newly explanted organ cultures of virginal mammary gland there is no detectable synthesis of these proteins. However, incubation of these cells with insulin eventually induces incorporation of ^{3}H-amino acids into proteins with the same electrophoretic mobility as the complex of proteins characteristic of differentiated cells. Synthesis of these proteins is induced several hours before initiation of DNA synthesis, and synthesis of these specific proteins continues in the differentiated daughter cells. Subsequent treatment of the daughter cells with hydrocortisone and prolactin does not substantially influence the synthesis of the acidic proteins. Therefore, those changes in acidic chromatin proteins which are characteristic of mammary cell differentiation occur independently of the influence of prolactin and hydrocortisone, hormones which induce other cytoplasmic changes characteristic of the differentiated secretory cells (Kadohama and Turkington, 1973a, Turkington et al., 1973).

IV. Role of the Acidic Chromatin Proteins in Hormonal Regulation

A stimulation of acidic chromatin protein synthesis has been observed in the course of action of various hormones. This has been particularly true for the action of steroid hormones which have been shown to exert an activation of transcription in their respective target cells. The administration of cortisol to adrenalectomized rats resulted in a stimulation of synthesis of a single non-histone acidic protein component in liver (Shelton and Allfrey, 1970). Teng and Hamilton (1970) administered 17β-estradiol to ovariectomized rats and observed a selective increase in the rate of labeling in a specific electrophoretic band of acidic chromatin proteins. This effect was observed in proteins prepared from the uterus, and no effect was observed on liver chromatin proteins. Previous studies in both of these systems have demonstrated a significant activation of transcriptional activity early in the course of the cellular response to hormonal stimulation. Similar specific alterations in the synthesis or phosphorylation of acidic nuclear proteins have been observed after stimulation of prostate cells by androgens (Ahmed, 1971) and after stimulation of insect chromosomes by ecdysone (Helmsing and Berendes, 1971). These results thus demonstrate a selective increase in the rate of formation of specific proteins at the time of gene activation.

Current evidence also favors the concept that steroid hormones also interact with the acidic components of chromatin as they act within the nucleus to stimulate transcription in their respective target cells. The initial action of steroid hormones is to bind to a specific cytoplasmic receptor, and cortisol receptors in liver and lymphoid cells, progesterone receptors in chick oviduct and uterus, dihydrotestosterone receptors in prostate, and aldosterone receptors in kidney have been extensively characterized. In each case, the hormone–receptor complex has been shown to enter the nucleus and bind to chromatin. O'Malley and co-workers (1971), working with the cytoplasmic progesterone receptor of chick oviduct, have demonstrated a more extensive binding of receptor–hormone complex to target tissue chromatin than to the purified DNA and in chromatin reconstitution studies have demonstrated binding in a specific fraction of acidic chromatin proteins which are present specifically in the target tissue. Although these data most consistently point to the presence of "acceptor" activity residing in specific sites on certain acidic chromatin proteins of oviduct chromatin it is not yet possible to rule out an alternative condition, that certain specific acidic proteins determine the conformation of DNA-chromatin necessary for accepting the hormone–receptor complex. Specific binding sites on target tissue chromatin have also been reported for the binding of aldosterone receptor to rat kidney chromatin (Swaneck *et al.*, 1970), for the binding of dihydrotestosterone receptor to rat ventral prostate chromatin (Bruchovsky and Wilson, 1968), and for the binding of estradiol receptor in rat uterus chromatin (King *et al.*, 1972). In each of these systems, an estimate of a limited number of binding sites, approximately 500 to 2000 sites per nucleus, has been predicted from binding activities. However, the role of the acidic chromatin proteins as a specific acceptor site for the binding of estradiol receptor has been called into question by Chamness *et al.*, (1973) who have demonstrated a high capacity, nonsaturable binding curve for the interaction of estradiol receptor with acidic chromatin proteins prepared from various target tissues.

Several experimental observations indicate that polypeptide hormones also influence the synthesis of acidic chromatin proteins. Turkington and Riddle (1969) demonstrated that insulin stimulates the phosphorylation of serine and threonine residues of the completed polypeptide chains of nuclear acidic proteins 8–10-fold in cultured mammary cells and that insulin and prolactin synergize to stimulate the rate of phosphorylation of nonhistone nuclear proteins in cultured mammary alveolar cells. Injection of glucagon into rats has been shown to increase the net rate of incorporation of [³H]leucine into two acidic chromatin proteins of molecular weight 60,000 and 80,000, respectively, in the rat liver (Enea and Allfrey, 1973). These proteins appear to be distinct from the specific acidic chromatin proteins of liver nuclei in which the net rate of labeling is augmented by either cortisol or insulin. Johnson and Allfrey (1972) have demonstrated that cyclic AMP also causes a rapid increase in the net rate of phosphorylation of specific nuclear proteins in rat liver and that cyclic AMP stimulates protein phosphorylation in isolated rat liver nuclei incubated with a soluble cyclic AMP-dependent protein kinase. Since the action of glucagon may be mediated by cyclic AMP, it is possible that the action of this hormone is mediated by such changes in synthesis and phosphorylation of acidic nuclear proteins. Buck and Schauder (1970) have also demonstrated an increase in the net radioactivity labeling of non-histone nuclear proteins of the rat liver five hours after an injection of insulin. Under the conditions of this experiment the net rate of incorporation of the single-label amino acid into histones was unchanged by insulin treatment, indicating a selective effect on the non-histone nuclear proteins.

V.   Studies on Acidic Chromatin Proteins in Breast Cancer Cells

A. Neoplastic Transformation and Progression

It is becoming increasingly more evident that the neoplastic transformation which gives rise to many different types of cancer involves a progression through one or more preneoplastic stages, and the cancer cells may continue to develop through multiple forms of the neoplastic state (Turkington, 1971a; Foulds, 1969). A well-studied model of neoplastic transformation and progression is the breast cancer system of the C3H mouse. A large body of evidence has demonstrated that the mammary adenocarcinomas of these mice do not arise directly from the normal epithelial cells of the mammary gland but arise instead from cell populations of a discrete preneoplastic lesion, the hyperplastic alveolar nodule (HAN). The formation of this lesion and its subsequent transformation to a rapidly growing adenocarcinoma is determined by a complex interaction among hereditary factors, hormonal stimulation, and the biological activities of the nodule-inducing virus and the mammary tumor virus. The hyperplastic alveolar nodules which arise from the glandular epithelium in older females of genetically predisposed mice are distinct by their morphological phenotype. They differ experimentally from normal cells also in terms of their apparently unlimited life span in serial transplantations (Daniel et al., 1968), their altered responsiveness to hormonal stimuli (Bern and Nandi, 1961; Nandi, 1966), as well as in their ability to produce mammary adenocarcinomas (DeOme et al., 1959a,b, 1962). Thus the transformation of normal gland cells into the preneoplastic HAN lesion and its subsequent neoplastic development have been regarded as obligatory successive steps in the development of mammary adenocarcinomas in the C3H mouse. Structural and functional changes in cell phenotype become apparent after the transition to adenocarcinoma cells, and this cell population exhibits another property of many cancer cells, a pleiotypic cell morphology. The neoplastic properties of this population of carcinoma cells may progress to the further acquisition of new, intrinsic characteristics of a more uniform population of cells which are selected and which survive serial transplantations. The C3HBA transplanted adenocarcinoma of the C3H mouse is an example of this progression leading to the presence of new morphological (Dunn, 1959; Pierce, 1965), biochemical (Turkington and Riddle, 1970a,b), and growth characteristics (McCredie *et al.,* 1965).

B. *Evidence of Altered Gene Expression*

It is an attractive hypothesis that the altered, pleiotypic phenotype of these cancer cells is determined by an altered pattern of gene expression. Several observations dealing with the synthesis of specific proteins in these mammary carcinoma cells support this hypophysis. Normal mammary epithelial cells in organ culture can be induced by the hormones insulin, hydrocortisone, and prolactin to differentiate into secretory alveolar cells, and the molecular mechanisms underlying this process have been extensively characterized (Turkington, 1968). The newly differentiated cells have the unique capacity to express the genetic information for the synthesis of the specific milk proteins, casein and α-lactalbumin. When tested by stimulation with the specific chemical inducers of cell differentiation, cells of the C3H mouse mammary carcinoma cannot respond by derepression of these genes with the synthesis of the specific milk proteins (Turkington and Riddle, 1970a). A second example of mammary carcinoma cell differentiation relates to the presence of an altered profile of enzymes for the methylation of specific bases in transfer RNA. The activities of these enzymes in the carcinoma cells were markedly increased above normal values both in terms of their specific activities and in proportion to the cellular content of transfer RNA. Extracts of the carcinoma cells contained a specific enzyme, transfer RNA guanine-7-methylase, an enzyme not detectable in normal mammary glands of the rat or mouse. Since this enzyme is a normal constituent of cells of the rodent liver, lung, spleen, and kidney, its presence in the mammary carcinoma cells suggest that the gene for this enzyme is normally repressed in mammary cells but becomes activated as a result of the neoplastic transformation (Turkington and Riddle, 1970b; Turkington, 1972).

If the genetic loci being transcribed in the neoplastic mammary cells were, in fact, different from those transcribed in the normal mammary cells, the nuclear RNA in the carcinoma cells would be expected to consist of different nucleotide sequences. This hypothesis has been tested by comparing the populations of nuclear RNA's to determine if they exhibited an altered pattern of gene transcription. These experiments were carried out by utilizing the techniques of RNA–DNA hybridization and hybridization–competition (Turkington and Self, 1970; Turkington, 1970, 1971a).

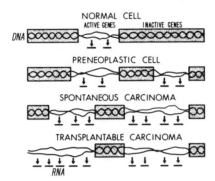

Fig. 1. Model diagram illustrating the activation of new genes during specific stages in the neoplastic development of mouse mammary cells.

Tissues from mouse or rat mammary glands or from HAN outgrowths or carcinomas were allowed to incorporate [³H]uridine or ³²P into nuclear RNA during a 30-minute incubation period *in vitro*. The nuclear RNA was purified highly ($E_{260}/E_{280} \geq 1.85$) and was then allowed to hybridize with species-homologous, thermally denatured DNA. At a point of relative saturation of the DNA, the addition of increasing amounts of competitor, nonradioactive nuclear RNA, from the same tissue caused a progressive decline in radioactivity of the labeled hybrid which closely approximated that which would be predicted from theoretical calculations for a competitor of similar base sequences. These RNA-driven reactions exhibited competition kinetics in proportion to the known genetic relatedness of the DNA's from which they were transcribed. The results of the hybridization–competition reactions with such RNA's demonstrated that each of the successive stages of neoplastic development, the preneoplastic HAN outgrowths, the spontaneously transformed cells, and the serially transplantable carcinoma cells were characterized by a discrete increment in the diversity of hybridizable nuclear RNA species formed. The changes in the numbers of transcribable genes which these populations of transcription products imply are diagrammed in the model shown in Fig. 1. These differences in RNA populations in comparison to the normal cell cannot be ascribed merely to the greater rates of cell proliferation in the carcinomas, since similar differences were observed in comparison to the rapidly proliferating mammary epithelial cells of pregnancy. Similar differences between the nuclear RNA's of mammary gland and of a transplantable mammary carcinoma have been observed in studies on the R3230AC transplantable carcinoma of the Fischer rat. Whereas the unlabeled mammary carcinoma RNA's competed with ³H-RNA from mammary carcinomas to 92% of the theoretical value for identical RNA populations, unlabeled mammary gland RNA competed with mammary carcinoma ^{3}H-RNA to only 52% of this value. A similar increase in the diversity of hybridizable nuclear RNA's in comparison to nonneoplastic cells has also been demonstrated in human chronic lymphocytic leukemia cells (Neiman and Henry, 1969), in minimal deviation Morris hepatomas (Mendecki *et al.*, 1969), in Yoshida ascites hepatoma cells (Chiarugi, 1969), and in the Walker 256 mammary carcinosarcoma (Kostraba and Wang, 1971). These concepts have been further extended by the experiments of Kostraba and Wang (1972b), who studied the RNA populations transcribed *in vitro* from chromatins derived from the Walker 256 mammary carcinoma or from rat mammary gland or rat liver. Experiments utilizing reciprocal double saturation hybridization of the transcribed RNA's demonstrated the presence of transcripts from Walker tumor chromatin which were not detectable in RNA populations transcribed from the chromatin of normal cells *in vitro*. Walker tumor chromatin was found to have the least template activity for RNA synthesis *in vitro*, and the RNA synthesized *in vitro* also showed the least saturation hybridization plateau in duplex formation with homologous DNA. These results are compatible with the concept that certain deoxynucleotide sequences which are transcribable in normal cells are not transcribable in the corresponding neoplastic cells, while certain genes which are repressed in the normal cells become derepressed in the neoplastic cells. The studies of Britten and Kohne (1966) and those of Melli and Bishop (1970) clearly indicate that because of the increased redundancy in mammalian chromatin structure only the most repetitive transcribable genome sequences may be detected under the experimental conditions used in these studies. The studies of Bishop (1972) have lent further reservations as to whether hybridization–competition experiments may be interpreted to represent qualitative or merely quantitative differences in the reactants compared. Within the experimental limitations of this method, however, the results of studies which compare populations of transcription products derived from normal or neoplastic cells have lent strong support to the concept that the transcription of new complementary RNA's and the possible restriction of certain other areas of the genome for transcription may lead to the altered functional properties expressed by neoplastic cells and may represent a fundamental characteristic of neoplastic cells. These results have also given a strong impetus to the search for factors that may regulate the activation of gene transcription during the normal differentiation of cells and during neoplastic transformation and progression.

C. Changes in Acidic Chromatin Proteins

In view of the large body of evidence implicating the acidic chromatin proteins in the restriction of template activity and in view of the results of our studies demonstrating changes in acidic chromatin proteins during mammary cell differentiation, it was of interest to analyze the acidic chromatin proteins of breast carcinoma cells to determine their possible participation in altering the pattern of gene expression in these cells. Several investigators had previously reported variations in the cellular content or rates of synthesis of acidic nuclear proteins in cancer cells. Steele and Busch (1963) reported that the synthesis of acidic nuclear proteins was less in normal rat liver in comparison to Walker 256 carcinosarcoma. Sporn and Dingman (1966) later found that hepatomas induced by chemical carcinogens contained higher amounts of acidic nuclear proteins than normal liver. However, another study (Grunicke et al., 1970) revealed no difference between the non-histone acidic protein contents of chromatins derived from rat liver or hepatomas 5123C and 7800. The template activities of chromatin from these hepatomas were found to be lower than the template activities of chromatin from their host livers. Consistent with this observation was the report that greater amounts of hepatoma chromatin are in the form of inactive heterochromatin in comparison to normal liver cells (Gellhorn et al., 1966; DeBellis et al., 1969). However, the interpretation of such results is subject to the limiting consideration that in an asynchronously dividing cell population various members of the population may contain different DNA cistrons in condensed or diffuse chromatin at any moment of the interphase period of the cell cycle. Also, fractionation methods for separating heterochromatin and euchromatin used in these studies were not sufficiently precise to provide clear fraction separations. Observations on preparations of acidic nuclear protein in human breast cancer cells were found not to yield in themselves a useful index for clinical prognosis (Smith et al., 1970), and further characterization of these proteins has not been carried out.

In an effort to determine the role of acidic chromatin proteins in the regulation of neoplastic breast cells, our studies were directed toward characterizing the acidic chromatin proteins of the normal and neoplastic breast tissues of C3H mice and of rats. Chromatin was prepared from highly purified nuclei, and the histones were selectively removed in 2 M sodium chloride at pH 6.0, according to the method of Spelsberg et al., (1971; Spelsberg and Hnilica, 1971). These procedures were chosen in an attempt to minimize proteolytic degradation and possible contamination with cytoplasm and nucleoplasmic proteins while avoiding the exposure of chromatin proteins to extreme conditions of pH or to solvent denaturation which may yield artifacts. Following the removal of histones, the residual acidic proteins were dissociated in 6 M urea and sodium dodecyl sulfate (SDS) and were then analyzed by electrophoresis in SDS–polyacrylamide gels.

Figure 2 shows the electrophoretic banding patterns of acidic chromatin proteins derived from the mouse mammary gland, spontaneous mammary carcinomas, and a transplantable mammary carcinoma. Each of the electrophoretic profiles showed a high degree of heterogeneity in the protein mixtures. The normal mammary gland proteins exhibited a complex of 6 high molecular weight proteins which represented a predominant and characteristic component. In comparison to this pattern of the normal tissue, the spontaneous tumors exhibited a relative deficiency of several of these bands, a greater predominance of several bands of intermediate molecular weight, the presence of several bands which were not detectable in the normal tissue, and a relative deficiency of at least one band of intermediate molecular weight present in the normal tissue. In comparison, the pattern of proteins derived from the transplantable mammary carcinoma exhibited a further deficiency of the high molecular weight proteins and increasing predominance of several specific proteins of intermediate molecular weight. These changes in the electrophoretic profiles could not be ascribed to differential proteolysis or to other artifacts in the extraction of individual preparations. Tests for proteolysis exhibited a minimal level of release of acid-soluble in [³H]tryptophan-labeled peptides, and admixtures of nuclei prepared from each of the various tissues yielded mixtures

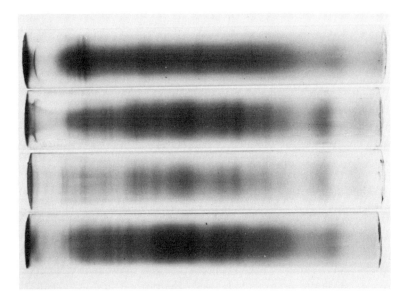

Fig. 2. Electrophoretograms of stained acidic chromatin proteins prepared from the following tissues: top, mouse lactational mammary gland; middle, preparations from two spontaneous mammary adenocarcinomas (type A) of the C3H mouse; bottom, transplantable C3HBA mammary adenocarcinoma of the C3H mouse.

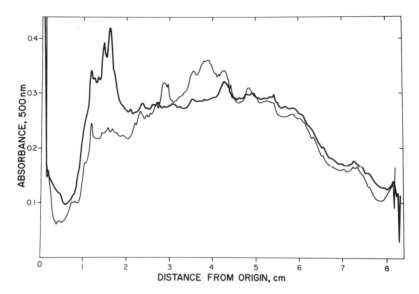

Fig. 3. Absorbance profiles of stained acidic chromatin proteins after electrophoresis in SDS–polyacrylamide gels. Samples were extracted from lactational C3H mouse mammary gland (heavy tracing) or from C3H mouse spontaneous mammary adenocarcinoma (light tracing). The front is at 8.0 cm. (Reproduced from *Cancer Res.* by permission.)

which were additive for all of the individual components. The electrophoretic banding profiles derived from normal or neoplastic tissues were also quantitatively compared by absorbance scanning of the stained gels. As shown by the absorbance tracings in Fig. 3, the proteins extracted from neoplastic mammary tissue exhibit a relative increase in proteins of intermediate electrophoretic mobility and a decrease in proteins of low electrophoretic mobility (high molecular weight) in comparison to the chromatin proteins of the normal tissue. The acidic chromatin proteins derived from normal and neoplastic mammary tissues were also characterized by amino acid analysis, and the histogram in Fig. 4 shows the relative amino acid compositions of these chromatins. The predominantly acidic nature of these proteins was indicated by the relatively high content of aspartic and glutamic acids and the relatively low content of the basic amino acids, lysine, histidine, and arginine. These results indicate a significant difference with respect to several amino acids between the normal and neoplastic tissues and further indicate that the differences in electrophoretic mobility among the acidic chromatin protein populations of normal and neoplastic tissues relate to differences in the polypeptide chains rather than merely to substituent modifications or to proteolytic effects.

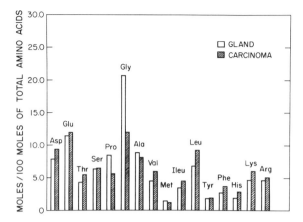

Fig. 4. Histogram showing the relative amino acid compositions of acidic chromatin proteins derived from lactational mammary gland (open bars) or from the C3HBA mammary adenocarcinoma (cross-hatched bars) of the C3H mouse.

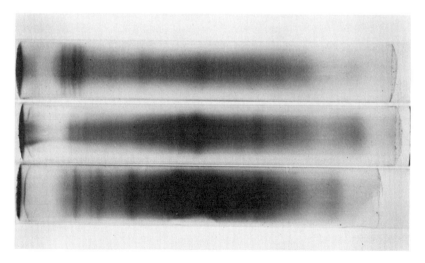

Fig. 5. Electrophoretograms of stained acidic chromatin proteins derived from the following tissues: top, lactational mammary gland of the Fischer rat; middle, transplantable R3230AC mammary carcinoma of Fischer rat; bottom, spontaneous DMBA-induced mammary adenocarcinoma of the Sprague-Dawley rat. The electrophoretogram of the acidic chromatin proteins derived from the lactational mammary gland of the Sprague-Dawley rat was indistinguishable from that of acidic chromatin proteins derived from the Fischer rat.

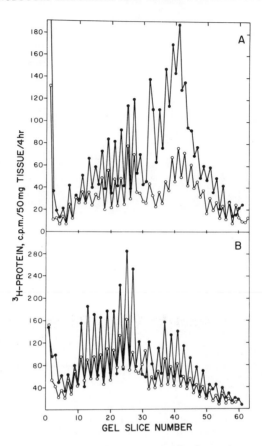

Fig. 6. Electrophoretic radioactivity patterns of acidic chromatin proteins synthesized by mouse mammary gland or mouse mammary transplantable carcinoma explants. Explants from lactational gland (A) or transplantable carcinoma (B) were allowed to incorporate [^{3}H]-aspartate and [^{3}H]leucine during the 0–4-hour period of incubation in organ culture. At the end of this labeling period one group of explants was analyzed for acidic chromatin proteins (closed circles). The other group was washed in medium 199 and transferred to nonisotopic medium for a 6-hour "chase." They were subsequently extracted of chromatin proteins, and acidic chromatin proteins were subjected to electrophoresis on polyacrylamide gels containing SDS (open circles). The front is at 6.1 cm. (Reproduced from *Cancer Res.* by permission.)

Similar studies have been carried out on two well-defined mammary carcinomas of the rat, the R323OAC transplantable adenocarcinoma in the Fischer rat, and the spontaneous DMBA-induced mammary adenocarcinoma of the Sprague-Dawley rat. Figure 5 shows the electrophoretic profile of stained acidic chromatin proteins derived from these tissues. As in the comparisons of the normal and neoplastic mouse tissues, these tumors exhibited a relative deficiency or loss of several of the high molecular weight species characteristic of the normal tissue, the appearance of protein bands which were undetectable in the preparation derived from the mammary gland, and a predominance of proteins of intermediate molecular weight. Quantitative differences in the absorbance profiles of the electrophoretic patterns and in the relative amino acid compositions of these preparations (Kadohama and Turkington, 1973b) were similar to those already described in the mouse system.

The acidic chromatin proteins in mammary carcinomas and in mammary gland have also been compared in terms of their relative rates of synthesis and turnover. Figure 6 compares the electrophoretic radioactivity profiles of ^{3}H-labeled acidic chromatin proteins of mouse carcinoma cells with those obtained from mammary gland following labeling under identical conditions in organ culture. The highest net rate of incorporation of amino acids was observed in protein constituents of intermediate electrophoretic mobility (gel slices 30–50) in the preparations derived from the normal mammary gland (panel A). These proteins also exhibited a relatively high rate of turnover, as indicated by the residual radioactivity (plotted as open circles) after a "chase" period of incubation on nonisotopic medium. In contrast to this result, the predominant radioactively labeled proteins in preparations from mouse mammary carcinoma (panel B) were of relatively high molecular weight (low electrophoretic mobility, gel slices 10–30). Similar differences in relative rates of synthesis of acidic chromatin proteins, as observed in electrophoretic radioactivity profiles, were also found in comparisons between normal and neoplastic mammary tissues of the rat (Kadohama and Turkington, 1973b).

The relative rates of phosphorylation of acidic chromatin proteins in normal and neoplastic mammary cells *in vitro* were also compared. Figure 7 shows the electrophoretic radioactivity patterns of the acidic chromatin proteins derived from normal or neoplastic rat mammary tissues after labeling with tritiated amino acids or ^{32}P under conditions of simultaneous labeling. As in the case of results in similar studies in the mouse system, significant labeling with ^{32}P was associated with a large number of protein peaks in all of the gel patterns, and in each preparation the majority of the ^{32}P-labeling was recovered as [^{32}P]phosphoserine and [^{32}P]phosphothreoninine. These patterns indicate a somewhat decreased net rate of phosphorylation of the acidic chromatin proteins of high molecular weight in the carcinoma cells as compared to the patterns observed with the normal rat mammary cells.

These studies comparing normal and neoplastic mammary cells in terms of their acidic chromatin proteins have documented definite differences in the qualitative and quantitative characteristics of the electrophoretic

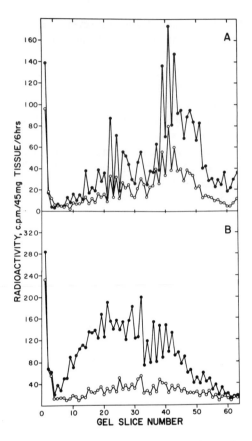

Fig. 7. Electrophoretic radioactivity patterns of acidic chromatin proteins labeled with [³H]aspartate and [³H]leucine or ³²P in rat mammary gland or rat mammary carcinoma explants. Explants from lactational gland (A) and rat mammary carcinoma R3230AC (B) were allowed to incorporate isotopic labels for four hours and were then extracted of acidic chromatin proteins. Closed circles, ³H; open circles, ³²P. The front is at 6.3 cm. (Reproduced from *Cancer Res.* by permission.)

profile, amino acid composition of the extracted acidic proteins, and relative rates of polypeptide synthesis and phosphorylation of these proteins. These differences do not relate merely to the physiological state of lactation in the normal tissue used for comparison, since significant differences in these parameters are also observed with epithelial cells derived from virginal, nonlactating mammary cells (Kadohama and Turkington, 1973a). The differences have been demonstrated for mammary carcinomas in two separate species, for a virus-associated as well as an apparently virus-independent neoplasm, and for spontaneous as well as transplantable carcinomas. The altered patterns of content and rates of synthesis of acidic chromatin proteins found in each of the model mammary cancers studied in these experiments were highly characteristic of the tumor type and were highly reproducible between tumors of the same type. Within the mouse system, progressive alterations in the content of acidic chromatin proteins was observed with progression to an advanced stage of neoplasia, the transplantable C3HBA carcinoma. These results suggest the likelihood that alterations in the acidic chromatin proteins may be a general characteristic of breast cancer cells and that differences in the acidic chromatin protein profiles may be anticipated between various human spontaneous breast cancers. Recently, Weisenthal and Ruddon (1972) have demonstrated distinct differences in the content of acidic nuclear proteins between various types of human leukemias, such as chronic granulocytic leukemia, chronic lymphocytic leukemia, lymphosarcoma, and acute monocytic leukemia. The profiles of non-histone proteins of the human leukemia cells could be distinguished from those of Burkitt's lymphoma cells, although the acidic nuclear protein from normal lymphocytes was indistinguishable from that obtained from chronic lymphocytic leukemia cells which were morphologically like mature lymphocytes. Stimulation of leukemic lymphocytes by the blastogenic agent phytohemagglutinin converted their nuclear acidic chromatin protein profiles to a pattern similar to that observed in Burkitt's lymphoma cells. These results provide further evidence for the possible participation of these proteins in the regulation of gene expression and suggest that these proteins may provide a valuable index for further characterizing the neoplastic development of other human cancers.

VI.   Concluding Comments

Further study of the acidic chromatin proteins is certain to provide fruitful information relating to their nature and their roles in nuclear and cellular physiology. It is likely that at least three classes of proteins will be identified according to functional properties. The first of these may include nuclear and chromatin proteins with an enzymatic function, such as the RNA polymerase enzymes, which are known constituents of the acidic chromatin protein fraction. A second class of proteins of potentially great significance will include those proteins which specifically interact with the DNA template to alter the transcriptive activities of genes in specific operons or other functional units. Studies on similar proteins in prokaryotic systems have demonstrated that the lac operon repressor as well as the lambda phage repressor are acidic proteins which regulate transcription of the DNA. It remains to be determined to what extent acidic chromatin proteins may represent the repressor activity of proteins which have been identified in nuclear transplantation experiments as primarily cytoplasmic repressors. It has been demonstrated in the nuclear transplantation studies of Gurdon (1962) that cytoplasmic influences may determine the pattern of gene expression in nuclei which are derived from highly differentiated cells and then transplanted into the cytoplasm of enucleate amphibian eggs. It is possible that such cytoplasmic proteins interact directly with acidic chromatin proteins or that certain chromatin proteins may in fact originate from the population of cytoplasmic repressor proteins. A third class of acidic chromatin proteins may be those contributing to the "structural"characteristics of chromatin. These proteins may be constituents of the nucleolus or chromosomes or of other intranuclear organelles which are as yet poorly defined. Advancement in two areas would appear to be required to attain this type of knowledge: improved techniques for the extraction and reconstitution of chromatin; and the purification of specific species of acidic chromatin proteins for the determination of their primary structure and the effect of their interaction with DNA on the template properties of specific deoxynucleotide sequences (operons and individual genes).

Knowledge relating to the effect of hormones on the nucleus may be advanced by further study of the acidic chromatin proteins. Identification of specific proteins which are activated or synthesized at a greater rate during the action of a specific hormone on its target cell may provide for the use of that protein as a molecular probe for identifying specific sites within the chromosome which are specifically activated by hormonal stimulation. In the field of cancer research, increasing knowledge relating to the acidic chromatin proteins of neoplastic cells may serve as a basis for characterizing and determining the neoplastic properties of cancer cells, not only in experimental models but also in dealing with clinical cancer as presented by the individual human patient with primary or metastatic disease. The acidic chromatin proteins may thus form a focal point bridging fundamental research on nuclear physiology and the application of fundamental concepts to important human problems.

ACKNOWLEDGMENT

Preparation of this manuscript was supported in part by Grants CA-12904 and HD-06215 from the U. S. Public Health Service and Grant VC-62B from the American Cancer Society.

REFERENCES

Ahmed, K. (1971). *Biochim. Biophys. Acta* **243**, 38–48.
Arnold, E. A., and Young, K. E. (1972). *Biochim. Biophys. Acta* **257**, 482–496.
Baserga, R., and Stein, G. (1971). *Fed. Proc., Fed. Amer. Soc. Exp. Biol.* **30**, 1752–1759.
Benjamin, W., and Gellhorn, A. (1968). *Proc. Nat. Acad. Sci. U.S.* **59**, 262–268.
Bern, H. A., and Nandi, S. (1961). *Progr. Exp. Tumor Res.* **2**, 90–144.

Bhorjee, J. S., and Pederson, T. (1972), *Proc. Nat. Acad. Sci. U.S.* **69**, 3345-3349.

Bishop, J. O. (1972). *In* "Gene Transcription in Reproductive Tissues" (E. Diczfalusy, ed.), pp. 247-276. Karolinska Institute, Stockholm.

Borun, T. W., and Stein, G. S. (1972). *J. Cell Biol.* **52**, 308-315.

Bouteille, M. (1972). *In* "Gene Transcription in Reproductive Tissues" (E. Diczfalusy, ed.), pp. 11-28. Karolinska Institute, Stockholm.

Britten, R. J., and Kohne, D. E. (1966). *Carnegie Inst. Yearb. Wash.*, **65**, 78-106.

Bruchovsky, N., and Wilson, J. D. (1968). *J. Biol. Chem.* **243**, 5953-5960.

Buck, M. D., and Schauder, P. (1970). *Biochim. Biophys. Acta* **224**, 644-646.

Busch, H. (1965). *In* "Histones and Other Nuclear Proteins," Chapter VIII, pp. 197-226. Academic Press, New York.

Chamness, G. C., Jennings, A. W., and McGuire, W. L. (1973). *Fed. Proc., Fed. Amer. Soc. Biol.* **32**, 230 (abstr.).

Chetsanga, C. J., Poccia, D. L., Hill, J., and Doty, P. (1970). *Cold Spring Harbor Symp. Quant. Biol.* **35**, 629-634.

Chiarugi, V. P. (1969). *Biochim. Biophys. Acta* **179**, 129-135.

Chytil, F., and Spelsberg, T. C. (1971). *Nature (London), New Biol.* **233**, 215-218.

Cognetti, G., Settineri, D., and Spinelli, G. (1972). *Exp. Cell Res.* **71**, 465-468.

Daniel, C. W., DeOme, K. B., Young, J. T., Blair, P. B., and Faulkin, L. J., Jr. (1968). *Proc. Nat. Acad. Sci. U.S.* **61**, 53-60.

DeBellis, R., Benjamin, W., and Gellhorn, A. (1969). *Biochem. Biophys. Res. Commun.* **36**, 166-173.

DeOme, K. B., Bern, H. A., Nandi, S., Pitelka, D. R., and Faulkin, L. J., Jr. (1959a). *In* "Genetics and Cancer," pp. 327-348. Univ. of Texas Press, Austin.

DeOme, K. B., Faulkin, L. J., Jr., Bern, H. A., and Blair, P. B. (1959b). *Cancer Res.*, **19**, 515-520.

DeOme, K. B., Nandi, S., Bern, H. A., Blair, P., and Pitelka, D. (1962). *In* "The Morphological Precursors of Cancer" (L. Severi, ed.), pp. 349-368. Perugia Univ. Press, Perugia, Italy.

Dijkstra, J., and Weide, S. S. (1972). *Exp. Cell Res.* **71**, 377-387.

Dounce, A. L., Chanda, S. K., Ickowicz, R., Volkman, D., and Palermiti, M. (1972). *In* "Gene Transcription in Reproductive Tissues" (E. Diczfalusy, ed.), pp. 86-111. Karolinska Institute, Stockholm.

Dunn, T. B. (1959). *In* "The Physiopathology of Cancer" (F. Homburger, ed.), pp. 123-148. Harper (Hoeber), New York.

Elgin, S. C. R., and Bonner, J. (1970). *Biochemistry* **9**, 4440-4447.

Elgin, S. C. R., Froehner, S. C., Smart, J. E., and Bonner, J. (1971). *Advan. Cell Mol. Biol.*, **1**, 1-57.

Enea, V., and Allfrey, V. G. (1973). *Nature (London)* **242**, 265-267.

Foulds, L. (1969). *In* "Neoplastic Development," Vol. 1, pp. 41-89. Academic Press, New York.

Gellhorn, A., Benjamin, W., Levander, O., and DeBellis, R. (1969). *Proc. Amer. Ass. Cancer Res.* **7**, 23.

Gershey, E. L., and Kleinsmith, L. J. (1969). *Biochim. Biophys. Acta* **194**, 331-334.

Gilmour, R. S., and Paul, J. (1969). *J. Mol. Biol.* **40**, 137-139.

Gilmour, R. S., and Paul, J. (1970). *FEBS Lett.* **9**, 242-244.

Graziano, S. L., and Huang, R. C. C. (1971). *Biochemistry* **10**, 4770-4777.

Grunicke, H., Potter, V. R., and Morris, H. P. (1970). *Cancer Res.* **30**, 776-787.

Gurdon, J. B. (1962). *J. Embryol. Exp. Morphol.* **10**, 622-640.

Helmsing, P. J., and Berendes, H. D. (1971). *J. Cell Biol.* **50**, 893-896.

Hill, R. J., Poccia, D. L., and Doty, P. (1971). *J. Mol. Biol.* **61**, 445–462.
Hnilica, L. S., and Johnson, A. W. (1970). *Exp. Cell. Res.* **63**, 261–270.
Johnson, E. M., and Allfrey, V. G. (1972). *Arch Biochem. Biophys.* **152**, 786–794.
Kadohama, N., and Turkington, R. W. (1973a). *Can. J. Biochem.* **51**, 1167–1176.
Kadohama, N., and Turkington, R. W. (1973b). *Cancer Res.* **33**, 1194–1201.
King, R. J., Gordon, J. B., and Steggles, A. W. (1972). *Biochem J.* **114**, 649–657.
Kleinsmith, L. J., and Allfrey, V. G. (1969). *Biochim. Biophys. Acta* **175**, 123–135.
Kleinsmith, L. J., Heidema, J., and Carroll, A. (1970). *Nature (London)* **266**, 1025–1026.
Kostraba, N. C., and Wang, T. Y. (1970). *Int. J. Biochem.* **1**, 327–334.
Kostraba, N. C., and Wang, T. Y. (1971). *Cancer Res.* **31**, 1663–1668.
Kostraba, N. C., and Wang, T. Y. (1972a). *Biochim. Biophys. Acta* **262**, 169–180.
Kostraba, N. C., and Wang, T. Y. (1972b). *Cancer Res.* **32**, 2348–2352.
Langan, T. (1967). *In* "Regulation of Nucleic Acid and Protein Synthesis" (V. V. Koningsberger and L. Bosch, eds.), pp. 233–241. Elsevier, Amsterdam.
LeStourgeon, W. M., and Rusch, H. P. (1971). *Science* **174**, 1233–1236.
LeStourgeon, W. M., and Rusch, H. P. (1973). *Arch. Biochem. Biophys.* **155**, 144–158.
Levy, S., Simpson, R. T., and Sober, H. A. (1972). *Biochemistry* **11**, 1547–1554.
Lilienfeld, L. (1893). *Z. Physiol. Chem.* **18**, 472–486.
Loeb, J. E., and Creuzet, C. (1970). *Bull. Soc. Chim. Biol.* **52**, 1007–1020.
McCredie, J. A., Inch, W. R., Kruuv, J., and Watson, T. A. (1965). *Growth* **29**, 331–347.
MacGillivray, A. J., Carroll, D., and Paul, J. (1971). *FEBS Lett.* **13**, 204–208.
MacGillivray, A. S., Paul, J., and Threlfall, G. (1972). *Advan. Cancer Res.* **15**, 93–162.
Marushige, K., and Ozaki, H. (1967). *Develop. Biol.* **16**, 474–488.
Marushige, K., Brutlag, D., and Bonner, J. (1968). *Biochemistry* **9**, 3149–3155.
Melli, M., and Bishop, J. O. (1970). *Biochem. J.* **120**, 225–235.
Mendecki, J., Minc. B., and Chorazy, M. (1969). *Biochem. Biophys. Res. Commun.* **36**, 494–501.
Nandi, S. (1966). *Proc. Can. Cancer Res. Conf.* **6**, 69–81.
Neiman, P. E., and Henry, P. H. (1969). *Biochemistry* **8**, 275–282.
O'Malley, B. W., Spelsberg, T. C., Schrader, W. T., Chytil, F., and Steggles, A. W. (1971). *Nature (London)* **235**, 141–144.
Panyim, S., Jensen, R. H., and Chalkley, R. (1968). *Biochim. Biophys. Acta* **160**, 252–255.
Patel, G., Patel, V., Wang, T. Y., and Zobel, C. R. (1968). *Arch. Biochem. Biophys.* **128**, 654–662.
Paul, J., and Gilmour, R. S. (1968). *J. Mol. Biol.* **34**, 305–316.
Paul, J., Gilmour, R. S., More, J. A. R., Threlfall, G., Wilkie, M., and Wilson, S. (1972). *In* "Gene Transcription in Reproductive Tissues" (E. Diczfalusy, ed.), pp. 277–297, Karolinska Institute, Stockholm.
Pierce, G. B., Jr. (1965). *Cancer Res.* **25**, 656–669.
Platz, R. D., Kish, V. M., and Kleinsmith, L. J. (1970). *FEBS Lett.* **12**, 38–40.
Richter, K. H., and Sekeris, C. E. (1972). *Arch. Biochem. Biophys.* **148**, 44–53.
Rovera, G., and Baserga, R. (1971). *J. Cell. Physiol.* **77**, 201–212.
Rovera, G., Baserga, R., and Defendi, V. (1972). *Nature (London), New Biol.* **237**, 240–241.
Shaw, L. M. J., and Huang, R. C. C. (1970). *Biochemistry* **9**, 4530–4542.
Shelton, K. R., and Allfrey, V. G. (1970). *Nature (London)* **228**, 132–134.
Shelton, K. R., and Neelin, J. M. (1971). *Biochemistry* **10**, 2343–2348.
Smith, J. A., King, R. J. B., Meggitt, B. F., and Allen, L. N. (1970). *Brit. Med. J.* **2**, 698–701.
Spelsberg, T. C., and Hnilica, L. S. (1971). *Biochim. Biophys. Acta* **228**, 202–211.
Spelsberg, T. C., Hnilica, L. S., and Ansevin, A. T. (1971). *Biochem. Biophys. Acta* **228**, 550–562.

Sporn, M. B., and Dingman, C. W. (1966). *Cancer Res.* **26,** 2488–2495.

Steele, W. J., and Busch, H. (1963). *Cancer Res.* **23,** 1153–1163.

Stein, G., and Baserga, R. (1970). *J. Biol. Chem.* **245,** 6097–6107.

Stein, G. S., and Borun, T. W. (1972). *J. Cell Biol.* **52,** 292–307.

Stellwagon, R. H., and Cole, R. D. (1969). *Annu. Rev. Biochem.* **38,** 951–989.

Swaneck, G. E., Chu, L. L. H., and Edelman, I. S. (1970). *J. Biol. Chem.* **245,** 5382–5389.

Teng, C. S., and Hamilton, T. H. (1969). *Proc. Nat. Acad. Sci. U.S.* **63,** 465–472.

Teng, C. S., and Hamilton, T. H. (1970). *Biochem. Biophys. Res. Commun.* **40,** 1231–1238.

Teng, C. S., Teng, C. T., and Allfrey, V. G. (1971). *J. Biol. Chem.* **246,** 3597–3609.

Teng, C. T., Teng, C. S., and Allfrey, V. G. (1970). *Biochem. Biophys. Res. Commun.* **41,** 690–696.

Tsuboi, A., and Baserga, R. (1972). *J. Cell. Physiol.* **80,** 107–118.

Turkington, R. W. (1968). *Curr. Top. Develop. Biol.* **3,** 199–218.

Turkington, R. W. (1970). *Biochim. Biophys. Acta* **213,** 484–494.

Turkington, R. W. (1971a). *Cancer Res.* **31,** 427–432.

Turkington, R. W. (1971b). *In* "Developmental Aspects of the Cell Cycle" (I. L. Cameron, G. M. Padilla, and A. Zimmerman, eds.), pp. 315–355. Academic Press, New York.

Turkington, R. W. (1972). *J. Nat. Cancer Inst.* **48,** 1231–1234.

Turkington, R. W., and Kadohama, N. (1972). *In* "Gene Transcription in Reproductive Tissues" (E. Diczfalusy, ed.), pp. 346–368. Karolinska Institute, Stockholm.

Turkington, R. W., and Riddle, M. (1969). *J. Biol. Chem.* **244,** 6040–6046.

Turkington, R. W., and Riddle, M. (1970a). *Cancer Res.* **30,** 127–132.

Turkington, R. W., and Riddle, M. (1970b). *Cancer Res.* **30,** 650–657.

Turkington, R. W., and Self, D. J. (1970). *Cancer Res.* **30,** 1833–1840.

Turkington, R. W., Majumder, G. C., Kadohama, N., MacIndoe, J. H., and Frantz, W. L. (1973). *Recent Progr. Horm. Res.* **29,** 417–449.

van den Broek, H. W. J., Nooden, L. D., Sevall, J. S., and Bonner, J. (1973). *Biochemistry* **12,** 229–236.

Wang, T. Y. (1966). *J. Biol. Chem.* **241,** 2913–2917.

Wang, T. Y. (1968). *Exp. Cell Res.* **53,** 288–291.

Wang, T. Y., and Johns, E. W. (1968). *Arch. Biochem. Biophys.* **124,** 176–183.

Weisenthal, L. M., and Ruddon, R. W. (1972). *Cancer Res.* **32,** 1009–1017.

Wilhelm, J. A., Groves, C. M., and Hnilica, L. S. (1972). *Experientia* **28,** 514–516.

Yoshida, M., and Shimura, (1972). *Biochim. Biophys. Acta* **263,** 690–695.

CHAPTER II

COMPARISON AMONG THE METABOLIC CHARACTERISTICS OF NORMAL, PRENEOPLASTIC, AND NEOPLASTIC MAMMARY TISSUES

S. ABRAHAM AND J. C. BARTLEY

I. Introduction

For many years we have investigated a mouse mammary gland system which is characterized by the occurrence of a recognizable preneoplastic tissue. We used the term preneoplastic as defined by DeOme and colleagues in 1961: "an identifiable part of the mammary gland which bears no morphological resemblance to mammary neoplasms, but which, nevertheless, is the site of the neoplastic transformation" (DeOme *et al.*, 1961). These preneoplastic structures are the hyperplastic alveolar nodules (HAN) found in the mammary glands of old virgin and old multiparous female mice.* HAN were first identified and described over sixty years ago (Apolant, 1906; Haaland, 1911) and have been repeatedly observed since that time (Gardner, 1942; Huseby and Bittner, 1946; Mühlbock, 1956, 1958; Squartini, 1956).

DeOme, Bern, and their co-workers (1958) have described the morphological and cytochemical characteristics of HAN. These nodules resemble the normal prelactating gland (DeOme *et al.*, 1958) in that the spacing and arrangement of the alveoli are the same and the cells possess simularly vacuolated cytoplasms. This morphology plus the presence of

---

* Subsequently, such hyperplasias have been identified and studied in other species such as dog (Cameron and Faulkin, 1971), rat (Beuving *et al.*, 1967), and even human (Wellings and Jentoft, 1972) breast tissue.

virus-like particles (Pitelka et al., 1958) in the nodules found in the mammary glands of C3H mice provided an indication of the preneoplastic nature of the HAN.

With the aid of a transplantation technique (DeOme et al., 1959), the increased neoplastic potential of these nodules over that of the normal gland has been repeatedly demonstrated (DeOme et al., 1959, 1961; Blair et al., 1962). After the mammary fat pads of female mice are cleared of their mammary elements, samples of HAN and normal gland of similar dimensions, when implanted into the cleared fat pad, will fill the pad within 3-4 months. Mammary adenocarcinomas appear more frequently and in a shorter time from the nodule than from the normal outgrowths (DeOme et al., 1959, 1961; Blair et al., 1962). In those cases where neoplasms did develop in normal outgrowths, the presence of HAN was detected in the transplanted tissue (DeOme et al., 1961). It appears clear, therefore, that the HAN is a good model for a naturally occurring preneoplastic state.

During the late nineteen-fifties and early nineteen-sixties, the influence of hormones on development and maintenace of nodules was extensively investigated by Bern, Nandi, and their colleagues (Bern et al., 1958; Bern, 1960; Bern and Nandi, 1961; DeOme et al., 1961). Those workers showed that a mixture of estradiol, a C-21 steroid, and growth hormone or prolactin could induce nodulogenesis in mice. This same mixture is responsible for normal lobuloalveolar development as well (Nandi, 1958). Ablation studies clearly demonstrated that a functional pituitary was required for the maintenance of established nodules (Bern et al., 1957). Additional studies, this time with hypophysectomized-ovariectomized-adrenalectomized mice, conclusively established that the pituitary factor required for such maintenance can be either growth hormone or prolactin and that steroids are not required to sustain the developed nodule (Nandi, 1958; Nandi and Bern, 1961). However, further studies and analysis of previous results led Bern (1960) to modify this view somewhat. Since the hormonal influence had more of the characteristics of a permissive effect than of an inductive one, Bern (1960) reasoned that sensitivity of some cells to the hormones responsible for development and maintenance of the normal gland may result in the development of preneoplastic nodules and subsequently to the production of neoplastic cells.

The importance of the transplantation technique cannot be overemphasized. This procedure for propagating the HAN in fat pads cleared of their glandular elements provided the means for demonstrating the preneoplastic nature of the nodule and allowed for an opportunity to study the hormonal requirements for development and maintenance. A further dividend from this technique is the availability of nodular tissue in amounts sufficient to allow metabolic and biochemical studies. In vivo propagation of the nodules in cleared fat pads of virgin mice will produce outgrowths of 50–100 mg in each pad. Therefore, we adapted techniques to this limited amount of tissue and have focused our attention on the biochemical and metabolic properties of these preneoplastic nodules, their normal precursors, and adenocarcinomas. However, the cellular components as well as the activity of the parenchymal cells of the gland are altered depending upon the physiological state of the female. Therefore, we have studied tissues from mice in all lactational stages: quiescent (virgin), prelactating, and lactating. Such an approach was taken partly to provide an adequate control tissue and partly to identify differences in cellular activity which accompany changes in the hormal environment of the cells.

II.   Metabolic Characteristics

A. Enzymology

In light of our recent studies demonstrating enzymological differences between spontaneous and transplanted mammary adenocarcinomas (Abraham et al., 1973), we should state that the studies on glycolytic and Krebs cycle enzymes were conducted with tumors arising spontaneously, either within normal glands or in transplanted HAN. In the other investigations discussed here, serially transplanted tumors were employed as indicated.

In these enzyme studies, and in others as well, the presence of milk in some tissues presented problems unique to mammary gland systems. Since enzyme activity is usually expressed per unit protein, it was essential to rid the tissues of all milk protein so that a proper assessment of the cellular activity could be made. It was also of importance to demonstrate that the tissue washing technique did not alter the concentration of cellular proteins. Lactose was the milk component chosen to measure the efficacy of the washing procedure. We could easily demonstrate that our routine procedure of washing tissue slices 4–5 times with the homogenizing solution removed all traces of lactose from the tissue (Kopelovich et al., 1966).

To provide additional proof for the reliability of the washing procedure, we compared the enzymatic activities of homogenates prepared (in 0.25 M sucrose) from washed slices with those from washed isolated cells. These cells were dissociated from the tissue with trypsin. No significant differences were observed between the specific activities of the enzymes studied in the two preparations (Kopelovich et al., 1966). Thus the washing procedure removed practically all soluble milk proteins from the slices. It is possible, of course, that the washing also removes proteins other than those of milk, but if a particular enzyme was preferentially lost, its specific activity in the washed slice homogenate fraction would have been lower than that in the cell homogenate fraction. It would appear that leakage of protein from the slices did not involve preferential loss of the enzymes we studied.

1. Subcellular Distribution

While glycolysis is usually confined to the so-called soluble fraction (cytosol) of most cells we could not assume that this would be the case in all tissues studied, particularly those which were preneoplastic and neoplastic. Therefore we examined the distribution of activity of various enzymes between three centrifically isolated subcellular fractions (Kopelovich *et al.*, 1966). With the exception of hexokinase (HK), 98% of the total enzyme activity could be recovered in the cytosol; the remainder being minor contaminations in the mitochondrial and microsomal fractions (Table I). However, when we localized cellular hexokinase activity, the lactating, normal gland and the adenocarcinoma contained appreciable activity associated with the mitochondrial fraction. To a much lesser extent, the gland from pregnant mice and the HAN also exhibited some mitochondrial hexokinase activity.

When we examined the intracellular distribution of the soluble enzymes acting on Krebs cycle intermediates, the distribution in the normal and abnormal tissues was also similar (Kopelovich *et al.*, 1967). Malic enzyme (ME), isocitrate dehydrogenase (NADPH) (ICDH), and citrate cleavage enzyme (CCE) were limited to the cytosol, whereas acontitase (AC) and malate dehydrogenase (NADH) (MDH) were present in both the mitochondrial fraction and the cytosol.

In the course of our studies on membrane proliferation by these mouse mammary tissues (Hillyard and Abraham, 1972) phosphodiesterase I (PDE I) and NADH–cytochrome c reductase (NCR) activities were used to establish the purity of the cell fractions isolated. The distribution of PDE I and NCR activities in the various subcellular fractions in normal glands from pregnant and lactating mice was similar (Table II). In tumor tissues, however, specific differences from the normal pattern were noted. For example, NCR activity was much higher in the cytosol and lower in the microsomal fraction obtained from tumor tissues than in these same fractions prepared from normal tissues. In addition, the percentage of the total PDE I activity in the tumor composite fraction was higher and that in the microsomal fraction was lower than in the corresponding fractions isolated from normal mammary tissues.

In order to determine whether the activities of PDE I and NCR in the cytosol were soluble or were bound to low-density particles, the supernatant

TABLE I

Hexokinase Activities in Homogenate Fractions of Normal Mammary Glands Taken from C3H Mice in Various Physiological States and HAN Outgrowths and Spontaneous Mammary Adenocarcinomas Excised from Virgin C3H Mice[a,b]

Tissue	State of mouse	Total activity in supernatant fraction from centrifugation			Specific activity in supernatant fraction from centrifugation			Distribution of total hexokinase		Specific activity of mitochondria
		5 minutes at 350 g	10 minutes at 10,000 g	60 minutes at 100,000 g	5 minutes at 350 g	10 minutes at 10,000 g	60 minutes at 100,000, (cytosol)	Particles (%)	Cytosol (%)	
Normal gland	Virgin (4)	0.78	0.76	0.75	9.6	16.7	22.0	4	96	0.6
Normal gland	Pregnant (4)	0.93	0.65	0.64	10.2	12.7	15.0	31	69	7.7
Normal gland	Lactating (4)	2.08	0.49	0.47	28.7	12.3	13.0	77	23	56.6
HAN outgrowth	Virgin (2)	0.80	0.64	0.58	10.4	19.6	19.0	27	73	3.4
Adenocarcinoma	Virgin (6)	1.94	1.04	1.00	30.2	27.7	27.7	48	52	36.3

[a] Taken from Kopelovich et al. (1966).

[b] Total activity is expressed as μmoles of NADPH formed/minute/gm wet weight of tissue, and specific activity as nmoles of reduced pyridine nucleotide formed/minute/mg protein of the homogenate fraction. The numbers of mice studied are given in parentheses.

TABLE II

Distribution of PDE I and NCR Activities among Subcellular Fractions of
Normal Mammary Glands and Mammary Adenocarcinomas in C3H Mice[a]

Tissue	State of mouse	Enzyme	Cell fraction			
			Mito-chondria[b]	Com-posite[c]	Microsome[d]	Cytosol
Normal	Pregnant	PDE I	3.8	12.9	70.8	12.6
		NCR	2.9	12.6	66.0	18.6
Normal	Lactating	PDE I	8.2	13.1	63.0	15.7
		NCR	9.1	14.1	60.2	16.7
Tumor	Virgin	PDE I	7.7	23.5	49.2	20.2
					(51.3)[e]	(17.1)[e]
		NCR	9.7	15.6	38.7	42.5
					(56.8)[e]	(11.4)[e]

[a] Taken from Hillyard and Abraham (1972).

[b] Particles sedimented at 8000 g for 10 minutes.

[c] Fraction sedimented at 15,000 g for 15 minutes.

[d] Particles sedimented at 100,000 g for 60 minutes.

[e] Values in parentheses, values obtained when these fractions were prepared by centrifugation at 100,000 g for 90 minutes instead of the usual 60 minutes.

fraction obtained after sedimentation of the composite fraction was centrifuged at 100,000 g for 90 minutes, rather than for the usual 60 minutes. The distribution of PDE I activity in normal and tumor tissues and NCR activity in normal tissues was not altered (Table II). In the tumors, however, the 90-minute centrifugation sedimented more NCR activity than did the 60-minute centrifugation, thereby reducing the NCR activity in the cytosol to a value similar to that found in normal tissues (11.4% versus 17.6% and 16.6%). It is apparent that homogenization of the mammary adenocarcinomas produced particles, derived from the endoplasmic reticulum, with a density distribution different than that produced from normal tissues.

The results of these studies show that the intracellular distribution of enzymes in the mammary adenocarcinoma and the HAN conforms to that in the tissue of origin. In addition our results confirmed reports from other laboratories that in neoplastic tissues the distribution of enzymes is not significantly altered from that of the normal (Lepage and Schneider, 1948; Paigen and Wenner, 1962; Blecher, 1963).

2. Isoenzyme Patterns

a. Hexokinase. We have recently investigated the binding properties and the isoenzymic identity of the mitochondrial-bound hexokinase in adenocarcinomas and in normal, lactating glands in C3H mice. The bound enzyme was solubilized from isolated mitochondria of both tissues by either glucose 6-phosphate or sodium chloride (pH 6.5) treatment as described by Rose and Warms (1967). By both procedures, the percentage of bound hexokinase released was slightly higher from tumor than from normal mitochondria. Increasing the magnesium concentration (Rose and Warms, 1967) facilitated rebinding in both cases. It was possible to bind tumor enzyme to normal mitochondria and normal enzyme to tumor mitochondria by means of the Mg^{2+} treatment. Furthermore, the change in the extent of rebinding with increasing Mg^{2+} concentration was similar in all cases.

With the use of DEAE columns (Shatton *et al.,* 1969), we separated the isoenzymes of hexokinase and found that the bound enzyme in both tissues consisted of a mixture of types I and II (J. C. Bartley, S. Barber, and S. Abraham, unpublished observations 1973). There was, however, a subtle difference between the tissues in the intracellular distribution of the isoenzymes. In the normal lactating gland, type II was the predominant isoenzyme in the cytosol and bound to the mitochondria; the reverse was true in the adenocarcinoma. In concurrence with Sato and associates (Sato *et al.,* 1969), we found no evidence of the unique appearance of Type III hexokinase in mammary adenocarcinomas, either ones carried by C3H (J. C. Bartley, S. Barber, and S. Abraham, unpublished observations, 1973) or by Balb/c mice (Abraham *et al.,* 1973), as has been reported in studies with rat tumors (Shatton *et al.,* 1969; Farron, 1972).

b. Glucose-6-phosphate Dehydrogenase. In these studies, the isoenzymes of glucose-6-phosphate dehydrogenase (GPDH) were separated by polyacrylamide gel electrophoresis according to the methods described by Hilf and co-workers (Richards and Hilf, 1972). We found that only two isoenzymes were prominent in normal mammary tissue taken from Balb/c mice, whether the animals were virgins or in the lactating condition (Hilf *et al.,* 1973). When we made a quantitative assessment of the activity of each isoenzyme, we found that the slowest migrating one (GPDH-3) represented over 80% of the total activity in the lactating gland while it was only 40% in the virginal tissue. Most of the remaining enzyme activity in both tissues was found to be in GPDH-2. On the other hand, in the experiments with the HAN outgrowths and adenocarcinomas carried by this strain of mouse, we detected the presence of a third distinct isoenzyme band (GPDH-1) which migrated much faster than GPDH-2. Furthermore, we could show that the preneoplastic HAN contained an immediate quantity in the GPDH-1 species—about 12%—while the adenocarcinoma possessed 35%. Thus, the preneoplastic and neoplastic mammary tissues can be distinguished from the normal gland by the presence of significant amounts of GPDH-1 and we suggest that its presence might even be used as a marker for predisposition toward neoplasia.

c. *Lactate Dehydrogenase.* All 5 isoenzymes of lactate dehydrogenase (LDH) were present in the cytosol prepared from virgin and lactating mammary glands of Balb/c mice, but LDH-1 and LDH-2 accounted for less than 3% of the total activity (Hilf *et al.*, 1973). On the other hand, the mammary adenocarcinoma contained a higher proportion of LDH-3 than did either normal tissue. The HAN outgrowth appeared to have an amount which was intermediate between the normal and the neoplastic tissue.

3. Changes in Enzyme Activity during Physiological Transformation

As pointed out previously (Abraham and Chaikoff, 1965; Kopelovich *et al.*, 1966, 1967; Pitelka *et al.*, 1969; Smith, and Abraham, 1970; Abraham *et al.*, 1972), a comparison of enzyme capacities of the mammary glands excised from virgin animals with those from pregnant and lactating animals must take into consideration the difference in the cell populations of these tissues. Only a small portion of the glands in virgins consist of parenchymal cells—about 9% of the defatted dry weight (Nicoll and Tucker, 1965). On the other hand, the gland in lactating animals contains a greater proportion of parenchymal cells than adipose cells; about 90% of the defatted dry weight are glandular elements. Thus, until preparations of mammary tissues in each of its physiological states essentially devoid of adipose cells can be obtained, all differences between virgin glands and pregnant or lactating glands might be due, in large part, to the differences in their cellular composition. The contents of adipose cells in the late pregnant and early lactating glands are more nearly alike, so that comparisons between these two tissues are likely to provide a reliable index of the metabolic differences among parenchymal cellular elements during transformation. In addition, recently we have shown that mammary glands from lactating mice can be dissociated into cell suspensions that are practically devoid of adipose cells (Pitelka *et al.*, 1969; Abraham *et al.*, 1972). With such preparations it was possible to demonstrate that the absence of adipocytes did not appreciably alter the metabolic characteristics of the lactating parenchymal cells.

The activity of soluble HK decreased during lactation (Tables I and III), and HK activity in the particulate fraction increased as the gland progressed from the pregnant to the lactating state (Kopelovich *et al.*,

TABLE III

Specific Activities of Glycolytic Enzymes in the Cytosols of Normal Mammary Glands and Adenocarcinomas Taken from C3H Mice in Various Stages of Development[a,b]

Enzyme[c]	State of mice from which normal glands were excised				Spontaneous tumors excised from mice in			Tumors that arose in HAN outgrowths in virgin mice (4)
	Virgin (4)	Pregnant (5)	Lactating (5)	Postlactating (4)	Virgin state (8)	Pregnancy (2)	Lactation (2)	
HK	28.3 ± 2.9	20.3 ± 2.2	10.5 ± 0.8	26.0 ± 1.8	20.1 ± 1.8	19.4	16.0	19.1 ± 1.5
PGM	35.5 ± 4.5	29.0 ± 2.0	26.0 ± 3.9	24.4 ± 4.5	37.0 ± 3.5	29.5	24.2	36.1 ± 2.9
PGI	2020 ± 64	1480 ± 39	4035 ± 50	1135 ± 61	3056 ± 37			2925 ± 49
PFK	187 ± 22	71 ± 9	83 ± 11		234 ± 9		215	
AL	1010 ± 30	663 ± 40	930 ± 20		674 ± 26		810	
α-GPDH	392 ± 19	147 ± 24	549 ± 25	126 ± 3	7.8 ± 0.5	8.6	34.5	8.6 ± 1.3
LDH	2020 ± 305	875 ± 145	1254 ± 95	833 ± 57	2278 ± 53	1880	2060	2205 ± 93
GPDH	197 ± 10	112 ± 11	623 ± 82	122 ± 5	48.7 ± 1.4	58.2	70.3	48.0 ± 2.5
6-PGDH	12.3 ± 1.2	10.6 ± 0.9	24.8 ± 2.2	9.8 ± 2.3	5.2 ± 0.4	8.2	11.0	5.9 ± 0.6
RP-GP	9.4 ± 1.8	4.4 ± 0.3	9.3 ± 2.6	3.9 ± 1.0	3.4 ± 0.4	3.8	6.3	2.9 ± 0.2
RP	14.0 ± 3.3	12.6 ± 0.9	23.0 ± 2.1		7.1 ± 1.1		12.2	6.9 ± 0.9

[a] Taken from Kopelovich et al. (1966).

[b] Specific activities are expressed as nmoles of pyridine nucleotide reduced or oxidized/mg protein/minute. Number of mice used is given in parentheses. Other details are given in Table I. The values are averages and their standard errors.

[c] HK, hexokinase; PGM, phosphoglucomutase; PGI, phosphoglucose isomerase; PFK, phosphofructokinase; AL, aldolase; α-GPDH, α-glycerophosphate dehydrogenase; LDH, lactate dehydrogenase; GPDH, glucose-6-phosphate dehydrogenase; 6-PGDH, 6-phosphogluconate dehydrogenase; RP-GP, the enzymes responsible for the breakdown of ribose-5-phosphate in the presence of added $NADP^+$; and RP, the enzymes involved in this breakdown in the presence of NADH.

1966). Since the intracellular distribution of HK in the normal lactating gland differed from that in the nonlactating gland, we also compared HK activity per gram wet tissue (Table I). These calculated results show that (a) the spontaneous neoplasm excised from virgin mice and normal lactating mammary tissues have similar activities for phosphorylating glucose; and (b) total HK activity in the adenocarcinoma was about twice that of normal gland in the nonlactating states (i.e., virgin and pregnant).

The value for the specific activity of soluble HK in the adenocarcinomas excised from virgin mice was about twice that in normal lactating glands (Table III). The specific activities of HK observed in the cytosol obtained from the normal glands excised from virgin, prepartum, and postlactating mice were similar to those found in the mammary tumor (Table III).

An increase in total HK activity of the normal rat mammary gland during lactation was demonstrated by McLean (1958) as well as by Baldwin and Milligan (1966). We have shown this to be true in mice. Thus, after 8–14 days of lactation, when glucose utilization by the mouse gland is high (Bartley et al., 1971), HK activity was greatest. During this period of glandular development, GPDH and 6-phosphogluconate dehydrogenase (6-PGDH), as well as the enzymes involved in ribose 5-phosphate breakdown via the pentose phosphate pathway, also showed highest activity. On the other hand, in the case of the tumors excised from virgin mice, even though total hexokinase activity was as high as that in normal lactating tissue, the activities of pentose phosphate pathway enzymes were low. This alteration in enzymatic profile of the neoplastic tissue may be of particular significance because of our finding that phosphoglucose isomerase (PGI) activity in the adenocarcinoma excised from the virgin animal is well within the range of that found in the normal lactating gland. These observations are consistent with the view that even though glucose utilization by the normal lactating tissue and the adenocarcinoma may be of the same order, the pathways of glucose utilization in these two tissues differ.

The activities of phosphoglucomutase (PGM) in the tumors did not differ from those in glands whether excised from pregnant, lactating. or weaned mice. The values for the ratio phosphofructokinase (PFK) activity/aldolase (AL) activity in tumors removed from virgin (0.35) and lactating mice (0.27) were higher than those for the normal glands excised from virgin mice (0.19), pregnant mice (0.11), and mice that had lactated from 11–15 days (0.10). These differences reflect the lower PFK activity and higher AL activity in the normal gland as compared to the adenocarcinoma.

The activities of α-glycerolphosphate dehydrogenase (α-GPDH) in these mouse mammary adenocarcinomas were much lower than those found in the normal glands regardless of physiological state, a finding consistent with that of Boxer and Shonk (1960). It is of interest to note, however, that although these neoplasms have lower α-GPDH activities, the levels of α-glycerolphosphate (GP) and dihydroxyacetone phosphate (DHAP) (Table IV) do not appear to be controlled by the activity of this enzyme (Rao and Abraham, 1973). It may be argued that the value for the substrate ratio, GP/DHAP, may be altered due to a change in the NADH levels in the tissue rather than from the difference in the levels of α-GPDH. However, when we measured the cytoplasmic redox state of the cells by estimating the content of lactate and pyruvate (Rao and Abraham, 1973), we found similar amounts of these two compounds in both normal and tumor tissues (Table IV). Thus the cellular contents of GP and DHAP did not correlate with the levels of enzyme activity and appeared to be independent of coenzyme levels as well. In this connection, it is of interest to note that the specific activity of LDH, another enzyme that requires NAD^+, was higher in the tumor—regardless of whether the host was in the virgin, pregnant, or lactating states—than in normal glands excised from pregnant, lactating, or postlactating mice.

The survey of the specific activity of some of the soluble Krebs cycle enzymes revealed that the activities of those enzymes which increased during transformation of the normal gland from the pregnant to the lactational state also increased in the adenocarcinoma (Table V). These differences were particularly obvious with those enzymes confined to the cytosol, i.e., ME and CCE. On the other hand, the activities of these two enzymes in all normal glands were much greater than those in the neoplasms. Aconitase activity did not differ among tumors excised from virgin, pregnant, and lactating mice but ICDH and MDH had lower specific activities in tumors from pregnant and lactating mice than in those from virgin mice. This pattern of activity was similar to that observed from these three enzymes when studied in homogenates prepared from normal glands.

4. Enzyme Activities in HAN Outgrowths

Only a portion of the HK activity was associated with the cytosol (Table I). Hence, comparisons of HK activities of HAN outgrowths with (a) those of normal glands and (b) those of mammary tumors should be based on total activities (μmoles of NADPH formed/gram tissue/minute). Although total HK activities in the HAN outgrowths did not differ from those in the normal glands excised from virgin and pregnant mice, they were less than half those of the normal lactating gland (Table I).

The activities of PGM, PGI, PFK, GPDH, and those enzymes responsible for pentose phosphate breakdown in the cytosol of the HAN outgrowth were within the range of those found in this fraction prepared from the normal mammary gland excised from the pregnant mouse (Tables

TABLE IV

α-Glycerolphosphate Dehydrogenase and Some Substrate Levels in Normal and Neoplastic Mammary Tissues of C3H Mice[a,b]

Tissue	α-GPDH activity	GP	DHAP	GP/DHAP	Lactate	Pyruvate	Lactate/pyruvate
Tumor	10 ± 0.5	135 ± 12	68 ± 2.5	2	5299 ± 184	112 ± 7	47
Lactating gland	372 ± 17	518 ± 41	36 ± 0.5	14	6000 ± 478	117 ± 6	51

[a] Taken from Rao and Abraham (1973).
[b] The results are given as averages and their standard errors of 4 experiments with tissues taken from different animals. α-GPDH activity is expressed as nmoles of NADH oxidized/minute/mg protein of the cytosol. The substrate concentrations are given as nmol/g wet weight tissue. GP, α-glycerolphosphate; DHAP, dihydroxy acetone phosphate.

TABLE V

Specific Activities of Some Krebs Cycle Enzymes in the Cytosols of Normal Mammary Glands and Adenocarcinomas Taken from C3H Mice in Various Stages of Development[a,b]

Enzyme[c]	State of mice from which normal glands were excised				Spontaneous tumors excised from mice in			Tumors that arose from HAN transplanted into virgin mice (4)
	Virgin (4)	Pregnant (5)	Lactating (5)	Postlactating (4)	Virgin state (8)	Pregnancy (3)	Lactation (3)	
AC (citrate)	10.8 ± 1.7	6.9 ± 0.8	8.2 ± 0.9	7.9 ± 1.2	7.2 ± 0.6	7.7 ± 0.9	7.5 ± 0.9	7.1 ± 0.5
AC (isocitrate)	19.4 ± 1.0	11.5 ± 1.5	17.5 ± 1.6	16.0 ± 1.7	12.6 ± 1.9	10.6 ± 1.1	11.5 ± 1.5	13.7 ± 1.1
ICDH (citrate)	13.7 ± 1.8	7.0 ± 1.1	6.2 ± 0.6	7.5 ± 1.3	7.0 ± 1.0	8.1 ± 1.2	7.6 ± 1.0	7.2 ± 1.1
ICDH (cis-aconitate)	19.4 ± 2.3	13.4 ± 1.4	17.0 ± 2.4	16.7 ± 1.6	17.4 ± 1.5	16.9 ± 1.9	14.3 ± 1.1	17.0 ± 1.9
ICDH (isocitrate)	133 ± 9	75.4 ± 7.0	31.3 ± 2.0	58.4 ± 3.9	61.8 ± 4.9	49.0 ± 3.8	48.3 ± 2.5	69.5 ± 6.3
MDH	3910 ± 96	1609 ± 119	2195 ± 97	3491 ± 183	3357 ± 151	2350 ± 131	2379 ± 91	3101 ± 101
ME	109 ± 10	29.1 ± 2.8	162 ± 23	45.9 ± 4.0	7.2 ± 1.1	5.0 ± 0.9	14.1 ± 1.6	7.4 ± 0.9
CCE	17.8 ± 1.8	10.1 ± 2.0	48.7 ± 5.1	6.6 ± 0.6	0.9 ± 0.2	0.9 ± 0.1	3.2 ± 0.5	0.8 ± 0.2

[a] Taken from Kopelovich et al. (1967).

[b] See Table III for expression of specific activity and other details. The values are averages and their standard errors.

[c] AC, aconitase (substrate used in assay given in parentheses); ICDH, isocitrate dehydrogenase (substrate used in assay given in parentheses); MDH, malate dehydrogenase; ME, malic enzyme; and CCE, citrate cleavage enzyme.

TABLE VI

Specific Activities of Enzymes in the Cytosol Fraction of HAN
Outgrowths in Gland-Free Fat Pads of Virgin C3H Mice[a,b]

Enzyme	Specific activity
Hexokinase	18.1 ± 1.9
Phosphoglucomutase	28.7 ± 1.5
Phosphoglucose isomerase	1390 ± 11
Phosphofructokinase	66.5 ± 7.3
Aldolase	211 ± 7
α-Glycerolphosphate dehydrogenase	94.1 ± 9.5
Lactic dehydrogenase	425 ± 25
Glucose-6-phosphate dehydrogenase	93.5 ± 8.6
6-Phosphogluconate dehydrogenase	13.8 ± 1.1
Ribose-5-phosphate breakdown ($NADP^+$)	7.0 ± 0.4
Ribose-5-phosphate breakdown (NADH)	14.1 ± 1.1
Aconitase (citrate)	6.5 ± 0.9
Aconitase (isocitrate)	13.7 ± 1.0
Isocitrate dehydrogenase (citrate)	4.8 ± 0.6
Isocitrate dehydrogenase (cis-aconitate)	14.8 ± 1.7
Isocitrate dehydrogenase (isocitrate)	100 ± 7
Malate dehydrogenase	1495 ± 145
Malic enzyme	28.5 ± 1.9
Citrate cleavage enzyme	9.6 ± 1.5

[a] Taken from Kopelovich et al. (1966, 1967).

[b] For expression of enzyme activities see Table III. Each value
is an average and its standard error of the results of 6 experiments
with different mice.

III, VI, and VII); aldolase activity was about three times greater in the latter than in the former tissue. Although the activities of α-GPDH and LDH
in HAN outgrowths were lower than those in normal glands, regardless of
the state of development, the values of the ratio LDH activity/α-GPDH
activity of the HAN outgrowths (about 4.5) were well within the normal
range (Table VI).

The specific activities of AC, ICDH, MDH, ME, and CCE in the
cytosol from the HAN outgrowths in gland-free mammary fat pads of
virgin mice are shown in Table VI. A comparison of the activities of these
enzymes in the HAN outgrowths with those of normal mammary glands
revealed that the activities of AC, ICDH, MDH, ME, and CCE in HAN
were well within the range of those found in normal pregnant mammary
tissue (Tables V, VI, and VII).

The enzymatic pattern of the preneoplastic tissue contrasts with that of the neoplastic tissue (Tables III and VI). Total HK activity in the preneoplastic tissue excised from the virgin mouse was less than half that of the adenocarcinoma excised from a virgin mouse. PFK and AL activities in the HAN outgrowth were about one-third those observed in the tumor. LDH and α-GPDH activities in the HAN outgrowths also differed from those of

TABLE VII

Comparison of Enzyme Activities of HAN
Outgrowths in Virgin C3H Mice and
Normal Glands in Pregnant C3H Mice[a,b]

Enzyme	Enzyme activities of HAN outgrowths in virgin mice/enzyme activities of normal glands in pregnant mice
HK	0.86
PGM	0.99
PGI	0.94
PFK	0.94
AL	0.32
α-GPDH	0.64
LDH	0.49
GPDH	0.83
6-PGDH	1.30
RP-GP	1.12
AC (citrate)	0.94
AC (isocitrate)	1.19
ICDH (citrate)	0.69
ICDH (cis-aconitate)	1.10
ICDH (isocitrate)	1.33
MDH	0.93
ME	0.98
CCE	0.96

[a] Taken from Kopelovich et al. (1966, 1967).

[b] The figures recorded above were calculated from the data given in Tables I, III, V and VI. The values for hexokinase were determined from the total activities given in Table I and those for the other enzymes were determined from the specific activities given in Tables III, V, and VI.

the tumor, i.e., lower LDH and higher α-GPDH activities were found in the HAN outgrowths (Tables III and VI).

The activities of the enzymes concerned with the pentose phosphate pathway of glucose metabolism, namely GPDH, 6-PGDH, RP-GP, and RP, in the HAN outgrowths excised from virgin mice were higher than those of the mammary tumors (Tables III and VI).

The pattern of soluble Krebs cycle enzymes in the preneoplastic tissue also differed strikingly from that in the tumor excised from a virginal animal, particularly with respect to malate utilization and CCE activity (Tables V and VI). While malate dehydrogenase activity in the HAN outgrowth was about half that in the tumor excised from a virgin mouse, the activity of malic enzyme in the former tissue was about 4 times that in the latter tissue. CCE activity in the HAN outgrowth was about 10 times that of the tumor excised from a virgin animal. Whereas aconitase activity (with citrate or isocitrate as substrate) in the HAN outgrowth was within the range found in the tumor, isocitrate dehydrogenase activity was about 40% higher in the HAN outgrowth than in the tumor (Tables V and VI).

In studies with enzymes of the endoplasmic reticulum (ER) (Hillyard and Abraham, 1972), we observed that the smooth (SER) and rough (RER) ER had markedly different PDE I activities in all mammary gland tissues studied (Table VIII). Total cellular activity in normal glands from pregnant and lactating mice was the same, whereas activity in HAN outgrowths was about 80% of that in normal glands of pregnancy. In tumor tissues, on the other hand, the activity of this enzyme was about 2.5 times greater. Total cellular NCR activity in tumors was the same as that in normal glands of pregnancy, whereas that in normal lactating glands and in HAN outgrowths was about two times higher.

The specific activities of NCR in the endoplasmic reticulum fractions did not parallel those for PDE I. The NCR-specific activities in RER were about twice that in SER for normal mammary tissues from both pregnant and lactating mice, as well as for tumors. In HAN outgrowths, on the other hand, the specific activity of NCR in SER was about twice that in RER.

5. Some Enzymes Involved in Nucleic Acid Metabolism

a. Xanthine Oxidase. Our interest in xanthine oxidase stems from the possibility that by removal of hypoxanthine and xanthine from the general pool in the form of uric acid, the activity of this enzyme could affect the overall rate of purine metabolism. This general concept has been discussed by Bergel et al. in 1956 (Bergel et al., 1957) and thereafter many workers have made quantitative assessments of xanthine oxidase activities in both

TABLE VIII

PDE I and NCR Activities in Normal Mammary Glands, HAN Outgrowths, and Mammary Adenocarcinomas[a,b]

Tissue	State of mouse	Enzyme	Whole homogenate		Endoplasmic reticulum	
			nmoles/min/ mg DNA	nmoles/min/ mg protein	Smooth (nmoles/min/ mg protein)	Rough (nmoles/min/ mg protein)
Normal	Pregnant (7)	PDE I	1327 ± 145	147.0 ± 10.6	1113 ± 153	331 ± 20
		NCR	90 ± 17	10.4 ± 1.3	57 ± 8	78 ± 6
Normal	Lactating (7)	PDE I	1432 ± 271	77.5 ± 4.9	817 ± 80	127 ± 9
		NCR	204 ± 18	8.8 ± 0.9	40 ± 2	84 ± 4
HAN outgrowth	Virgin (20)	PDE I	1035 ± 188	98.1 ± 15.6	1107 ± 147	236 ± 4
		NCR	200 ± 29	24.2 ± 1.8	125 ± 19	63 ± 6
Tumor	Virgin (9)	PDE I	3129 ± 237	178.6 ± 9.0	934 ± 68	191 ± 24
		NCR	90 ± 3	5.4 ± 0.3	20 ± 2	34 ± 2

[a] Taken from Hillyard and Abraham (1972).
[b] Tissues from individual mice (C3H) were analyzed separately, except in the experiments with the HAN outgrowth. In these latter experiments, 4 pools composed of tissues from 5 mice each were analyzed. The values are given as averages and their standard errors and the number of mice used is given in parentheses.

normal and abnormal tissues. For example Bergel *et al.* (1957) and deLa-mirande and Allard (1957) have shown the virtual absence of xanthine oxi-dase activity in breast tumors and hepatomas, respectively. In addition Lewin *et al.* (1957) have demonstrated that the activity of this enzyme was fourfold lower in mouse mammary adenocarcinomas than in virgin mouse breast tissue. However it has been known for some time now that xanthine oxidase activity of mammary tissue increases with the onset of lactation (Ling *et al.*, 1961) and one might therefore question the validity of a com-parison between virginal mammary tissue with its preponderance of adi-pose cells and mammary adenocarcinoma with its neoplastic parenchymal cells.

Thus, just as in our other studies, we looked at xanthine oxidase ac-tivities in all physiological conditions (S. Abraham, T. Hall, and B. Hacker, unpublished observations, 1973). Because of the small sample size and the need to measure low activities, the procedure used was the radio-active assay method developed by al-Khalidi and Chaglassian (1965) wherein the conversion of [8-^{14}C]xanthine to uric acid is followed chromatographically. The mice selected for this study were the Balb/c strain which do not possess either the mammary tumor or nodule inducing virus.

Contrary to the data presented by Lewin *et al.* (1957) with mice of the C strain or by Sheth *et al.* (1968) who used C3H (JAX) and ICRC mice, we observed that tumors in virgin mice had higher xanthine oxidase activity than did the normal mammary glands. Furthermore, xanthine oxidase activity in the tumors and the HAN outgrowths (Table IX) responded to the physiological state of the mouse just as it did in the normal tissues (Table IX; Lewin *et al.*, 1957). From our study it is clear that low xanthine oxidase activity is not associated with all tumors. In addition, our results indicate that the gland, when excised from pregnant or lactating mice that carry either the tumor or the HAN outgrowth, contains higher xanthine oxidase activity (Table IX).

b. tRNA Methylases. For some time now numerous investigators (Ber-quist and Mathews, 1962; Tsutsui *et al.*, 1966; Mittelman *et al.*, 1967; Silber *et al.*, 1967; Hancock, 1968; McFarlane and Shaw, 1968; Baliga *et al.*, 1969) have observed a higher level of activity of a unique group of enzymes in tumors than in normal tissues. These enzymes, tRNA methylases catalyze the transfer of methyl groups from methyl-*S*-adenosylmethionine to specific locations on the bases of tRNA at the macromolecular level (Fleissner and Borek, 1963). At the present time, al-though the exact function of these bases remains obscure, changes in tRNA methylase activities have been correlated with tissue differentiation and shifts in control mechanisms (Fleissner and Borek, 1963; Kaye *et al.*, 1966;

TABLE IX

Xanthine Oxidase Activities in Normal Mammary Glands, HAN Outgrowths, and Mammary Adenocarcinomas Taken from BALB/c Mice in Various Physiological States[a,b]

State of mouse	Tissue			Normal tissue in mice	
	Normal	HAN	Tumor	Bearing HAN	Bearing tumor
Virgin	0.78 ± 0.14	0.51 ± 0.20	6.95 ± 3.81	0.63 ± 0.43	0.55 ± 0.31
Pregnant	8.84 ± 4.13	4.52 ± 3.84		15.0 ± 13.2	
Lactating	18.5 ± 1.9	3.21 ± 2.64	30.4 ± 7.3	24.2 ± 2.8	39.3 ± 7.7

[a] Taken from S. Abraham, T. Hall, and B. Hacker, unpublished observations (1973).

[b] Specific activities are expressed as nmoles of uric acid formed from xanthine per mg cytosol protein per 30 minutes and are recorded below as the averages and standard errors of at least 6 determinations.

Wainfan *et al.*, 1966; Hancock *et al.*, 1967; Simon *et al.*, 1967; Kerr and Dische, 1970). Indeed, Waalkes *et al.* (1971) have observed that the activity of this class of enzymes is severalfold higher in hepatomas induced in monkeys by the administration of *N*-nitrosodiethylamine than in normal livers. In addition, they were able to show that premalignant liver also exhibited an elevated level of tRNA methylase activity.

In limited studies of this enzyme system in Balb/c mice, we (S. Abraham, T. Hall, and B. Hacker, unpublished observations, 1973) found that methylating activity of normal glands was 70 and 120 pmoles of the ^{14}C-methyl groups of [^{14}C]methyl-*S*-adenosylmethionine incorporated into *Escherichia coli* β tRNA/mg protein/30 minutes (Bradford *et al.*, 1972) for virgins and midlactating mice, respectively. In tumors, the values were 319 and 350 for virgins and lactators, respectively, whereas the values for HAN outgrowths were not different from those observed in normal mammary tissues. Thus, although we did observe that neoplasms had elevated activities, we could not confirm (in a naturally occurring preneoplastic tissue) the findings of Waalkes *et al.* (1971).

B. Substrate Utilization and Product Formation

Enzyme activities measured under optimum conditions are usually interpreted as an indication of the maximum potential of a pathway and yield little information concerning the actual metabolic fate of a substrate or its rate of utilization under physiological conditions. We have, therefore, attempted to correlate changes in enzyme activity with actual changes in "metabolic throughput." Thus we compared the data obtained from our enzyme studies of these tissues with data obtained from experiments with slices incubated with specifically labeled precursors of the products which are characteristic of these mammary tissues.

Our enzyme studies have revealed that the preneoplastic tissues of the mammary gland are metabolically responsive to changes in the physiological state of the animal and, hence, are under some neurohormonal influence. Furthermore, the levels of enzymatic activity in the outgrowth of the HAN were closer to that of normal lactating gland than to that of the adenocarcinoma and were distinguishable from that of normal gland from a pregnant mouse in only three enzymes (AL, α-GPDH, and LDH) whose activities are usually not considered rate limiting in any pathway.

Pregnant and lactating mice were used to compare the response of the preneoplastic and neoplastic tissues with that of normal mammary gland. Normal outgrowths and the tissues from glands with seared nipples provided controls for comparison with the hyperplastic alveolar outgrowths. In these tissues, the hormonal environment would be the same and, in addition, the biosynthetic products produced within the tissues could not be removed by means of suckling.

In order to compare the metabolic activities between the various mammary tissues, one must consider the differences in the relative amounts of protein in each tissue type. Thus, for facilitation of comparisons between tissues, the uptake and conversion of isotopically labeled glucose and acetate to metabolic products have been expressed in terms of the amount of substrate taken up or product formed per milligram protein. Since the utilization of glucose per milligram protein by each tissue type did not differ to any large degree (Table X), the conclusions based on the nmoles of substrate converted to product per milligram protein and those derived from calculations based on the uptake of glucose would be similar.

1. Tissue Composition

Normal mammary outgrowth had the highest and mammary adenocarcinoma had the lowest lipid content of all tissues (Table XI). Whereas the protein content of the normal outgrowths was somewhat lower than that of either the tumors or the normal lactating glands, the values obtained with the normal lactating glands and the HAN outgrowths were similar. The

TABLE X

Uptake of Glucose and of Acetate by Slices of Normal Mammary Gland, HAN, and Adenocarcinoma Prepared from Lactating C3H Mice[a,b]

Tissue	Glucose uptake in presence of acetate	Acetate uptake in presence of	
		No added substrate	Glucose
Normal gland	556 ± 32	357 ± 32	492 ± 24
Normal outgrowth	624 ± 45	323 ± 32	355 ± 43
HAN outgrowth	627 ± 43	373 ± 17	432 ± 25
Adenocarcinoma	453 ± 20	313 ± 13	307 ± 20

[a] Taken from Bartley et al. (1971).

[b] Experimental details are given in Bartley et al. (1971). Each value recorded above is the average and its standard error of the results of triplicate determinations on 4 to 7 experiments with tissues from separate mice and is presented as nmoles of added substrate taken up per mg protein.

TABLE XI

Composition of Normal Mammary Glands, HAN, and
Adenocarcinomas from Lactating C3H Mice[a,b]

	Percent of wet weight		
Kind of tissue	Lipid	Protein	Water
Lactating gland	10.6 ± 0.1	12.6 ± 0.8	76.7 ± 0.9
Normal outgrowth	24.7 ± 0.7	9.3 ± 1.3	66.0 ± 2.0
HAN outgrowth	7.2 ± 1.6	11.8 ± 1.8	81.0 ± 3.4
Adenocarcinoma	3.2 ± 0.7	15.0 ± 0.7	81.8 ± 1.4

[a] Taken from Bartley et al. (1971).
[b] Each value recorded above is the average and its standard
error from 3 to 5 separate determinations.

relatively high lipid and low protein contents of the normal outgrowths may
be a reflection of the presence of a greater number of adipose cells in the
tissues, relative to that found in the HAN outgrowths (Bartley et al., 1971).

The DNA contents of the normal glands, whether from pregnant or lactating mice, and of the HAN outgrowths were very similar, but the adeno-
carinoma contained almost twice as much as these other tissues (Table
XII). Whether this greater amount of DNA per gram of tissue is a
reflection of the polyploidy of the adenocarcinoma (Banerjee and DeOme,
1963) or is due to a greater cell density has not been ascertained. The RNA
contents of these tissues, on the other hand, did not show any distinct patterns in that the tumors and the lactating normal tissues were the highest
and the HAN and the pregnant, the lowest (Table XII).

2. Protein Synthesis

We have also measured protein synthesis, in the normal (Pitelka et al.,
1969; Abraham et al., 1972; Hillyard and Abraham, 1972; J. C. Bartley, S.
Barber, and S. Abraham, unpublished observations, 1973), preneoplastic
(Hillyard and Abraham, 1972; J. C. Bartley, S. Barber, and S. Abraham,
unpublished observations, 1973), and neoplastic mammary tissues (Hillyard
and Abraham, 1972; J. C. Bartley, S. Barber, and S. Abraham,
unpublished observations, 1973). The rate of ^{14}C-labeled L-leucine incorporation into protein by intact mammary gland cells from lactating mice was
similar (27 μmoles/mg protein/hour) in all studies. The rate of protein syn-

thesis in glandular tissue from pregnant mice was 3-fold higher (J. C. Bartley, S. Barber and S. Abraham, unpublished observations, 1973). Considering the high rate of synthesis of milk components, it is surprising that the rate of protein synthesis is higher in pregnant than in lactating glands. As expected, RNA synthesis showed a similar pattern (J. C. Bartley, S. Barber and S. Abraham, unpublished observations, 1973).

The rate of protein synthesis in the HAN and the tumor was greater than that of lactating gland and slightly less than that of the pregnant. A similar relationship was observed in the case of phosphatidylcholine synthesis (Hillyard and Abraham, 1972). Changes in the physiological state of the host had no effect on the rate of protein synthesis in either the HAN outgrowths or the adenocarcinomas (J. C. Bartley, S. Barber, and S. Abraham, unpublished observations, 1973).

3. Lactose Synthesis

Lactose is a unique carbohydrate which is synthesized only in mammary glands. The enzyme system responsible for its synthesis, lactose synthetase, is composed of two subunits, both of which are required (Brodbeck et al., 1967). The A component is nonspecific and has N-acetyllactosamine synthetase activity (transfers galactose from UDP galactose to N-acetylglucosamine) (Brew et al., 1968). The B component is responsible for the specific transfer of galactose from UDP galactose to glucose, and is identical to the common milk protein α-lactalbumin

TABLE XII

DNA and RNA Contents of Normal Mammary Glands in Pregnant and Lactating C3H Mice and in HAN Outgrowths and Adenocarcinomas in Virgin C3H Mice[a,b]

Tissue	State of mouse	DNA (mg/gm tissue)	RNA (mg/gm tissue)	RNA/DNA
Normal	Pregnant (7)	2.9 ± 0.3	8.4 ± 0.6	2.9 ± 0.7
Normal	Lactating (6)	2.4 ± 0.2	18.5 ± 1.1	7.7 ± 0.6
HAN outgrowth	Virgin (10)	2.4	6.2	3.6
Tumor	Virgin (7)	4.4 ± 0.7	11.4 ± 0.8	2.6 ± 0.1

[a] Taken from Hillyard and Abraham (1972).

[b] Tissues from individual mice were analyzed separately except for the experiments with HAN outgrowths. In these experiments, 2 pools (each composed of tissue from 5 mice) were used. The values represent the averages and standard errors. Number of mice used is given in parentheses.

TABLE XIII

Lactose Synthesized from Glucose by Mammary Gland
Slices and Isolated Parenchymal Cells from C3H Mice[a,b]

| Substrate | Lactose synthesized by | |
	Slices	Cells
[1-¹⁴C]Glucose	42.5 ± 10.9	143 ± 5
[6-¹⁴C]Glucose	46.0 ± 9.6	147 ± 12

[a] Taken from Abraham et al. (1972).
[b] Slices or cell suspensions were incubated with [1-¹⁴C]
or [6-¹⁴C] glucose as described in Abraham et al. (1972).
The results are given as the average number of nmoles
of glucose converted to lactose per mg protein with
standard errors from 6 experiments.

(Brodbeck et al., 1967). The recent work of Palmitier (1969) has
demonstrated that the same hormones necessary for differentiation of the
mammary gland (Juergens et al., 1965; Lockwood et al., 1966) are also
responsible for augmentation of lactose synthetase activity when the animal
goes from the pregnant to the lactating state. Both subunits can be induced
in tissue culture by insulin, hydrocortisone, and prolactin (Palmitier, 1969).

Whereas the normal lactating mouse mammary gland is capable of
lactose synthesis from glucose (Table XIII) by the mechanism outlined previously (Bartley et al., 1966), all attempts to demonstrate such production
from adenocarcinomas proved unsuccessful. Whether this lack of lactose
synthesis represents a deletion of the A or B component or both of lactose
synthetase has not, as yet, been determined.

4. Glucose and Acetate Uptake by Tissues from Lactating Mice

The disappearance of glucose from the medium containing slices prepared from the adenocarcinomas was significantly lower than that
containing slices from any of the other tissues (Table X) (Bartley et al.,
1971). The glucose uptakes by HAN and normal outgrowths and by
normal lactating glands were similar. This relationship does not agree with
that of the total hexokinase activity found in these same tissues. This
dichotomy is a good example of the enzyme capabilility having little
relevance to actual tissue performance. Obviously, other factors are involved among which are availability of cofactors or presence of activators
or inhibitors.

Acetate uptake in the absence of glucose was similar in all tissues. Only in slices from normal glands did the addition of glucose increase the disappearance of acetate from the medium.

5. Conversion of Glucose to Carbon Dioxide, Fatty Acids, and Lactate

Comparing the conversion of the isotopes of [1-^{14}C]glucose, [6-^{14}C]glucose, and [6-^{3}H] glucose to fatty acids reveals that the activity of the HAN outgrowths resembled that of the normal outgrowths, both of which were 15 to 25 times more active than the adenocarcinomas (Bartley et al., 1971). The normal lactating mammary gland was 2 to 3 times more active in this regard than either outgrowth (Table XIV). The incorporation into fatty acids of ^{3}H from carbon-6 of glucose relative to that of ^{14}C from the same carbon was similar in all four tissues.

Carbon dioxide production from [1-^{14}C]glucose by the HAN outgrowths and the normal outgrowths was also nearly the same (Table XIV). On the other hand, the $^{14}CO_2$ yields from this glucose carbon in the experiments with normal lactating tissue were about twice as high as those with either outgrowth and about 5 times as high as those with the adenocarcinoma. Slices prepared from normal lactating gland oxidized almost 3 times as much of carbon-6 of glucose as did the slices from the tumor, whereas the conversion of [6-^{14}C]glucose to $^{14}CO_2$ by slices from the normal outgrowths and from the HAN outgrowths was not significantly different from that by the normal tissues (Table XIV). Such results indicate lowered Krebs cycle activity in frank tumors. Therefore, when we investigated the production of lactate from glands by these same tissues, we were not surprised to find that mammary tumor produced 2–5 times more lactate from glucose than did the normal lactating gland (Table XV). In contrast, both outgrowths, the normal as well as the HAN, converted glucose carbon to lactate carbon slightly more actively than did the tumors.

The incorporation of tritium on carbon-6 of glucose into fatty acids relative to that of ^{14}C was the same in the preneoplastic tissue, the neoplastic tissue, and the normal lactating gland (Table XIV). Such a finding provides evidence not only that glucose is catabolized to triose phosphate via the same pathways but that similar mechanisms operate at each step in all three tissues.

That there is a difference in the utilization of the triose phosphates is obvious from lactate accumulation in all tissues except the normal, suckled gland. It is well known that lactate production is high in many tumors, so it is not surprising that the preneoplastic tissues shows the same characteristic. However, the normal, unsuckled tissue in the lactating mouse shows the same tendency toward lactate production. Hence, increased lactate production cannot be used as a criterion of neoplasia in mammary

TABLE XIV

Incorporation of Labeled Glucose and Acetate into Fatty Acids and CO$_2$ by Slices of Normal Mammary Glands, HAN, and Adenocarcinomas from Lactating C3H Mice[a,b]

| Substrates | | Normal lactating gland | | Outgrowths | | | | | |
| | | | | Normal gland | | HAN | | Adenocarcinoma | |
Labeled	Unlabeled	CO$_2$	Fatty acids	CO$_2$	Fatty acids	CO$_2$	Fatty acids	CO$_2$	Fatty acids
[1-^{14}C]Glucose	Acetate	200.0 ± 15.1	104.0 ± 3.2	123.7 ± 15.0	66.7 ± 11.8	104.2 ± 6.8	67.8 ± 11.0	41.3 ± 6.0	4.0 ± 0.6
[6-^{14}C]Glucose	Acetate	57.9 ± 4.8	219.0 ± 18.3	43.0 ± 5.4	90.3 ± 15.0	48.3 ± 4.2	89.8 ± 18.6	20.0 ± 3.3	4.7 ± 0.6
[6-^{3}H]Glucose	Acetate		71.4 ± 7.2		32.3 ± 8.6		39.0 ± 10.2		2.0 ± 0.2
[1-^{14}C]Acetate	None	118.3 ± 10.3	13.5 ± 5.6	153.8 ± 25.8	7.5 ± 1.1	195.8 ± 11.9	8.5 ± 1.7	105.3 ± 14.0	2.0 ± 0.1
[1-^{14}C]Acetate	Glucose	96.8 ± 5.6	174.6 ± 12.7	124.7 ± 20.4	62.4 ± 8.6	159.3 ± 7.7	61.0 ± 13.6	84.0 ± 14.0	8.0 ± 0.7

[a] Taken from Bartley et al. (1971).
[b] Each value is the average and its standard error of results from 10 to 12 experiments with different mice and is presented as nmoles of added labeled compound converted to CO$_2$ and fatty acids per mg of protein.

gland. This point has been clearly made by Weinhouse (1956) for many other tumors.

Of the various pathways of glucose catabolism studied, two have been most intensively investigated in mammalian tissues, the Embden-Meyerhof (EMP) and the pentose phosphate pathways (PPP). For the most part, only these two pathways of carbohydrate catabolism have been demonstrated in mammary glands and tumors (Abraham and Chaikoff, 1959, 1965). An estimate of the extent of operation of these major pathways can be made from the data in Table XIV. Carbon-1 of glucose is converted to CO_2 in the PPP and in the EMP via the tricarboxylic acid cycle, whereas carbon-6 of glucose is converted to CO_2 solely in the tricarboxylic acid cycle. Hence, a comparison of $^{14}CO_2$ derived from [1-^{14}C]glucose in the various tissues indicates the relative extent of PPP activity (Abraham et al., 1963) since, except for the adenocarcinoma, the $^{14}CO_2$ yield from carbon-6 was similar in all tissues examined. Clearly, the two outgrowths exhibited very similar patterns of glucose degradation. The normal lactating gland has more extensive PPP activity than the two outgrowths, and the tumor possesses the least.

This pattern of PPP activity conforms to the pattern that would be predicted based on our enzyme studies. The normal lactating gland exhibited the highest activity of PPP enzymes, the adenocarcinoma the lowest, and the pregnant gland and the HAN together in the middle ground. It is interesting to note that here we have a correlation between enzyme activity and metabolic throughput.

The proportion of glucose carbon appearing in fatty acids and lactate after traversing the PPP can also be estimated (Abraham and Chaikoff, 1959) if certain assumptions are made (Katz, 1961). The same pattern is

TABLE XV

Incorporation of ^{14}C-Labeled Glucoses into Lactate by Slices of Normal Mammary Glands, HAN, and Adenocarcinomas from Lactating C3H Mice[a,b]

Substrate	Normal lactating gland	Outgrowths of		
		Normal gland	HAN	Adenocarcinoma
[1-^{14}C]Glucose	32.5 ± 8.0	240.9 ± 21.5	194.9 ± 11.0	168.0 ± 16.0
[6-^{14}C]Glucose	73.8 ± 21.4	310.8 ± 24.8	255.1 ± 14.4	182.6 ± 20.6

[a] Taken from Bartley et al. (1971).

[b] Each value recorded above is the average and its standard error of results from 7 to 9 experiments with different mice and is presented as nmoles of added labeled glucose converted to lactate per mg of protein.

revealed. Similar routes of conversion of glucose carbon to fatty acids and lactate operate to similar extents in both outgrowths; the normal suckled gland has the higher PPP contribution, and the adenocarcinoma has the lower. It would appear that the EMP is the only pathway of glucose catabolism operative in the tumor.

6. Conversion of Acetate to Fatty Acids and Carbon Dioxide

The recovery of the isotope of [1-^{14}C]acetate in fatty acids was studied both in the absence and presence of glucose. As in the experiments with labeled glucose, the activity of the HAN outgrowth closely resembled that of the normal outgrowth (Table XIV). When glucose was added to the incubation medium, the conversion of acetate to fatty acids by normal lactating mammary gland was about 2 times greater than by either outgrowth. Such conversion by both outgrowths exceeded that observed with tumors by about 10-fold.

Omission of glucose from the incubation medium decreased the incorporation of acetate into fatty acids by all tissues (Table XIV). Again, slices of the normal and preoplastic outgrowths exhibited similar incorporation rates. The conversion of acetate to fatty acids by slices from normal lactating glands exceeded that by the outgrowths. In the absence of glucose, slices of the adenocarcinoma converted about 25% as much acetate to fatty acids as did the normal and HAN outgrowths.

Glucose did not affect the oxidation of acetate by the normal lactating gland slices (Table XIV). Oxidation by slices prepared from the normal outgrowth and the HAN outgrowth were similar to one another but significantly higher than by the other two tissues. Upon the addition of glucose to the incubation medium, these comparative relationships were maintained, as acetate oxidation to CO_2 decreased to a similar extent in both outgrowth tissues and the tumor.

The conversion of [1-^{14}C]acetate in the presence of glucose to CO_2 and fatty acids by tissues from mice in the last trimester of pregnancy was lower than that from the same tissue types from lactating mice (Table XVI). In these pregnant mice, the slices of the normal tissue and the HAN outgrowth had virtually identical patterns, that into CO_2 being 3- to 4-fold that into fatty acids. The recovery of labeled CO_2 and fatty acids from the tumor was much lower than in the other two tissues, a finding similar to that in the studies with lactating mice. Incorporation into fatty acids was less than 10% that in the other two tissues. The HAN outgrowth and adenocarcinoma did respond to the onset of lactation by increasing synthesis of fatty acids from acetate by 3- to 4-fold (Tables XIV and XVI). The magnitude of this increase was similar to that observed in the enzymatic studies with adenocarcinomas excised from pregnant and lactating mice.

7. Glucose Stimulation of Acetate Incorporation into Fatty Acids

The effect of glucose on the conversion of acetate to fatty acids by normal mammary gland slices prepared from lactating and nonlactating rats has been studied by many workers (Balmain et al., 1952; Hirsch et al., 1954; Abraham and Chaikoff, 1959). In studies with lactating glands, glucose increased incorporation of ^{14}C of [1-^{14}C]acetate about 15-fold, whereas its effect in nonlactating glands was only about 3-fold (Abraham and Chaikoff, 1959). With mice, the presence of glucose caused a 13-fold stimulation of lipogenesis from acetate in the normal gland. The extent of the stimulatory effect was slightly less in the outgrowths, namely, 8-fold with the normal and 7-fold with the HAN. The adenocarcinoma did respond to the addition of glucose, but the extent was only one-third that observed with the normal mammary gland.

Clearly, preneoplastic tissue and even neoplastic tissue can alter lipogenic capacity in respc ise to glucose concentration. The fact that the extent of stimulation varied between tissues might be related to the metabolic basis for the response. It has been suggested that glucose diverts acetyl units from oxidation toward fatty acid synthesis (Balmain et al., 1952; Hirsch et al., 1954). The correlation between (a) the total conversion to CO_2 or to fatty acids and (b) the extent of glucose stimulation was calculated for all tissues (Bartley et al., 1971). In each case, the ability of glucose to divert acetyl units toward the synthesis of fatty acids was related directly to the lipogenic capacity of the tissues as indicated by the total incorporation into fatty acids and indirectly to the oxidative capacity as measured by conversion of both substances to CO_2.

TABLE XVI

Incorporation of [1-^{14}C]Acetate into CO_2 and Fatty Acids by Slices of Normal Mammary Gland, HAN, and Adenocarcinomas from Pregnant C3H Mice[a,b]

Tissue	CO_2	Fatty acids
Normal gland (5)	109 ± 8.1	33 ± 4.0
HAN outgrowth (3)	112 ± 10.3	27 ± 0.3
Adenocarcinoma (2)	32	2

[a] Taken from Bartley et al. (1971).

[b] Each value is the average and its standard error. The number of experiments is given in parentheses. Units are expressed as nmoles of added labeled acetate converted to carbon dioxide and fatty acids per mg protein.

TABLE XVII

Incorporation of [1-^{14}C]Acetate into Various Classes of Lipids by Normal Mammary
Gland, HAN, and Adenocarcinomas from Pregnant and Lactating C3H Mice[a,b]

Lipid class	Pregnant mice		Lactating mice		
	Normal gland (13)	Outgrowth of HAN (3)	Suckled gland (4)	Nonsuckled gland (4)	Outgrowth of HAN (2)
Cholesterol ester	0.2	0.2	0.1	0.2	0.3
Triglyceride	46.8	40.2	82.3	86.2	79.9
Fatty acid	5.6	5.4	10.3	4.9	10.1
Diglyceride	24.4	29.1	4.8	5.4	6.9
Cholesterol	1.3	1.5	0.2	0.3	0.4
Monoglyceride	10.4	12.2	1.3	0.5	1.6
Phospholipid	10.9	11.4	1.0	2.3	0.8

[a] Taken from Bartley et al. (1971).

[b] The results are expressed as the percentage of radioactivity in each lipid class. Each
value is the average of the number of experiments listed in parentheses.

While we do not know the precise mechanism for this effect, the
availability of oxalacetate as a carrier of acetyl units out of the mitochondria in the form of citrate (Bartley et al., 1965) could influence both oxidation and lipogenesis. Whatever the control mechanism is, it does operate
in both preneoplastic and neoplastic tissues.

8. Type of Lipids Synthesized

The predominant type of lipid synthesized from acetate by slices of HAN
outgrowth from pregnant mice was identical with that by normal glandular
tissue from the same mice (Table XVII). Triglycerides constituted 40 to
50% of the labeled lipid, diglyceride, and cholesterol together accounted for
about 25%, and phospholipid constituted about 11%.

When the normal and preneoplastic tissues were taken from lactating
mice, the synthesis of triglyceride from acetate was two times that observed
in tissues from pregnant mice. Whether the normal tissue was suckled or
not made no difference in the type of lipid synthesized.

9. Type of Fatty Acids Synthesized

Glands of normal pregnant mice synthesized more fatty acids of medium
chain length, C_{12} and C_{14}, than did HAN outgrowths, but the differences
were not outstanding (Table XVIII). During lactation, the fatty acids

TABLE XVIII

Incorporation of [1-^{14}C]Acetate into Individual Fatty Acids by Normal Mammary Gland, HAN, and Adeno-carcinomas from Pregnant and Lactating C3H Mice[a,b]

Chain length of fatty acid	Pregnant mice			Lactating mice			
	Normal gland (6)	Outgrowth of HAN (4)	Tumor (1)	Suckled gland (4)	Nonsuckled gland (2)	Outgrowth of HAN (2)	Tumor (3)
8	0.7	2.5	0	2.0	1.0	1.1	0.1
10	3.7	1.4	0.3	25.7	13.8	6.9	2.6
12	11.2	6.0	1.4	29.0	20.8	9.0	6.5
14	18.5	8.6	13.6	19.1	19.3	14.8	13.5
16	45.8	52.6	57.2	16.3	29.0	54.5	54.3
18	13.6	14.3	15.0	4.6	8.8	9.2	16.5
>18	5.7	14.2	12.5	3.3	5.7	4.3	6.5

[a] Taken from Bartley et al. (1971).

[b] The tissues were incubated with labeled acetate and unlabeled glucose as described by Bartley et al. (1971). The results are expressed as the percentage of the total ^{14}C recovered in each fatty acid fraction. Each value is the average of the number of experiments listed in parentheses.

synthesized *in vitro* by normal glands were predominantly 10 to 12 carbons long, whereas those by outgrowths of HAN were the same as those synthesized by the preneoplastic outgrowths in pregnant mice. The HAN outgrowth did not respond to lactation as did the normal tissue. While the nonsuckled mammary gland excised from lactating mice synthesized less C_{10} and more C_{16} than suckled tissue, the pattern of fatty acids synthesized by the nonsuckled tissue was clearly different from that of its preneoplastic counterpart. The pattern of synthesis of fatty acids by the adenocarcinomas was similar to that of the HAN outgrowths and, hence, was distinctly different from that of normal mammary tissue. The physiological (hormonal) state of the mouse had much less effect on the individual fatty acids synthesized by the adenocarcinoma than by the other tissues.

10. Pathway of Incorporation of Carbon into Fatty Acids

The incorporation of acetate into fatty acids in the presence of glucose was less in nonsuckled tissue, whether normal or preneoplastic outgrowth, than in suckled tissue (Table XIV). This difference could be explained by a difference in the extent of operation of the two pathways of fatty acid synthesis, i.e., *de novo* or elongation. The functioning of these pathways can be discerned from degradation studies performed on the fatty acids produced from [1-^{14}C]acetate. Evaluation of the extent of *de novo* synthesis in normal gland, both suckled and nonsuckled, and in HAN outgrowth again revealed no differences between the preneoplastic tissue and its non-suckled, normal counterpart (Bartley *et al.*, 1971).

11. Conversion of Glutamate Carbon to Fatty Acids via Citrate

Evidence that the Krebs cycle can operate in a reverse manner in a number of tissues has been presented (D'Adamo and Haft, 1962, 1965; Abraham *et al.*, 1964; Madsen *et al.*, 1964a, b; Kopelovich, 1970; Kopelovich and McGrath, 1970; Sabine *et al.*, 1973). For example, D'Adamo and Haft (1962, 1965) have shown that, in the perfused rat liver, glutamate contributes carbon to the glucose molecule by a pathway which involves a backward operation of the cycle. This pathway has been described as α-ketoglutarate $\rightarrow$ isocitrate $\rightarrow$ *cis*-aconitate $\rightarrow$ citrate which is cleaved to form acetyl-CoA and oxalacetate. The oxalacetate is converted to pyruvate which acts as a substrate for glucose synthesis while acetyl-CoA is the substrate for fatty acid formation. The functional operation of such a backward pathway has also been demonstrated and quantitated in lactating rat mammary glands (Abraham *et al.*, 1964; Madsen *et al.*, 1964a) and rat epididymal adipose tissue (Madsen *et al.*, 1964b) by the conversion of [2-^{14}C]glutamate and [5-^{14}C]glutamate to ^{14}C-fatty acids. Furthermore, we have shown that the presence of glucose in the incubation medium will facilitate the operation of this backward pathway (Madsen *et al.*, 1964a, b,) in slices of these tissues. Recently, the occurrence of this pathway was also demonstrated in slices prepared from HAN outgrowths (Kopelovich and McGrath, 1970) and adenocarcinomas (Kopelovich, 1970) carried by virgin C3H mice as well as in slices prepared from transplanted rat hepatomas (Sabine *et al.*, 1973). The operation of this pathway in the preneoplastic and neoplastic mammary tissues is, of course, not unexpected when one considers our previous results on the enzyme levels in these tissues. All the enzymes needed to carry out this backward pathway are present in these abnormal tissues.

C. Mitochondria: Function and Activity

In 1965, we reported our initial studies on the conversion of three carbons of lactate to carbon dioxide and fatty acids by normal mammary glands and by the Barrett adenocarcinoma (C3HBA) carried by lactating C3H mice (Abraham and Chaikoff, 1965). Those investigations revealed that lactate utilization by the neoplastic tissue was lower than that of the normal tissue. Since the production of CO_2 from succinate carbons by tumor slices was not lower than that from normal tissue slices, it was inferred that the defect in the tumor resided at the level of entry of lactate carbon into the Krebs cycle. Thus, at that time, we suggested that decreased lactate utilization and hence lactate accumulation in the adenocarcinoma could be due to a deficiency in the mechanisms responsible for (a) pyruvate decarboxylation or (b) condensation of the resulting acetyl-CoA with oxalacetate to form citrate. Recently, this property of mammary tumors has been confirmed (Kopelovich, 1973a) and demonstrated to occur in the same HAN outgrowths (Kopelovich, 1973b) and resulting adenocarcinomas already described in this chapter.

It is well known that the enzyme systems catalyzing both reactions reside within the mitochondria and therefore a more detailed study of them was conducted with the isolated organelles (Mehard *et al.*, 1971). Functional mitochondria could be obtained from the normal mammary glands* only when milk was not present in the tissue prior to homogenization and when bovine serum albumin was added to the isolation medium (Mehard *et al.*, 1971). Albumin also protected tumor mitochondria from destructive fac-

---

* Free fatty acids have been shown to be responsible for uncoupled oxidative phosphorylation and to induce swelling in isolated mitochondria (Emmelot, 1962). Since lipoprotein lipase activity in mammary glands increases during lactation (McBride and Korn, 1963) and has also been demonstrated in milk (Korn, 1962), we have suggested that the ultrastructural and functional damage we observed when intact mitochondria were exposed to milk might result from the free fatty acids released by the action of this hydrolytic enzyme (Mehard *et al.*, 1971).

TABLE XIX

Mouse Mammary Gland and Tumor Mitochondrial Activity with
Different Substrates[a,b]

	Q_{O_2} (natoms oxygen/minute/mg protein)			
Substrate	Pregnant	Lactating	Lactating (NS)[c] gland	Tumor
Pyruvate	15	7	12	18
Malate	12	10	26	22
Aspartate	17	10	20	26
Glutamate	43	11	29	39
β-Hydroxybutyrate	50	15	33	31
Succinate	79	75	92	72
Ascorbate + tetramethylphenylene-diamine	91	93	91	90

[a] Taken from Mehard *et al.* (1971).

[b] Mitochondria were obtained from mammary glands of normal lactating and pregnant C3H mice and from tumors excised from virgin C3H mice. Other glands taken from lactating C3H mice whose nipples were closed (NS)[c] were also used for the isolation of mitochondria. Mitochondria were assayed for oxygen utilization as given in Mehard *et al.* (1971). Substrates were added as sodium salts to a final concentration of 1.4 mM and ADP was added to give a final concentration of 0.14 mM.

[c] Glands taken from lactating mice, 14 to 18 days postpartum, in which the nipples on the left side had been closed by electrocautery 1 to 6 days before parturition. The normal, undisturbed nipples on the right side of the animals delivered enough milk to sustain at least 6 healthy pups per dam for the entire postpartum period.

tors released into the homogenate by disruption of the adenocarcinoma cells. Only in the presence of bovine serum albumin did the mitochondria isolated from the neoplasm exhibit good respiratory control, show proper ADP:O ratios, exhibit energized phosphate transport, and appear to have intact ultrastructure.

Thus it is very clear that studies which involve the measurements of enzyme activities within organelles, particularly mitochondria, isolated from either normal or neoplastic mammary tissues, must be interpreted with considerable caution. It is imperative that data be presented which conclusively prove the functional integrity of such particles before valid comparisons can be made.

When functionally intact mitochondria were isolated from normal and neoplastic mouse mammary gland tissues, no major differences in the rate of substrate oxidation (Table XIX), phosphorylation (Table XX) or, phosphate ion transport (Mehard et al., 1971) could be demonstrated between them. In addition, when mitochondrial swelling in KCl or sucrose was tested in the presence of digitonin and phosphate, no difference could be detected (Table XXI). No significant differences could be demonstrated in cytochrome content of the intact organelles from normal and tumor tissues (Table XXII). However, we could show that the tumor contained less mitochondria per gram tissue since the total cytochrome oxidase activities, exclusively present in the mitochondria of those tissues, was 50% lower in tumors than in normal lactating glands (Mehard et al., 1971). Thus we have concluded that although the normal lactating mammary gland and the adenocarcinoma mitochondria oxidize pyruvate at about the same rate when compared per milligram mitochondrial protein, the difference in lactate utilization observed in tissue slice experiments is likely to result from the lower number of mitochondria per gram of tumor rather than from a defect within the organelle itself (Mehard et al., 1971).

D. DNA and RNA Synthesis

As shown above, the biosynthetic activities of HAN outgrowths and adenocarcinomas increase with the onset of lactation but to a lesser extent

TABLE XX

Mouse Mammary Gland and Tumor Mitochondrial Phosphorylation and RCR[a,b]

Substrate	Pregnant		Lactating (NS)[c]		Tumor	
	ADP:O	RCR[b]	ADP:O	RCR[b]	ADP:O	RCR[b]
Pyruvate	2.5	4.6	2.2	3.6	2.2	2.5
Malate	1.5	1.8	1.5	3.1	2.7	2.2
Aspartate	2.0	3.5	1.8	2.5	2.5	3.3
Glutamate	1.7	2.2	1.8	2.0	2.3	3.5
β-Hydroxybutyrate	2.6	3.1	2.7	3.1	2.3	3.7
Succinate	1.6	3.2	1.7	2.6	2.0	3.4
Ascorbate + tetramethyl- phenylenediamine	0.7	1.5	0.7	1.6	1.0	2.3

[a] Mitochondria were assayed for oxygen utilization (Mehard et al., 1971). Other experimental details are given in Table XIX.

[b] Ratio between state 3 and state 4 respiration.

[c] Nonsuckled glands from lactating mice, see Table XIX for details.

TABLE XXI

The Response of Mammary Gland and Mammary
Tumor Mitochondria to Swelling Agents[a,b]

Medium	Agent added	% Absorbance change	
		Lactating (NS)[c]	Tumor
Sucrose	None	3	0
Sucrose	Digitonin	24	22
Sucrose	Phosphate	5	4
KCl	None	16	12
KCl	Digitonin	22	26
KCl	Phosphate	18	16

[a] Taken from Mehard et al. (1971).

[b] Mitochondria were incubated at 22°C for 60 minutes in 0.3 M sucrose or 0.125 M KCl each containing 20 mM Tris-HCl, pH 7.4. Additions of either $4 \times 10^{-4} M$ sodium phosphate or $5 \times 10^{-5} M$ digitonin, at pH 7.4, were made to induce swelling. The change in absorbance at 520 nm was measured with a Cary Model 14 recording spectrophotometer. Enough mitochondria were added to each cuvette to give an initial absorbance between 0.5 and 0.6. See Table XIX for other details.

[c] Nonsuckled glands from lactating mice, see Table XIX for details.

than the normal gland. While the gland may not be actively synthesizing milk components during pregnancy, it is active: proliferating (Bresciani, 1971) and differentiating (Owens et al., 1973). These changes in activity are under different hormonal influences (Bresciani, 1971; Denamur, 1971; Owens et al., 1973) and are expressed by differences in the rates of synthesis of RNA and DNA (Stellwagen and Cole, 1969; Banerjee et al., 1971). With this in mind, we examined the rates of synthesis of DNA and RNA in HAN outgrowths and tumors from pregnant and lactating mice (J.C. Bartley, S. Barber, and S. Abraham, unpublished observations, 1973).

The incorporations of thymidine and uridine into nucleic acids were used as indicators of DNA and RNA synthesis, respectively. Tritium-labeled substrates of the highest possible specific activity were used so that the small, intracellular pools of the nucleosides and their corresponding triphosphorylated derivatives would not be altered. Any change in the concentration of the precursors could influence the rate of incorporation into nucleic acids.

TABLE XXII

Concentration of Cytochromes in Mouse Mammary Gland and
Tumor Mitochondria[a,b]

Tissue	State of mouse	Cytochrome			
		a	b	c_1	c
Tumor	Virgin	0.158	0.125	0.059	0.059
Nonlactating	Pregnant	0.151	0.152	0.065	0.091
Nonsuckled	Lactating	0.159	0.139	0.044	0.079

[a] Taken from Mehard et al. (1971).

[b] The cytochrome contents of isolated mitochondria were determined with a Cary Model 14 spectrophotometer. The results are presented as nmoles of cytochrome per mg of mitochondrial protein and are given as the average of 3 preparations. See Table XIX for other details.

TABLE XXIII

Synthesis of Nucleic Acids and Protein by Normal Mammary Glands, HAN, and
Tumors from Pregnant and Lactating C3H Mice[a,b]

Tissue	State of mouse	Conversion of substrate to		
		Protein[c]	RNA[d]	DNA[d]
Normal	Pregnant	14.5 ± 2.5	0.077 ± 0.010	0.093 ± 0.011
	Lactating	4.3 ± 0.6	0.047 ± 0.008	0.011 ± 0.001
HAN	Pregnant	10.0 ± 1.5	0.116 ± 0.028	0.074 ± 0.023
	Lactating	9.5 ± 2.5	0.055 ± 0.011	0.047 ± 0.013
	Hypox	5.5 ± 2.9	0.145 ± 0.028	0.010 ± 0.006
Tumor	Pregnant	6.0 ± 2.5	0.062 ± 0.026	0.037 ± 0.018
	Lactating	7.5 ± 1.0	0.058 ± 0.010	0.064 ± 0.013
	Hypox	6.0	0.063	0.010

[a] J. C. Bartley, S. Barber, and S. Abraham (unpublished observations, 1973).

[b] Tissues were incubated with either [3H]methylthymidine (6 Ci/mm) or with [5-3H] uridine (8 Ci/mm) and 5 mM 14C-R-L-leucine both in 1 ml of buffer containing 10mM glucose. The hypophysectomized (hypox) mice were virgins bearing either HAN or tumors. The pituitary was removed 5–7 days prior to the experiment. With the exception of a single tumor from a hypophysectomized mouse, the results are expressed as averages and standard errors of 5–10 experiments with each tissue.

[c] Units, nmoles/minute/100 mg wet weight.

[d] Units, percent added isotope incorporated/minute/100 mg wet weight.

The normal gland responds dramatically to the transition from the pregnant to the lactating state (Stellwagen and Cole, 1969; Banerjee *et al.*, 1971) and we have confirmed this result (Table XXIII). The rate of synthesis of DNA was sharply curtailed, indicating less new cell formation, during lactation. In light of the high biosynthetic capacity of the lactating gland, it is surprising that the rates of synthesis of RNA were somewhat lower in glands from lactating than from pregnant mice. Evidently, the rate of RNA synthesis needed to meet the needs of milk formation is lower than that necessary for synthesis and repair of new cells in the developing gland of the pregnant animal. On the other hand, the HAN and the adenocarcinoma exhibited little difference in the rates of synthesis of DNA and RNA due to the change in physiological state of the mouse (Table XXIII). This refractory nature of DNA and RNA synthesis in the abnormal tissue is in sharp contrast to other metabolic characteristics—lipogenesis and enzymatic activity, among others—that are influenced by the physiological state of the animal.

The results of experiments with hypophysectomized mice clearly indicated that the lack of response by abnormal tissues is not due to insensitivity to hormones. In the absence of pituitary hormones, the rate of DNA synthesis dropped dramatically in tumors and in HAN outgrowths (Table XXIII). It is significant, that in both abnormal tissues, DNA synthesis was altered without concomitantly affecting RNA synthesis. Clearly, an early effect of hormone withdrawal is specifically directed toward DNA synthesis.

E. Membrane Phospholipid Synthesis

The rate of incorporation of [^{14}C]methylcholine into the phosphatidylcholine of microsomes, mitochondria, and cytosol fractions of various mammary tissues, both normal and abnormal, taken from C3H mice are shown in Table XXIV. Phosphatidylcholine synthesis in normal mammary glands in lactating animals is only 11% of that in the glands of pregnant animals. Since there is little growth or proliferation of the endoplasmic reticulum in the lactating mammary gland one week postpartum, the reduced rate of choline incorporation into microsome phosphatidylcholine may be a reflection of this reduction in membrane production (Hillyard and Abraham, 1972). The rates for tumor and for HAN were somewhat less than those for the normal gland during pregnancy but were much greater than those for the lactating mammary gland.

It is generally accepted that the rate of thymidine incorporation into DNA is representative of cell growth. Therefore, we compared the relative rates of incorporation of leucine into protein and of choline into

TABLE XXIV

Incorporation of [^{14}C]Methylcholine into Phosphatidylcholine of Normal Mammary Glands, HAN Outgrowths, and Mammary Adenocarcinomas from C3H Mice[a,b]

Tissue	State of mouse	No. of experiments	[^{14}C]Phosphatidylcholine found in			
			Whole tissue	Microsomes	Mitochondria	Cytosol
Normal	Pregnant	4 (4)	10.5 ± 0.6	10.7 ± 1.0	8.4 ± 1.7	11.7 ± 1.9
Normal	Lactating	4 (4)	1.1 ± 0.1	1.3 ± 0.1	0.7 ± 0.1	1.1 ± 0.3
HAN outgrowth	Virgin	2 (18)	8.9	9.4	7.4	9.2
Tumor	Virgin	4 (2)	5.9 ± 1.0	6.4 ± 1.3	4.7 ± 0.4	6.9 ± 0.6

[a] Taken from Hillyard and Abraham (1972).

[b] The results are the average and standard error and are expressed as nmoles of [^{14}C] methylcholine incorporated per hour per μmole phospholipid phosphorus. See Hillyard and Abraham (1972) for further details. Numbers in parentheses represent the number of pools of tissues from individual mice used in each experiment.

TABLE XXV

The Relative Rates of Incorporation of L-Leucine into Protein, of Choline
into Phosphatidylcholine, and of Thymidine into DNA of Normal
Mammary Glands, HAN Outgrowths, and Mammary
Adenocarcinomas from C3H Mice[a,b]

		Relative rates of incorporation of		
Tissue	State of mouse	Leucine	Choline	Thymidine
Normal	Pregnant	100	100	100
Normal	Lactating	80	11	11
HAN outgrowth	Virgin	151	85	64
Tumor	Virgin	56	56	40

[a] Taken from Hillyard and Abraham (1972).

[b] The results are expressed as a percentage of the values found for the normal
gland in pregnant mice. Details of these experiments are given by Hillyard and
Abraham (1972).

phosphatidylcholine with those of thymidine incorporation (Table XV). It
is obvious that for each tissue the choline incorporation rates corresponded
more closely to the thymidine rates than did the leucine incorporation rates.
These results show that [^{14}C]methylcholine incorporation into
phosphatidylcholine can be correlated with the rate of cell replication and,
thus, provides an additional tool for such studies.

III. Conclusions

In any study of carcinogenesis, we feel that the proper question to ask is
"What are the changes which had to occur that allow transformation of a
single normal cell into a neoplastic cell?"; and not, as is so often asked,
"How does the tumor differ from the normal tissue?" The preneoplastic
HAN, naturally occurring in mammary glands, is an excellent model for
answering such questions regarding the irreversible changes characteristic
of the neoplastic process. The HAN must have undergone some
transformation, however minimal, since this unique tissue is not a normal
tissue nor is it a tumor.

Our studies, which attempt to define biochemical changes taking place
early in the carcinogenic process, have initially concentrated on the differences between normal and HAN. A most difficult problem, then, is to
establish the condition of the host animal from which to take the normal

tissue. In the mammary system,* the complement of hormones impinging on responsive cells during pregnancy is quite different from that during lactation. The hormonal environment during pregnancy promotes active proliferation and differentiation of the parenchymal cells with less emphasis on the actual formation of milk components; the reverse is true during lactation. Thus, when studying carcinogenesis, normal and abnormal tissue should best be obtained from hosts in the same physiological state. One should also keep in mind that the removal of milk from a lactating gland contributes to the metabolic characteristics of the tissue (Bartley *et al.*, 1971). Thus, an added control tissue must be considered: the nonsuckled gland taken from a lactating animal.

TABLE XXVI

Evaluation of Deviation of Abnormal Tissues from the Normal Gland[a]

		Tissue comparison		
Measurement	State of mouse	HAN to normal	Tumor to normal	From Table
Protein synthesis	Pregnant	=	−	XXIII
	Lactating	+	+	XXIII
Xanthine oxidase activity	Virgin	−	+ + + +	IX
	Pregnant	−		IX
	Lactating	− − −	+	IX
Fatty acid synthesis	Pregnant	=	− − −	XVI
	Lactating	− −	− − −	XIV
	Lactating (NS)	=	− − −	XIV
Class of lipid[b]	Pregnant	=		XVII
	Lactating	=		XVII
	Lactating (NS)	=		XVII
Length of C-chain of fatty acid[c]	Pregnant	−	− −	XVIII
	Lactating	−	− −	XVIII
	Lactating (NS)	−	− −	XVIII

[a] Activities in HAN and tumor are expressed as being greater than (+), less than (−), or equal to (=) those in normal glands taken from mice in the same physiological state. The designated differences are statistically significant ($P < 0.05$).

[b] Triglyceride; as percentage of total synthesized lipid.

[c] Percentage of synthesized fatty acids of 14 carbons or less.

* A similar dilemma occurs in studies with hepatomas, since, as many workers have shown, the nutritional state of the host influences the biochemical activities of the hepatocytes.

TABLE XXVII

Response of Normal Gland, HAN, and Tumor to Transition from
Pregnancy to Lactation[a]

Measurement	Tissues			From Table(s)
	Normal gland	HAN	Tumor	
Protein synthesis	$P \gg L$	$P = L$	$P = L$	XXIII
RNA synthesis	$P > L$	$P < L$	$P = L$	XXIII
DNA synthesis	$P \ggg L$	$P = L$	$P = L$	XXIII
Xanthine oxidase activity	$P < L$	$P = L$		IX
Fatty acid synthesis	$P \ll L$	$P < L$	$P < L$	XIV + XVI
Class of lipid[b]	$P < L$	$P < L$		XVII
Chain length[c]	$P < L$	$P < L$	$P < L$	XVIII

[a] Activities in tissues from pregnant mice (P) are expressed as greater than ($>$), less than ($<$), or equal to ($=$) those in tissues from lactating mice (L). The designated differences are statistically significant ($P < 0.05$).

[b] Triglyceride; as percentage of total synthesized lipid.

[c] Percentage of synthesized fatty acids of 14 carbons or less.

In the light of these considerations, we can conclude that the metabolic activity of HAN is very similar to that of normal, particularly glands from pregnant mice and nonsuckled glands from lactating mice (Table XXVI). Although the length of the carbon chain of the fatty acids synthesized by HAN was consistently different from that of normal gland in all three control conditions, in each case, the differences were quantitative, not qualitative. The HAN possesses the ability to produce medium chain length fatty acids; its capacity, however, in the same physiological condition is not as great as that of the normal gland.* Only in the activity of xanthine oxidase did the HAN differ from the normal in all conditions examined. While the fundamental significance of this finding is not apparent at this time, the level of enzyme activity might be used to distinguish between normal gland and preneoplastic nodule.

* Recently we have shown that the multienzyme complex responsible for fatty acid synthesis from malonyl-CoA and acetyl-CoA isolated from the mammary glands of lactating mice is immunologically identical to that of the mammary adenocarcinoma (Lin et al., 1973). Since these tissues synthesize fatty acids with widely differing chain lengths (Bartley et al., 1971), it is obvious that the synthetase enzyme is not the sole determinant of chain length. It is possible that a factor (protein ?) present in the normal lactating cell is not operative or not present in the neoplastic cell.

A comparison of the tumor with the normal gland on this same basis shows that the abnormal tissue differs from the normal in all metabolic parameters evaluated (Table XXVI). Thus, the HAN falls between the normal and the neoplastic metabolically, just as it does morphologically (Bern *et al.*, 1958; DeOme *et al.*, 1958). Such findings are consistent with the idea of a minimal deviation of this tissue from the normal gland.

With respect to hormonal sensitivity, we have evaluated the responses of these tissues to the transition of the host from pregnancy to lactation and have found additional differences between the HAN and the normal gland (Table XXVII). HAN and normal respond similarly in only three of the parameters measured: RNA synthesis, type of lipid formed, and the length of the synthesized fatty acids. In all other aspects, particularly DNA synthesis, the response of the HAN was more like that of the tumor than that of the normal gland.

Evaluation of the response of the abnormal tissues to the change in the hormonal environment (Table XXVII), leads to conflicting conclusions. On the one hand, the lack of change in protein synthesis, DNA synthesis, and xanthine oxidase activity suggests that the abnormal tissues are not hormonally responsive. On the other hand, the alterations in the extent and type of lipid synthesized, as well as the fatty acids formed, indicate that the neoplastic and preneoplastic tissues are influenced by the hormonal complement of the host. Our results with hypophysectomized mice have resolved this conflict. The rate of DNA synthesis, in both HAN and tumors, decreased dramatically when hormonal support was withdrawn by means of hypophysectomy (Table XXIII) (J.C. Bartley, S. Barber, and S. Abraham, unpublished observations, 1973). Clearly, these tissues are hormonally responsive. It is significant that, in both abnormal tissues, DNA synthesis was altered without concomitantly affecting the synthesis of RNA or protein. Which specific hormones are involved in maintaining DNA synthesis in these preneoplastic and neoplastic tissues and, how their effect is translated into biosynthetic activity, remains to be determined.

ACKNOWLEDGMENTS

This report is not intended to be a complete review of this field but a compilation of the results obtained in our laboratories. Investigations by other workers which relate directly to the studies reported here are also included.

We acknowledge support from the National Institutes of Health (CA-11736 and RR-05733) and the Anita Oliver Lunn Foundation.

REFERENCES

Abraham, S., and Chaikoff, I. L. (1959). *J. Biol. Chem.* **234,** 2246–2253.
Abraham, S., and Chaikoff, I. L. (1965). *Cancer Res.* **25,** 647–655.
Abraham, S., Katz, J., Bartley, J. C., and Chaikoff, I. L. (1963). *Biochim. Biophys. Acta* **70,** 690–693.

Abraham, S., Madsen, J., and Chaikoff, I. L. (1964). *J. Biol. Chem.* **239**, 855–864.

Abraham, S., Kerkof, P. R., and Smith, S. (1972). *Biochim. Biophys. Acta* **261**, 205–218.

Abraham, S., Bartley, J., DeOme, K. B., Faulkin, L. J., and Medina, D. (1973). *J. Nat. Cancer Inst.* **51**, 251–256.

al-Khalidi, U. A. S., and Chaglassian, T. H. (1965). *Biochem. J.* **97**, 318–320.

Apolant, H. (1906). *Arb. Kgl. Inst. Exp. Ther., Frankfurt* **1**, 7–64.

Baldwin, R. L., and Milligan, L. P. (1966). *J. Biol. Chem.* **241**, 2058–2066.

Baliga, B. S., Borek, E., Weinstein, I. B., and Srinivasan, P. R. (1969). *Proc. Nat. Acad. Sci. U.S.* **62**, 899–905.

Balmain, J. H., Folley, S. J., and Glascock, R. F. (1952). *Biochem. J.* **52**, 301–306.

Banerjee, M. R., and DeOme, K. B. (1963). *Cancer Res.* **23**, 546–550.

Banerjee, M. R., Wagner, J. E., and Kinder, D. L. (1971). *Life Sci.* **10**, 867–877.

Bartley, J. C., Abraham, S., and Chaikoff, I. L. (1965). *Biochem. Biophys. Res. Commun.* **19**, 770–776.

Bartley, J. C., Abraham, S., and Chaikoff, I. L. (1966). *J. Biol. Chem.* **241**, 1132–1137.

Bartley, J. C., McGrath, H., and Abraham, S. (1971). *Cancer Res.* **31**, 527–537.

Bergel, F., Bray, R. C., Haddow, A., and Lewin, I. (1957). *Chem. Biol. Purines, Ciba Found. Symp., 1956* pp. 256–269.

Bergquist, P. L., and Mathews, R. E. F. (1962). *Biochem. J.* **85**, 305–313.

Bern, H. A. (1960). *Science* **131**, 1039–1040.

Bern, H. A., and Nandi, S. (1961). *Progr. Exp. Tumor Res.* **2**, 90–144.

Bern, H. A., Nandi, S., and DeOme, K. B. (1957). *Proc. Amer. Ass. Cancer Res.* **2**, 187–188.

Bern, H. A., DeOme, K. B., Alfert, M., and Pitelka, D. R. (1958). *Int. Symp. Mammary Cancer, Proc., 2nd, 1957* pp. 565–573.

Beuving, L. J., Faulkin, L. J., DeOme, K. B., and Bergs, V. V. (1967). *J. Nat. Cancer Inst.* **39**, 423–429.

Blair, P. B., DeOme, K. B., and Nandi, S. (1962). *Biol. Interactions Norm. Neoplastic Growth, Contrib. Host-Tumor Probl., Symp., 1961* pp. 371–389.

Blecher, M. (1963). *J. Biol. Chem.* **238**, 513–516.

Boxer, G. E., and Shonk, C. E. (1960). *Cancer Res.* **20**, 85–91.

Bradford, D. S., Hacker, B., and Clark, I. (1972).*Biochem. J.* **126**, 1057–1066.

Bresciani, F. (1971). *In* "Basic Actions of Sex Steroids on Target Organs" (P. O. Hubinont, F. Leroy, and P. Garland, eds.), pp. 130–159. Karger, Basel.

Brew, K., Vanaman, T. L., and Hill, R. L. (1968). *Proc. Nat. Acad. Sci. U.S.* **59**, 491–497.

Brodbeck, U., Denton, W. L., Tanahashi, N., and Ebner, K. E. (1967). *J. Biol. Chem.* **242**, 1391–1397.

Cameron, A. M., and Faulkin, L. J. (1971). *Proc. Amer. Ass. Cancer Res.* **12**, 101.

D'Adamo, A. F., and Haft, D. E. (1962). *Fed. Proc., Fed. Amer. Soc. Exp. Biol.* **21**, 6.

D'Adamo, A. F., and Haft, D. E. (1965). *J. Biol. Chem.* **240**, 613–617.

deLamirande, G., and Allard, C. (1957). *Proc. Amer. Ass. Cancer Res.* **2**, 224.

Denamur, R. (1971). *J. Dairy Res.* **38**, 237–264.

DeOme, K. B., Bern, H. A., Elias, J. J., Nandi, S., and Faulkin, L. J. (1958). *Int. Symp. Mammary Cancer, Proc., 2nd, 1957* pp. 595–604.

DeOme, K. B., Faulkin, L. J., Bern, H. A., and Blair, P. (1959). *Cancer Res.* **19**, 515–520.

DeOme, K. B., Nandi, S., Bern, H. A., Blair, P., and Pitelka, D. (1961). *In* "The Morphological Precursors of Cancer" (L. Severi, ed.), pp. 349–368. Perugia Univ. Press, Perugia, Italy.

Emmelot, P. (1962). *Cancer Res.* **22**, 38–48.

Farron, F. (1972). *Enzyme* **13**, 233–237.

Fleissner, E., and Borek, E. (1963). *Biochemistry* **2**, 1093–1100.

Gardner, W. U. (1942). *Cancer Res.* **2**, 476–488.

Haaland, M. (1911). *Sci. Rep. Imp. Cancer Res. Fund, 4th, 1910* pp. 1–111.

Hancock, R. L. (1968). *Biochem. Biophys. Res. Commun.* **31**, 77–81.

Hancock, R. L., McFarland, P., and Fox, R. B. (1967). *Experientia* **23**, 806–807.

Hilf, R., Rector, W., and Abraham, S. (1973). *J. Nat. Cancer Inst.* **50**, 1395–1398.

Hillyard, L. A., and Abraham, S. (1972). *Cancer Res.* **32**, 2834–2841.

Hirsch, P. F., Baruch, H., and Chaikoff, I. L. (1954). *J. Biol. Chem.* **210**, 785–797.

Huseby, R. A., and Bittner, J. J. (1946). *Cancer Res.* **6**, 240–255.

Juergens, W. G., Stockdale, F. E., Topper, Y. J., and Elias, J. J. (1965). *Proc. Nat. Acad. Sci. U.S.* **54**, 629–634.

Katz, J. (1961). *In* "Radioactive Isotopes in Physiology, Diagnostics, and Therapy" (H. Schwiegk and F. Turba, eds.), pp. 705–751. Springer-Verlag, Berlin and New York.

Kaye, A. M., Friedlender, B., and Soloman, R. (1966). *Isr. J. Chem.* **3**, 78.

Kerr, S. J., and Dische, Z. (1970). *J. Invest. Ophthalmol.* **9**, 286.

Kopelovich, L. (1970). *Biochim. Biophys. Acta* **210**, 241–249.

Kopelovich, L. (1973a). *Proc. Soc. Exp. Biol. Med.* **142**, 954–962.

Kopelovich, L. (1973b). *Proc. Soc. Exp. Biol. Med.* **142**, 936–967.

Kopelovich, L., and McGrath, H. (1970). *Biochim. Biophys. Acta* **218**, 18–28.

Kopelovich, L., Abraham, S., McGrath, H., DeOme, K. B., and Chaikoff, I. L. (1966). *Cancer Res.* **26**, 1534–1546.

Kopelovich, L., Abraham, S., McGrath, H., and Chaikoff, I. L. (1967). *Cancer Res.* **27**, 800–805.

Korn, E. D. (1962). *J. Lipid Res.* **3**, 246–250.

Lepage, G. A., and Schneider, W. C. (1948). *J. Biol. Chem.* **176**, 1021–1027.

Lewin, I., Lewin, R., and Bray, R. C. (1957). *Nature (London)* **180**, 763–764.

Lin, C. Y., Smith, S., and Abraham, S. (1973). *Pac. Slope Biochem. Conf. 1973* No. 31, p. 16.

Ling, E. R., Kon, S. K., and Porter, J. W. G. (1961). *In* "Milk" (S. K. Kon and A. T. Cowie, eds.), Vol. 2 pp. 195–263. Academic Press, New York.

Lockwood, D. H., Turkington, R. W., and Topper, Y. J. (1966). *Biochim. Biophys. Acta* **130**, 493–501.

McBride, O. W., and Korn, E. D. (1963). *J. Lipid Res.* **4**, 17–20.

McFarlane, E. S., and Shaw, G. T. (1968). *Can. J. Microbiol.* **14**, 499–502.

McLean, P. (1958). *Biochim. Biophys. Acta* **30**, 303–315.

Madsen, J., Abraham, S., and Chaikoff, I. L. (1964a) *J. Biol. Chem.* **239**, 1305–1309.

Madsen, J., Abraham, S., and Chaikoff, I. L. (1964b). *J. Lipid Res.* **5**, 548–553.

Mehard, C. W., Packer, L., and Abraham, S. (1971). *Cancer Res.* **31**, 2148–2160.

Mittelman, A., Hall, R. H., Yohn, D. S., and Grace, J. T. (1967). *Cancer Res.* **27**, 1409–1414.

Mühlbock, O. (1956). *Advan. Cancer Res.* **4**, 371–391.

Mühlbock, O. (1958). *Int. Symp. Mammary Cancer, Proc., 2nd, 1957* pp. 811–816.

Nandi, S. (1958). *Science* **128**, 772–774.

Nandi, S., and Bern, H. A. (1961). *J. Nat. Cancer Inst.* **27**, 173–185.

Nicoll, C., and Tucker, A. (1965). *Life Sci.* **4**, 993–1002.

Owens, I. S., Vonderhaar, B. K., and Topper, Y. J. (1973). *J. Biol. Chem.* **248**, 472–477.

Paigen, K., and Wenner, C. E. (1962). *Arch. Biochem. Biophys.* **97**, 213–216.

Palmitier, R. D. (1969). *Biochem. J.* **113**, 409–417.

Pitelka, D. R., Bern, H. A., DeOme, K. B., Schooley, C. N., and Wellings, S. R. (1958). *J. Nat. Cancer Inst.* **20**, 541–553.

Pitelka, D. R., Kerkof, P. R., Gagné, H. T., Smith, S., and Abraham, S. (1969). *Exp. Cell Res.* **57**, 43–62.

Rao, G. A., and Abraham, S. (1973). *Lipids* **4**, 232–234.

Richards, A. H., and Hilf, R. (1972). *Endocrinology* **91,** 287–295.

Rose, I. A., and Warms, J. V. B. (1967). *J. Biol. Chem.* **242,** 1635–1645.

Sabine, J. R., Kopelovich, L., Abraham, S., and Morris, H. P. (1973). *Biochim. Biophys. Acta* **296,** 493–498.

Sato, S., Matsushima, T., and Sugimura, T. (1969). *Cancer Res.* **29,** 1437–1446.

Shatton, J. B., Morris, H. P., and Weinhouse, S. (1969). *Cancer Res.* **29,** 1161–1172.

Sheth, N. A., Bhide, S. V., and Ranadive, K. J. (1968). *Brit. J. Cancer* **22,** 833–838.

Silber, R., Goldstein, B., Berman, E., Decter, J., and Friend, C. (1967). *Cancer Res.* **27,** 1264–1269.

Simon, L. N., Glasky, A. J., and Rejal, T. H. (1967). *Biochim. Biophys. Acta* **142,** 99–104.

Smith, S., and Abraham, S. (1970). *Arch. Biochem. Biophys.* **136,** 112–121.

Squartini, F. (1956). *Lav. Anat. Pathol. Perguia* **16,** 211–269.

Stellwagen, R. H., and Cole, R. D. (1969). *J. Biol. Chem.* **244,** 4878–4887.

Tsutsui, E., Srinivasan, P. R., and Borek, E. (1966). *Proc. Nat. Acad. Sci. U.S.* **56,** 1003–1009.

Waalkes, T. P., Adamson, R. H., O'Gara, R. W., and Gallo, R. C. (1971). *Cancer* **8,** 1069–1073.

Wainfan, E., Srinivasan, P. R., and Borek, E. (1966). *J. Mol. Biol.* **22,** 349–353.

Weinhouse, S. (1956). *Science* **124,** 267–269.

Wellings, S. R., and Jentoft, V. L. (1972). *J. Nat. Cancer Inst.* **49,** 329–338.

CHAPTER III

SUBCELLULAR BIOCHEMISTRY OF
ESTROGEN IN BREAST CANCER

WILLIAM L. MCGUIRE, GARY C. CHAMNESS, MARK E. COSTLOW, AND ROGER E. SHEPHERD

The first demonstration that the growth of a human cancer could be dramatically influenced by endocrine secretions was made by Beatson (1896) who observed the regression of metastatic breast cancer lesions following ovariectomy. More than 75 years later, the biochemical mechanism of this phenomenon remains incompletely understood. Part of the difficulty has been that approximately one-third of patients with metastatic breast cancer respond to either ovariectomy, adrenalectomy, or hypophysectomy with objective regression of the cancer. This observation has led to experiments designed to see whether the hormones which are of primary importance in breast tumor regressions are ovarian, adrenal, or pituitary in origin. In view of the uncertainty of the role of any particular hormone, tumors which respond to any endocrine therapy have been labeled with the ambiguous but accurate term "hormone-dependent." It is the purpose of this review to examine the role of estrogen, a principle hormone implicated in tumor regression, in light of recent advances in endocrinology, especially in the biochemistry of estrogen action. Wherever possible, data derived from human mammary tumors will be cited, but most of the studies in hormone-dependent breast carcinoma are derived from carcinogen-induced rat breast tumors which regress after endocrine ablative surgery. The methods of induction and ablation and the endocrine aspects of these tumors have been extensively reviewed (Huggins *et al.,* 1961; Dao, 1964).

I.   Biological Effects of Estrogen on Breast Tumors

Estrogen has clearly been shown to act directly on the normal mammary gland to promote growth and differentiation (Lyons *et al.,* 1958). However, estrogen stimulates the release of pituitary prolactin which also acts on the mammary cell (Mcites and Nicoll, 1966). Since estrogen cannot support mammary tumor growth in the absence of a pituitary (Sterental *et al.,* 1963), whereas prolactin reportedly supports mammary tumor growth in the absence of ovaries and adrenals (Pearson *et al.,* 1969), estrogen is considered by many to play only a secondary role in tumor growth and regression. In this regard, however, it may be significant that experiments showing prolactin stimulation of tumor growth in the absence of ovarian steroids were of brief duration and that if dimethylbenzanthrene (DMBA) tumor-bearing rats are ovariectomized and simultaneous lesions are placed in the median eminence to increase prolactin release, these tumors grow at an accelerated pace for only 10 to 12 days and then regress, even though prolactin levels remain elevated (Clemens *et al.,* 1968; Sinha *et al.,* 1973). Furthermore, it has been reported that the transplantation survival of the MTW9 rat mammary tumor is dependent on ovarian hormones (Murota and Hollander, 1971), and MTW9 tumors transplated to rats immunized with estradiol–BSA conjugates will grow less well than in untreated controls (Caldwell *et al.,* 1971).

One might summarize the evidence bearing on the role of physiological estrogen levels as follows: estrogens are probably essential but not sufficient for growth of certain mammary tumors. The role of prolactin in breast cancer growth and regression has been extensively reviewed elsewhere (Meites, 1972; Pearson *et al.,* 1972).

Another important effect of estrogen is the regression of some mammary tumors following pharmacological doses of estrogen (Pearson and Nasr, 1971). This paradoxical effect of estrogen appears to act by interfering with the prolactin stimulation of growth, since the effect can be overcome by increasing endogenous or exogenous prolactin (Meites *et al.,* 1971; Nagasawa and Yanai, 1971).

There is considerable current information on portions of the intracellular estrogen response mechanism in both rat mammary tumor systems and human breast cancer. We now turn to examine aspects of this mechanism and to assess their roles in the full set of endocrine controls over mammary cancer cells.

II. Subcellular Biochemistry of Estrogen Action

A. *Localization of Estrogens in Target Tissues*

In 1959, Glascock and Hoekstra reported that tritium-labeled hexestrol injected into immature female goats and sheep was localized in highest concentrations in the organs which respond to estrogen or excrete it. Simultaneously, Jensen and Jacobson (1960) reported indentical results in the rat and further demonstrated that a majority of the injected tritiated estradiol (^{3}H-E) was retained in the target tissue as unmetabolized 17β-estradiol (E). Soon after, tritiated hexestrol was administered to human subjects with breast cancer just prior to adrenalectomy (Folca *et al.*, 1961). It was discovered that the tumor metastases of patients responding to adrenalectomy concentrated a larger fraction of [^{3}H]hexestrol than those of patients who failed to respond. Other investigators subsequently studied the *in vivo* uptake of ^{3}H-E into human mammary tumor tissue and a recent report suggests that there is a general correlation between the uptake of E by malignant breast tissue and the response to endocrine therapy, but the correlation is not sufficiently strong to be useful for predicting response in an individual patient (Braunsberg *et al.*, 1973).

With this background several laboratories began to study uptake of estrogen by tumor using the DMBA-induced rat mammary carcinoma. King and co-workers (1965, 1966) in England demonstrated the rapid accumulation of ^{3}H-E in the nuclei of mammary tumors one hour after injection. They confirmed that the majority of the tritium counts were associated with unmetabolized E. Most of the E could be extracted from the nuclei with high molar salt solutions and was recovered bound to a macromolecule as evidenced by G-100 Sephadex chromatography. A key observation made by Mobbs (1966, 1969) and later confirmed by Sander and Attramadal (1968) and Terenius (1972) indicated that hormone-dependent tumors took up more E *in vitro* than autonomous tumors. In addition Mobbs demonstrated that the occasional spontaneous regression of DMBA tumors was not the result of loss of E uptake.

Simultaneously, Jensen and co-workers (1967) in the United States showed that the uptake of ^{3}H-E by tumor slices could be competitively inhibited by synthetic estrogen analogs. That the low uptake of ^{3}H-E by other tissues, such as muscle, could not be inhibited, indicated specificity of the uptake into tumors. Jensen proposed that the *in vitro* slice technique might be extended to human tissue to predict the response to adrenalectomy.

Terenius (1968) confirmed Jensen's data with the *in vitro* slice technique, demonstrating the selectivity of E uptake and further showing that more potent estrogens were taken up more avidly than less potent estrogens.

B. Estrogen Receptors

The concentration of estrogen by target tissues has been shown to result from the presence of a very high affinity estrogen-binding protein. This receptor protein is found in the cytoplasm of target tissue cells but not in nontarget cells. On binding estrogen, the receptor enters the nucleus, where it may be associated with one or more components of chromatin. It can be released by 0.3 *M* salt, still carrying the unmodified estrogen molecule. These results, obtained primarily in experiments with rat and calf uterus, have been extensively reviewed (Gorski *et al.*, 1968; Jensen and DeSombre, 1972; Mueller *et al.*, 1972). The mechanism by which the receptor initiates a specific synthetic sequence of RNA's and proteins (Hamilton, 1968; Barnea and Gorski, 1970; Baulieu *et al.*, 1972; Mohla *et al.*, 1972) is under intensive investigation.

The presence of receptor in induced hormone dependent rat mammary tumors was first demonstrated in the laboratories of King *et al.*, (1965) and Jensen *et al.*, (1967). We have studied the presence and behavior of the receptor in several mammary tumor model systems. The remainder of this chapter will be devoted largely to the results of these studies.

III.   Rat Mammary Carcinoma

A. Hormone-Dependent Rat Mammary Tumors

All of our hormone-dependent rat tumors have been induced with dimethylbenzanthracene (DMBA) by standard methods (McGuire and Julian, 1971). Since DMBA-induced tumors often are autonomous, it is necessary to define criteria of hormone dependence. When tumors appear they are measured approximately three times a week with calipers and the tumor length times the width is plotted on a growth chart. Hormone dependence is then determined by performing an ovariectomy and observing the changing size of the tumor following the procedure. Figure 1 demonstrates three types of response that can be distinguished. In the first, rapidly growing tumors rapidly regress following ovariectomy. This is our definition of a hormone-dependent tumor. On the other hand, some tumors fail to regress after ovariectomy and continue to grow to enormous size. This is our definition of an autonomous tumor. Finally, in a significant number of cases, an intermediate response is observed, in which tumor growth is static or erratic or has an equivocal response to ovariectomy. This potentially interesting group of tumor responses we have omitted from present consideration because of our inability to classify the tumor accurately.

We first demonstrated estrogen receptor (R) in the cytoplasm of hormone-dependent tumors by incubating the cytosol fraction with tritiated estradiol (^{3}H-E) and applying it to a Sephadex G-100 column. A majority of the ^{3}H-E was eluted bound to the macromolecular fraction. Sucrose gradient centrifugation of these cytosols usually revealed two peaks of radioactivity—one at 8 S and another at 4 S (Fig. 2). Whereas the 8 S binding peak always represents specific R-E interaction, the 4 S peak may contain both specific and nonspecific binding components.

In 0.3 M KCl, bound ^{3}H-E in either uterus or tumor cytosol migrates exclusively at 4 S, suggesting that the 8 S binding molecules dissociate into subunits at high ionic strength. The sedimentation of uterine R-E in the presence of polyanions ranges between 4 S and 8 S, depending on polyanion concentration (Chamness and McGuire, 1972). If rat uterine cytosol is centrifuged either at physiological ionic strength (0.15 M salt) or in the actual "press juice" of the organ, the receptor sediments at 6 S (Reti and Erdos, 1971). Although the 8 S sedimenting species obtained in low salt gradients is

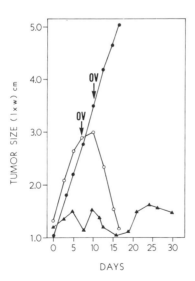

Fig. 1. Growth patterns of DMBA-induced rat mammary carcinoma. Tumor size is obtained by caliper measurements. The assessment of hormone dependency is provided by the growth response to ovariectomy (OV).

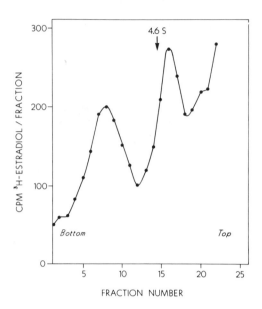

Fig. 2. Sucrose gradient centrifugation of a DMBA-induced rat mammary carcinoma cytosol incubated with [³H]estradiol. The sedimentation value of 4.6 S is obtained with a bovine serum albumin standard.

therefore probably a nonphysiological form, it is a fortuitous one where separating specific receptor is concerned since all proteins which bind estradiol nonspecifically sediment at 4.6 S or less.

Evaluation of the affinity of receptor for E requires a method for separating bound from free estradiol. The dextran-coated charcoal method (Korenman, 1969) as recently modified (McGuire, 1973) has proved both accurate and convenient for this purpose. A single class of high affinity binding sites with a K_d of the order of 2×10^{-10} *M* has been found in hormone-dependent DMBA induced tumors (McGuire *et al.,* 1971). The binding of ³H-E is estrogen specific, since it is inhibited by low concentrations of unlabeled E but not by 1000- to 10,000-fold excesses of hydrocortisone, progesterone, or testosterone.

Hormone-dependent mammary tumors also accumulate E in their nuclei. One hour after *in vivo* injection of radioactive E, the hormone can be recovered from the nuclei of dependent tumors in a form sedimenting at approximately 5 S (McGuire and Julian, 1971). We will discuss the nuclear binding of E in more detail later.

Clearly, then, hormone-dependent rat mammary tumors contain the cytoplasmic estrogen receptor. Like that described in uterus, this receptor sediments primarily at 8 S in low salt and 4 S in high salt sucrose gradients, binds E with a K_d of approximately 2×10^{-10} M, exhibits stringent structural ligand requirements, and is found with E in the nucleus after exposure of the tissue to the hormone.

B. Autonomous Rat Mammary Carcinoma

In this laboratory we have used the R3230AC transplantable mammary carcinoma described in detail by Hilf *et al.* (1967) as one example of a breast tumor that does not regress after ovariectomy.

We first found that nuclei from this tumor do not concentrate ³H-E injected *in vivo* (McGuire and Chamness, 1973). This was attributed to the very low level of cytoplasmic receptor: Figure 3 shows 10-fold lower E-binding capacity in R3230AC cytosol than in a representative hormone-dependent DMBA tumor cytosol, though the affinities are equal. The R3230AC 8 S receptor revealed by sucrose gradient sedimentation was also very low (McGuire *et al.*, 1971).

We also considered the possibility that R3230AC might have lost the ability to bind R-E to chromatin, providing another reason for its autonomy. We therefore prepared chromatin from purified R3230AC nuclei and measured the ability of cytosols containing various amounts of R to bind E to chromatin. In Fig. 4 we see that cytoplasm from R3230AC tumor, muscle, or brain failed to bind E to the tumor chromatin. This failure is due to the paucity or total lack of R in these tissues. However, we see that the complex of E with rat uterine cytosol, which contains abundant R, demonstrated remarkable binding to R3230AC chromatin. These results indicate that chromatin of these autonomous cells possesses the capacity for extensive interaction with R-E. Consequently, the failure of R3230AC nuclei to accumulate E *in vivo* can be localized to a deficiency of R in the cytoplasm (McGuire *et al.*, 1972a).

C. Temperature-Dependent Binding of Estrogen Receptor to Chromatin

Most investigators have found the nuclear accumulation of E to be temperature dependent, the translocation of R-E from the cytoplasm to the nucleus appearing to be the critical temperature-dependent step (Jensen *et al.*, 1968; Shyamala and Gorski, 1969; Giannopoulos and Gorski, 1971). However, Williams and Gorski (1971) recently provided convincing evidence that the entry of E into the cell was the initial and perhaps even the exclusive temperature-dependent step. We had studied R-E behavior in mammary carcinoma tissue and had preliminary evidence that, in a cell-free system, the binding of R-E to chromatin (C) was directly influenced by temperature. We explored this interaction in more detail.

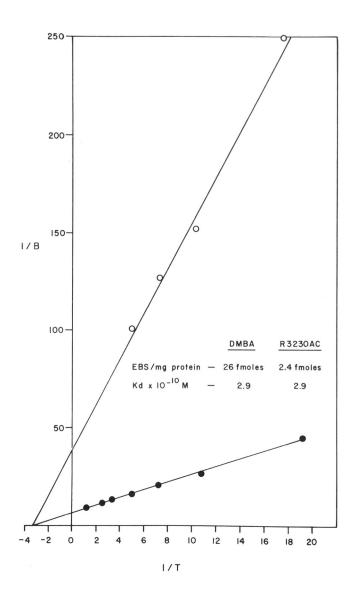

Fig. 3. Quantitation of estradiol-binding sites in a hormone-dependent DMBA-induced rat mammary tumor cytosol ●——●——● and in an autonomous transplantable rat mammary tumor cytosol R3230AC ○——○——○. The numbers of estradiol-binding sites (EBS) and dissociation constants (K_d) of the interaction are determined by a Lineweaver-Burk plot of the data from a dextran-coated charcoal assay.

We first investigated whether the effect of warming was to induce a permanent conformational change in R-E such that the complex now recognized certain C acceptor sites (Jensen *et al.*, 1971a), or conversely whether the C sites themselves might undergo such a change. Figure 5 shows, however, that preincubation of R-E at 21°C was ineffective for enhancement of 4°C binding; only when the components were warmed together to 21°C did significant binding of R-E to C occur. Similarly, 21°C preincubation of the chromatin component alone did not enhance the 4°C binding.

This result seemed to eliminate the possibility that the 21°C effect was to induce a permanent conformational change in any of the individual components. Rather it suggested either that some *reversible* enzymatic or conformational event was occurring at the actual time of binding, or that the 21°C effect was simply affecting the *rate* of binding independent of other effects. The finding that the rate of binding of R-E to C was directly

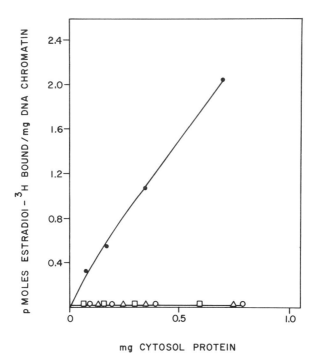

Fig. 4. Binding to rat mammary tumor chromatin (R3230AC) of [^{3}H]estradiol in the presence of increasing concentrations of cytosol from rat uterus ●——●——●, R3230AC ○——○——○, rat brain □-□-□, and rat muscle △-△-△.

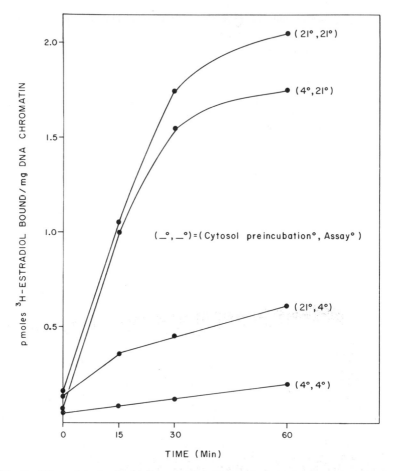

Fig. 5. Effect of preincubating the estradiol–receptor complex at 4° and 21°C on subsequent binding to R3230AC chromatin. The first in each pair of temperatures is the estradiol–cytosol incubation temperature, the latter is the chromatin-binding temperature.

proportional to the increase in temperature between 4° and 21°C, rather than increasing abruptly at some critical temperature, seemed to support the second hypothesis. We also found that incubation at 4°C, carried out for sufficient time, produced as much binding as incubation at the higher temperature. This again suggested a primary effect of temperature on reaction rate (McGuire *et al.,* 1972b).

It is noteworthy that other investigators studying C-receptor–steroid hormone interaction have not reported the influence of temperature on their systems and have incubated the components for only one hour at 4°C (Mainwaring and Peterken, 1971; Spelsberg *et al.*, 1971; Steggles *et al.*, 1971). Our data would suggest that incubation at 4°C for one hour would not permit sufficient interaction and would lead to an underestimation of the number of C acceptor sites. This might be important since experiments designed to demonstrate the specificity of receptor–steroid–chromatin binding have largely depended upon a comparison of the number of chromatin acceptor sites in various tissues.

D. Nuclear Acceptor Activity

The finding that chromatin from the autonomous R3230AC tumor binds receptor led to an investigation of receptor binding by nuclei of other tissues. As indicated above only target cells for estrogen possess the specific cytoplasmic estrogen receptor, and there have been suggestions that nuclear acceptor sites for estrogen receptor are likewise found only in target cells (Jensen *et al.*, 1969; Musliner *et al.*, 1970; Gschwendt and Hamilton, 1972; King *et al.*, 1971). In questioning these latter suggestions, we determined quantitative receptor binding to nuclei prepared from several different tissues and also examined the recovered receptor qualitatively by sucrose sedimentation (Chamness *et al.*, 1973).

When cytoplasmic estrogen receptor was prepared from rat uterus and charged with ^{3}H-E at 4°C before incubating at 25°C with crude nuclear pellets from various rat tissues (Fig. 6), we found that nuclei from stomach, liver, or R3230AC mammary tumor retained as much receptor-bound estradiol as nuclei from uterus, while spleen nuclei retained only a little less. Highly purified liver nuclei showed the same binding as the crude liver nuclear pellets. Assuming about 6 pg of DNA per diploid nucleus in the rat (Davidson, 1969) all tissues tested bound at least 3000–4000 estradiol molecules per nucleus.

Receptors recovered from these nuclei by salt extraction showed similar sucrose gradient sedimentation patterns in all cases, so that there were no apparent qualitative differences resulting from binding to target as opposed to nontarget nuclei. The appearance of a binding peak at 3 S in these nuclei along with the 4–5 S nuclear receptor peak found in uteri *in vivo* was shown to result from binding of untransformed receptor under the artificial condition of cell-free incubation. Where the cytoplasmic receptor was transformed by warming (Jensen and DeSombre, 1972) before incubation with nuclei, the 3 S peak did not appear, and there were still no significant differences in estrogen receptor binding to target and nontarget nuclei.

Results so far published for progesterone binding to chromatin (Spelsberg *et al.*, 1971; Steggles *et al.*, 1971; O'Malley *et al.*, 1972) and androgen receptor binding to whole nuclei (Fang and Liao, 1971) or chromatin

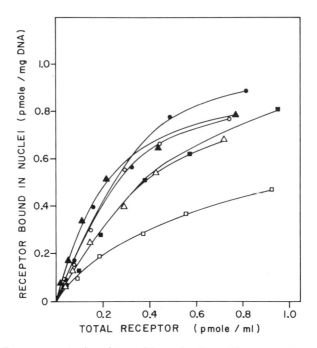

Fig. 6. Estrogen receptor bound to nuclei as a function of the concentration of estradiol-charged receptor. The nuclei were prepared from rat uterus O——O——O, R3230AC mammary tumor ●——●——●, spleen □-□-□, stomach ■-■-■, and liver (crude pellet △-△-△, sucrose purified ▲-▲-▲).

(Mainwaring and Peterken, 1971) have suggested that more receptor is bound by target than nontarget nuclear components in those systems. But significant binding to nontarget nuclei or chromatin is present in those systems as well. Even though we have questioned the evidence that binding sites for estrogen receptor are restricted to target tissue nuclei, the basic concept of steroid hormone initial action is essentially unchanged and the cytoplasmic receptor remains the primary determinant of tissue responsiveness.

We then investigated the binding sites involved in nuclear acceptor activity. Either of two types of sites might account for receptor binding. Type I sites would be limited in number and would bind receptor with very high affinity; individual sites would retain the receptor for extended periods, and saturation and competition for binding should be observed. Type II sites would have lower affinity but much higher total numbers, so that as much receptor would bind to nuclei as with type I sites but without demonstrating saturation or competition.

Williams and Gorski (1972) have reported that nuclear binding of receptor *in vivo* or in whole tissue incubations is apparently all of type II. To examine this question in isolated nuclei, we prepared a partially purified, concentrated R-E and incubated it with purified nuclei under a variety of conditions. Figure 7 shows one such experiment. There is no difference in binding to nuclei of uterus, kidney, or spleen, and there is no evidence of saturation of sites as expected for type I binding. In other experiments we observed hyperphysiological receptor binding up to 5–10 times the level present in nuclei at maximal estrogen stimulation *in vivo,* still strictly proportional to the input of E-R. Nor did direct competition experiments reveal any competible type I binding (Chamness *et al.,* 1974).

Further evidence against type I binding sites for receptor in the nucleus comes from experiments in which we treated rats *in vivo* with increasing doses of nonradioactive estradiol (Shepherd *et al.,* 1974). One hour later, we isolated the uterine nuclei and showed by a nuclear exchange assay

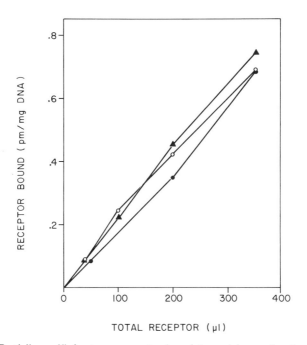

Fig. 7. Partially purified estrogen receptor bound to nuclei as a function of receptor concentration. Receptor-containing cytosol was charged with ³H-E, gently precipitated with 30% ammonium sulfate, and redissolved for incubation with sucrose purified nuclei from uterus ●——●——●, spleen ▲-▲-▲, kidney O——O——O. Each dose of receptor was diluted to 500 μl with a similarly treated cytosol not containing receptor.

(Anderson *et al.*, 1972) that these nuclei contained increasing concentrations of E-R. The nuclei were then incubated with an exogenous source of E-R to determine if the nuclei containing increasing amounts of *in vivo* bound E-R would have a decreased capacity to subsequently bind E-R *in vitro*. The result was that all groups of nuclei bound the same amount of exogenous E-R. Competition was not observed. Unless E-R binds to totally different classes of nuclear sites *in vitro* and *in vivo*, the *in vivo* nuclear binding of E-R must be a nonsaturable process at physiological receptor levels.

Though we cannot exclude the presence of a very few type I binding sites, as was suggested by Baulieu *et al.*, (1972), these experiments indicate that most if not all of the receptor bound to nuclei is associated with sites of type II. It seems likely that some mechanism other than long-term binding to a small number of specific sites must be found to explain the action of estrogen receptor in target cell and tumor nuclei. Of course, this does not preclude a transcriptional level of action for the receptor. Many mechanisms of transcriptional control might be proposed, for example an enzymatic action of receptor on certain chromatin proteins or a modification of RNA polymerase activities, which would not require type I binding sites. But it is also important to recall that binding of R-E in the nucleus has not yet been rigorously proved to be directly involved in mediating the hormone responses. Undetected activities of R-E in the nucleus or even in the cytoplasm may have major roles in determining these responses.

IV.   Human Mammary Carcinoma

The concluding part of this chapter will deal with characteristics of R in human breast cancer. It will become obvious that, although our understanding of the hormone dependence is far from complete, the information derived from the experimental rat tumor systems regarding the estrogen receptor may well have clinical relevance.

We have previously shown that E-R in human mammary tumor cytosol is excluded in G-100 Sephadex chromatography, sediments at 8 S and 4 S in low ionic strength sucrose gradient centrifugation, precipitates with protamine sulfate, and demonstrates stringent ligand requirements (McGuire and DeLaGarza, 1973). We have used these observations to assay E-R in human breast cancer specimens obtained at surgery.

A. *Evaluation of Receptor*

Both sucrose gradient centrifugation and quantitative E binding assays are used for the evaluation of estrogen receptor in our human breast tumors. Figure 8 presents sucrose gradient centrifugation of a human tumor cytosol containing R. The characteristic 8 S and 4 S peaks are clearly shown. The 8 S peak always indicates specific R but the 4 S peak could be nonspecific E binding, so a preincubation of a portion of the same cytosol with a 100-fold excess of unlabeled estradiol is always included. Figure 8 shows that the unlabeled estradiol predictably eliminated all the 8 S peak of [3H]-E and also the majority of the 4 S peak. Therefore, in this particular

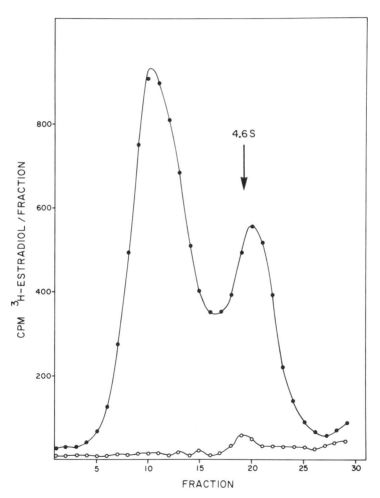

Fig. 8. Sucrose gradient centrifugation of a human mammary tumor cytosol incubated with [3H]estradiol in the presence O——O——O or absence ●——●——● of a 100-fold excess of nonradioactive estradiol.

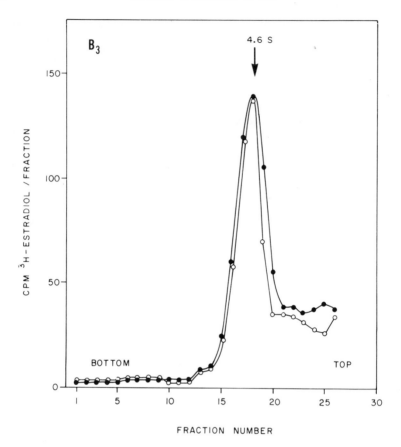

Fig. 9. Sucrose gradient centrifugation of a different human mammary tumor cytosol incubated with [³H]estradiol in the presence O——O——O or absence ●——●——● of a 100-fold excess of nonradioactive estradiol.

cytosol, the majority of the 4 S peak represented specific ³H-E binding. Figure 9 reveals a tumor cytosol which lacked an 8 S peak, but had an appreciable 4 S peak. In this instance, the 4 S peak was unaffected by nonradioactive estradiol preincubation. Hence, all of the ³H-E binding observed in this tumor cytosol was nonspecific, emphasizing the need for proof of specificity in measuring R.

In order to quantitate R, a slightly modified version of the dextran-coated charcoal (DCC) method originally described by Korenman and Dukes (1970) is used (McGuire, 1973). The addition of DCC to a preincubated mixture of cytosol and ³H-E removes the nonbound ³H-E and leaves the bound ³H-E in the supernatant for measurement. Since the ³H-E left in the supernatant may be bound either to R or to nonspecific proteins, it is important to incubate cytosols with very low quantities of ^{3}H-E ($< 1 \times 10^{-9}$ M) to minimize nonspecific binding. Figure 10 shows a representative DCC binding curve of human mammary carcinoma cytosol, plotted according to Scatchard (1949). The linear relationship that results indicates a single class of high affinity binding sites with a capacity, in this particular case, of 53 fmoles per mg cytosol protein. At higher dose levels of ^{3}H-E, nonspecific binding would become appreciable and the Scatchard plot would no longer be linear. Another advantage of the Scatchard plot is that an estimate of the dissociation constant (K_d) is readily obtained. This in turn reflects the specificity of the cytosol-^{3}H-E interaction, since nonspecific interactions yield

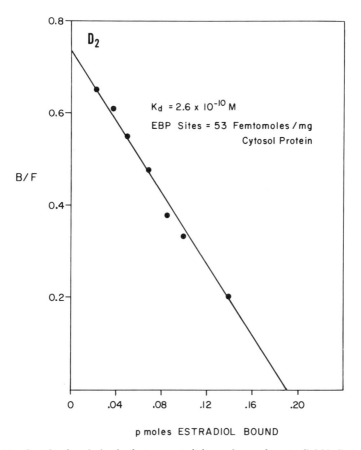

$K_d = 2.6 \times 10^{-10}$ M

EBP Sites = 53 Femtomoles / mg
Cytosol Protein

B/F

p moles ESTRADIOL BOUND

Fig. 10. Scatchard analysis of a dextran-coated charcoal assay for estradiol-binding sites in a human mammary tumor cytosol. The number of sites (EBP) and dissociation constant (K_d) are calculated by methods described in the text references.

K_d's several orders of magnitude higher than the 2.6×10^{-10} M seen here, which is typical for specific E binding in human tumors.

B. A Spectrum of Receptor Concentrations in a Series of Human Breast Tumors

Jensen's original suggestion that the presence of R in a breast tumor might indicate that the tumor was hormone dependent and could therefore be made to regress following appropriate endocrine therapy is now supported by experimental data (Jensen *et al.*, 1971b). To further correlate the presence of R in human breast tumors with the biological behavior of the tumor and the response to endocrine therapy, we have begun a prospective study using both the DCC technique and the sucrose gradient technique described above to provide specific quantitative results. In Table I can be seen a range of values from 0 to 612 fmoles R per mg cytosol protein in 43 primary tumors. With the exception of the highest value, the numbers of sites fall in a rather continuous spectrum. As expected, an 8–10 S peak is present in those cytosols with the greater amounts of R. In Table II are the data from 21 metastatic tumors. Again, a wide continuous range of values can be seen with the higher R concentrations associated with an 8–10 S peak. Considering both Tables I and II, it appears that an R concentration of at least 9 fmoles/mg of cytosol protein is necessary for a detectable 8–10 S peak by sucrose gradient centrifugation.

Although it is not known what factors account for the wide range of R concentration found here and elsewhere, there are several possibilities. First, since tumors contain various cell types, the R concentration might be expected to vary inversely with the proportion of non-epithelial connective cells present. This is supported by the observation that although normal breast epithelial cells contain R (Puca and Bresciani, 1969; Shyamala and Nandi, 1972; Wittliff *et al.*, 1972a) the abundance of non-epithelial cells in a random sample of normal breast prevents detection of specific R (Korenman and Dukes, 1970; Feherty *et al.*, 1971; Hähnel *et al.*, 1971). Yet this problem has been investigated in breast cancer specimens and no obvious correlation exists between the histology of a tumor and its ability to bind E (Sander, 1968; Johansson *et al.*, 1970; Feherty *et al.*, 1971; Wittliff *et al.*, 1972b).

Second, endogenous tumor estradiol must be considered, since available methods only measure that R which is unoccupied by endogenous estradiol. Limited data on this point (Korenman and Dukes, 1970) indicate that endogenous E can be determined in certain breast tumors, but since it is present in exceedingly low levels, only assays on tumors with very low R would be significantly influenced.

Finally, if we consider only the epithelial cells, the concentrations of R may vary from cell to cell within a tumor, since the measured R concentration is an integrated value for the whole tumor. As a special case, let us consider a model in which R is either present or absent in a given cell. (It is important to emphasize that we are using R to indicate the presence in the cell of the entire endocrine regulatory unit to be discussed

TABLE I

Estrogen Receptors in Human Primary
Mammary Carcinoma

Code	EBP sites (fmoles/mg cytosol protein)	8–10 S binding[a]
B	612	+
D_3	96.2	+
K_1	78	+
D_2	54	+
Y_2	50	+
E_1	42	+
K_3	28.4	+
T_2	20.8	+
L	20.5	ND
E	15.3	0
S	11.3	ND
T_1	9.8	0
Z_2	9.0	+
N	8.0	ND
C_1	6.2	0
K_2	5.1	0
Z	4.9	0
S_1	4.6	0
J_3	4.4	0
U_1	3.8	0
F_1	2.4	0
K	1.3	ND
P_2	1.0	0
S_2	0.6	0
19 Patients	0.0	0

[a] The + represents definite binding of [³H]-estradiol in the 8–10 S region of the sucrose gradient centrifugation while 0 indicates a lack of such binding. ND indicates not done.

TABLE II

Estrogen Receptors in Human Metastatic Mammary Carcinoma

Code	EBP sites (fmoles/mg cytosol protein)	8–10 S binding[a]	Site of biopsy
H_1	185	+	Breast
L_1	91	+	Lymph node
R_1	46	+	Breast
V	44	ND	Ovary
N_1	28	+	Breast
F_2	11.6	+	Lymph node
J_1	11.0	0	Breast
G_1	9.4	0	Breast
M_1	9.0	0	Lymph node
Y_1	8.2	0	Breast
V_1	8.0	0	Liver
D_1	7.0	0	Liver
W_1	5.0	0	Bone
R_2	1.8	0	Lymph node
7 Patients	0	0	

[a] The + represents definite binding of [³H]estradiol in the 8–10 S region of the sucrose gradient centrifugation while 0 indicates a lack of such binding. ND indicates not done.

later.) The percentage of cells in a tumor that contain R would vary from zero (all R−) to 100% (all R+). R+ cells might regress after appropriate hormone therapy whereas R− cells would not regress. Now certain predictions regarding tumor regression can be made. If the percentage of R+ is zero, then endocrine ablation would have zero effect on tumor growth. Our quantitative data in human tumors indicate that this would be a frequent situation. If the percentage R+ is 100%, then regression would be prompt and theoretically indefinite. Observed breast cancer regressions more commonly behave as though an intermediate percentage of cells were R+. If this value were 75%, then endocrine therapy would cause a regression of cells comprising 75% of the tumor while 25% of the cells would continue to grow. The net result would be a measurable decrease in tumor size (objective remission). After a period of time, the influence of the original 25% R− cells would be noticed as the tumor began again to increase in size. This pattern of regression and regrowth is the actual sequence observed in nature. One could further predict that the percentage R+ cells would correlate with the extent and duration of the tumor regression.

Using this hypothesis, one might anticipate that a tumor regrowing after an endocrine-induced remission should be comprised entirely of R− cells. The situation is more complex, however, since we frequently observe that if a tumor responds to endocrine therapy (e.g., ovariectomy) but after a period of time regrows, then a second endocrine therapy (e.g., adrenalectomy or hypophysectomy) will again cause the tumor to regress. According to the hypothesis, tumor regrowth in this instance would include both R− and R+ cells, with adrenal androstenedione converted to estrone in peripheral tissues (Longcope, 1971; Kirschner and Taylor, 1972; Grodin et al., 1973) allowing R+ cells to participate. Now adrenalectomy directly or hypophysectomy would eliminate the adrenal source of estrogen precursors and the R+ cells would again regress. As an alternative explanation, the second endocrine therapy might be affecting a different part of the endocrine regulatory unit to achieve another regression of the tumor. And of course, in reality, cells may contain intermediate levels of R or of other components of the regulatory unit, further complicating the interpretation.

C. Anti-Estrogens in Analysis and Therapy

Anti-estrogens have recently been employed experimentally in therapy, following long use in laboratory investigations of hormone dependence. There are several types of anti-estrogen, distinguished by the point at which they interfere with estrogen action. The compounds pertinent to this discussion act by direct competition with active estrogens for the receptor binding sites. These compounds have been used extensively to differentiate specific from nonspecific binding in the slice uptake assay of receptor; binding which is not prevented by a large excess of competing anti-estrogen is considered to be nonspecific. For example, Terenius (1971) showed clomiphene and U-11, 100A inhibition of estradiol uptake in both human breast cancer slices and rat mammary tumor slices in order to demonstrate specific estrogen binding in these tissues.

The finding that competing anti-estrogens could cause a dose-dependent growth arrest or even regression in DMBA mammary tumors has been confirmed by Schulz and Wüstenberg (1971). More recently Heuson et al. (1972) have reported the use of U-11, 100A (Nafoxidine) in the treatment of human breast cancer. The administration of 60 mg of U-11, 100A three times daily resulted in objective remissions in 8 out of 23 patients with breast cancer. The only side effect was photosensitivity.

It has been suggested that the weakly uterotrophic steroid estriol has significant anti-carcinogenic properties because it is able to act as an anti-estrogen by competing with estradiol for the cytoplasmic receptor sites in mammary tissues (Lemon et al., 1971). The increased estriol excretion during pregnancy would then be related to the protective effect of early

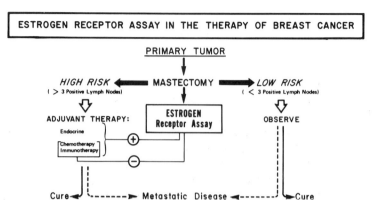

Fig. 11. A scheme for using estrogen receptor data as a guide to adjuvant therapy at the time of mastectomy.

pregnancy against development of breast cancer (MacMahon *et al.*, 1973). This latter hypothesis seems unlikely because the weak binding of estriol to the receptor compared to estradiol would require the presence of large amounts of estriol to compete successfully, while it has recently been shown that there is more unconjugated estradiol than estriol present during pregnancy (Lipsett, 1971; Loriaux *et al.*, 1972). In addition it has been found that estriol itself is able to enter target cell nuclei and to induce the synthesis of an estrogen-specific protein in the rat uterus. The degree of stimulation is proportional to the amount of estriol bound to the cytoplasmic receptor or the amount of estriol found in the nucleus (Ruh *et al.*, 1973).

D. Receptor Levels as a Guide to Therapy

As more extensive data are obtained to support Jensen's observation on the usefulness of receptor assays in prognosticating tumor response to endocrine therapy, these assays will come to play a role in the design of the overall therapeutic regimen. Here we consider a scheme for the use of estrogen receptor assays in a clinical setting. In Fig. 11, we suggest that the receptor assays be done on all primary breast tumors at the time of original surgery. Based on several criteria, including the number of tumor-containing lymph nodes in the mastectomy specimen, the patients are divided into low and high risk groups with regard to the likelihood of tumor recurrence. The first group is watched, while the high risk group is evaluated for adjuvant therapy. It has been proposed that combinations of endocrine therapy, chemotherapy, and immunotherapy given at the time of original surgery might favorably influence survival in this high risk group (Fisher, 1972). Early reduction of the metastatic tumor cell population at a time when the numbers of metastatic sites are few and the tumor cells are still likely to be hormone dependent might enable the immune surveillance of the host, especially with the appropriate stimuli, to act effectively against the metastases. The result of the estrogen receptor assay in this instance would determine the inclusion of an anti-estrogen in the adjuvant therapy.

In the case of metastatic disease (Fig. 12) an attempt to repeat the receptor assay on a metastatic tissue specimen would be made. If receptor is present in the metastatic lesion the patient's therapy would include a form of endocrine therapy; if receptor is absent the patient would receive nonendocrine therapy. If the metastatic lesion cannot be assayed (e.g., pulmonary nodule, bone lesion) but the primary tumor had contained appreciable receptor, the patient would still receive endocrine therapy. The reasoning here is that responses to hormonal therapies are achieved in 20–40% of *unselected* cases. Since the best estimate from the data of all laboratories is that at least one-half of all primary tumors do not contain appreciable receptor, then a preliminary selection of patients based on receptor assays should at least double the response rate obtained in unselected patients, assuming of course that the development of metastases is independent of the presence or absence of receptor in the original tumor. If the patient did not have receptor in the primary tumor and tumor later recurs, the patient would receive nonendocrine therapy.

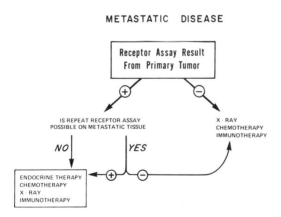

Fig. 12. A scheme for using estrogen receptor data as a guide in the therapy of metastatic breast cancer.

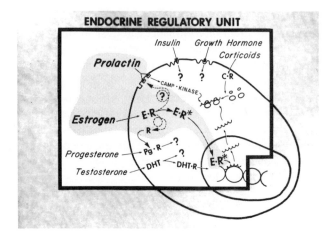

Fig. 13. The endocrine regulatory unit of the normal mammary cell. It is postulated that part or all of the endocrine regulatory unit may sometimes be lost as a mammary cell undergoes malignant transformation.

V.   The Endocrine Regulatory System

We have described estrogen binding to receptor in target cell cytoplasm, the subsequent binding of receptor in the nucleus, and the properties and significance of receptor in mammary tumors. But other hormones besides estrogen exercise control over the growth and function of mammary cells, and we would now like to formalize our concept of the complete endocrine regulatory unit in these cells and to examine how it may be related to the regression of hormone-dependent mammary tumors. Figure 13 is our schematic representation of the endocrine regulatory unit. The estrogen portion is derived from information concerning normal estrogen target tissue, largely from the laboratories of Jensen and DeSombre (1972), Gorski *et al.* (1968), Mueller *et al.* (1972), and Baulieu *et al.* (1972). It begins with the entry of estrogen into the target cell and ends with the induction of specific RNA and protein synthesis by receptor in the nucleus. We must also include in our endocrine regulatory unit the actions of prolactin, androgens, progesterone, corticoids, insulin, and growth hormone. For example, synthesis of the cytoplasmic receptor for progesterone appears to be dependent on estrogens (Feil *et al.*, 1972). It is useful to consider the endocrine regulatory unit as being present in the normal mammary cell and having the potential of being present totally or in part in the mammary carcinoma cell, where it can superimpose its control mechanism over the inherent unrestrained growth and function of the cancer cell.

How then might we relate the estrogen receptor to the prediction of hormone-dependent tumor regression? Since R is an essential component of the mammary endocrine regulatory unit, the disappearance of R from a tumor cell is one indication of the relative departure from normality that has occured and may, therefore, be useful in predicting hormone dependence. But since all the components are probably necessary for full hormonal regulation of cell growth and function, we would predict that other lesions in the unit could sometimes lead to autonomy even in the presence of measurable cytoplasmic R. We have examples of transplantable tumors in our laboratory that have significant cytoplasmic R but do not regress after ovariectomy. Shyamala (1972) has also reported an example of an autonomous mouse mammary tumor which appeared to contain R but failed to translocate it into the nucleus; the level of R was only 10% of that in a normal mammary cell, however. Our full appreciation of the endocrine regulation in a given mammary tumor cell must await our ability to measure precisely estrogen, progesterone, androgen, and corticoid receptors inside the cell as well as prolactin, growth hormone, and insulin receptors on the cell surface. When we can measure the ability of a hormone to interact with target cell receptor and trigger off a chain of biochemical events, we will be able to discuss "hormone-dependent" mammary carcinoma in a meaningful way.

ACKNOWLEDGMENTS

These studies were supported in part by grants and contracts from the USPHS (CA11378, G-72-3862) and The American Cancer Society (BC23B).

REFERENCES

Anderson, J., Clark, J. H., and Peck, E. J. (1972). *Biochem. J.* **126,** 561.

Barnea, A., and Gorski, J. (1970). *Biochemistry* **9,** 1899.

Baulieu, E. E., Alberga, A., Raynaud-Jammet, C., and Wira, C. R. (1972). *Nature (London)* **236,** 236.

Beatson, G. T. (1896). *Lancet* **2,** 104 and 162.

Braunsberg, H., James, V. H. T., Irvine, W. T., James, F., Jamieson, C. W.,Sellwood, R. A., Carter, A. E., and Hullbert, M. (1973). *Lancet* **1,** 163.

Caldwell, B. V., Tillson, S. A., Esber, H., and Thorneycroft, I. H. (1971). *Nature (London)* **231,** 118.

Chamness, G. C., and McGuire, W. L. (1972). *Biochemistry* **11,** 2466.

Chamness, G. C., Jennings, A. W., and McGuire, W. L. (1973). *Nature (London)* **241,** 458.

Chamness, G. C., Jennings, A. W., and McGuire, W. L. (1974). *Biochemistry* **13,** 327.

Clemens, J. A., Welsch, C. W., and Meites, J. (1968). *Proc. Soc. Exp. Biol. Med.* **127,** 969.

Dao, T. L. (1964). *Progr. Exp. Tumor Res.* **5,** 157.

Davidson, J. N. (1969). "The Biochemistry of the Nucleic Acids," 6th ed., p. 325. Methuen, London.

Fang, S., and Liao, S. (1971). *J. Biol. Chem.* **246,** 16.

Feherty, P., Farrer-Brown, G., and Kellie, A. E. (1971). *Brit. J. Cancer* **25,** 697.

Feil, P. D., Glasser, S. R., Toft, D. O., and O'Malley, B. W. (1972). *Endocrinology* **91**, 738.

Fisher, B. (1972). *Cancer* **30**, 1556.

Folca, P. J., Glascock, R. F., and Irvine, W. T. (1961). *Lancet* **2**, 796.

Giannopoulos, G., and Gorski, J. (1971). *J. Biol. Chem.* **246**, 2530.

Glascock, R. F., and Hoekstra, W. G. (1959). *Biochem. J.* **72**, 673.

Gorski, J., Toft, D., Shyamala, G., Smith, D., and Notides, A. (1968). *Recent Progr. Horm. Res.* **24**, 45.

Grodin, J. M., Siiteri, P. K., and MacDonald, P. C. (1973). *J. Clin. Endocrinol. Metab.* **36**, 207.

Gschwendt, M., and Hamilton, T. H. (1972). *Biochem. J.* **128**, 611.

Hähnel, R., Twaddle, E., and Vivian, A. B. (1971). *Steroids* **18**, 681.

Hamilton, T. H. (1968). *Science* **161**, 649.

Heuson, J. C., Coume A., and Staquet, M. (1972). *Eur. J. Cancer* **8**, 387.

Hilf, R., Michel, I., and Bell, C. (1967). *Recent Progr. Horm. Res.* **23**, 229.

Huggins, C., Grand, L. D., and Brillantes, F. P. (1961). *Nature (London)* **189**, 204.

Jensen, E. V., and DeSombre, E. R. (1972). *Ann. Rev. Biochem.* **41**, 203.

Jensen, E. V., and Jacobson, H. I. (1960). *In* "Biological Activities of Steroids in Relation to Cancer" (G. Pincus and E. P. Vollmer, eds.), p. 191. Academic Press, New York.

Jensen, E. V., DeSombre, E. R., and Jungblut, P. W. (1967). *In* "Endogenous Factors Influencing Host-Tumor Balance" (R. W. Wissler, T. L. Dao, and S. Wood, Jr., eds.), p. 15. Univ. of Chicago Press, Chicago, Illinois.

Jensen, E. V., Suzuki, T., Kawashima, T., Stumpf, W. E., Jungblut, P. W., and DeSombre, E. R. (1968). *Proc. Nat. Acad. Sci. U.S.* **59**, 632.

Jensen, E. V., Numata, M., Smith, S., Suzuki, T., Brecher, P. I., and DeSombre, E. R. (1969). *Symp. Soc. Develop. Biol.* **28**, 151.

Jensen, E. V., Numata, M., Brecher, P. I., and DeSombre, E. R. (1971a). *Biochem. Soc. Symp.* **32**, 133.

Jensen, E. V., Block, G. E., Smith, S., Kyser, K., and DeSombre, E. R. (1971b). *Nat. Cancer Inst. Monogr.* **34**, 55.

Johansson, H., Terenius, L., and Thoren, L. (1970). *Cancer Res.* **30**, 692.

King, R. J. B., Cowan, D. M., and Inman, D. R. (1965). *J. Endocrinol.* **32**, 83.

King, R. J. B., Gordon, J., Cowan, D. M., and Inman, D. R. (1966). *J. Endocrinol.* **36**, 139.

King, R. J. B., Beard, V., Gordon, J., Pooley, A. S., Smith, J. A., Steggles, A. W., and Vertes, M. (1971). *Advan. Biosc.* **7**, 21.

Kirschner, M. A., and Taylor, J. P. (1972). *J. Clin. Endocrinol. Metab.* **35**, 513.

Korenman, S. G. (1969). *Steroids* **13**, 163.

Korenman, S. G., and Dukes, B. A. (1970). *J. Clin. Endocrinol. Metab.* **30**, 639.

Lemon, H. M., Miller, D. M., and Foley, J. F. (1971). *Nat. Cancer Inst. Monogr.* **34**, 77.

Lipsett, M. B. (1971). *Lancet* **2**, 1378.

Longcope, C. (1971). *Amer. J. Obstet. Gynecol.* **111**, 778.

Loriaux, D. L., Ruder, H. J., Knab, D. R., and Lipsett, M. B. (1972). *J. Clin. Endocrinol. Metab.* **35**, 887.

Lyons, W. R., Li, C. H., and Johnson, R. E. (1958). *Recent Progr. Horm. Res.* **14**, 219.

McGuire, W. L. (1973). *J. Clin. Invest.* **52**, 73.

McGuire, W. L., and Chamness, G. C. (1973). *In* "Receptors for Reproductive Hormones" (B. W. O'Malley and A. R. Means, eds.). Plenum, New York.

McGuire, W. L., and DeLaGarza, M. (1973). *J. Clin. Endocrinol. Metab.* **36**, 548.

McGuire, W. L., and Julian, J. A. (1971). *Cancer Res.* **31**, 1440.

McGuire, W. L., Julian, J., and Chamness, G. C. (1971). *Endocrinology* **89**, 969.

McGuire, W. L., Huff, K., Jennings, A., and Chamness, G. C. (1972a). *Science* **175**, 335.

McGuire, W. L., Huff, K., and Chamness, G. C. (1972b). *Biochemistry* **11**, 4562.

MacMahon, B., Cole, P., and Brown, J. (1973). *J. Nat. Cancer Inst.* **50**, 21.

Mainwaring, W. I. P., and Peterken, B. M. (1971). *Biochem. J.* **125**, 285.

Meites, J. (1972). *J. Nat. Cancer Inst.* **48**, 1217.

Meites, J., and Nicoll, C. S. (1966). *Annu. Rev. Physiol.* **28**, 57.

Meites, J., Cassell, E., and Clark, J. (1971). *Proc. Soc. Exp. Biol. Med.* **137**, 1225.

Mobbs, B. G. (1966). *J. Endocrinol.* **36**, 409.

Mobbs, B. G. (1969). *J. Endocrinol.* **44**, 463.

Mohla, S., DeSombre, E. R., and Jensen, E. V. (1972). *Biochem. Biophys. Res. Commun.* **46**, 661.

Mueller, G. C., Vonderhaar, B., Kim, U. H., and Mahieu, M. L. (1972). *Recent Progr. Horm. Res.* **28**, 1.

Murota, S., and Hollander, V. P. (1971). *Endocrinology* **89**, 560.

Musliner, T. A., Chader, G. J., and Villee, C. A. (1970). *Biochemistry* **9**, 4448.

Nagasawa, H., and Yanai, R. (1971). *Int. J. Cancer* **8**, 463.

O'Malley, B. W., Spelsberg, T. C., Schrader, W. T., Chytil, F., and Steggles, A. W. (1972). *Nature (London)* **235**, 141.

Pearson, O. H., and Nasr, H. (1971). *Horm. Steroids, Proc. Int. Congr., 3rd, 1970* Int. Congr. Ser. No. 219, p. 602.

Pearson, O. H., Llerena, O., Llerena, L., Molina, A., and Butler, T. (1969). *Trans. Ass. Amer. Physicians* **82**, 225.

Pearson, O. H., Murray, R., Mozaffarian, G., and Pensky, J. (1972). *In* "Prolactin and Carcinogenesis" (A. R. Boyns and K. Griffiths, eds.), p. 154. Alpha Omega Alpha Publ., Cardiff, Wales.

Puca, G. A., and Bresciani, F. (1969). *Endocrinology* **85**, 1.

Reti, I., and Erdos, T. (1971). *Biochimie* **53**, 435.

Ruh, T. S., Katzenellenbogen, B. S., Katzenellenbogen, J. A., and Gorski, J. (1973). *Endocrinology* **92**, 125.

Sander, S. (1968). *Acta Pathol. Microbiol. Scand.* **74**, 301.

Sander, S., and Attramadal, A. (1968). *Acta Pathol. Microbiol. Scand.* **74**, 169.

Scatchard, G. (1949). *Ann. N.Y. Acad. Sci.* **51**, 660.

Schulz, K.D., and Wüstenberg, B. (1971). *Horm. Metab. Res.* **3**, 295.

Shepherd, R. E., Huff, K., and McGuire, W. L. (1974). *Endocr. Res. Commun.* **1**, 73.

Shyamala, G. (1972). *Biochem. Biophys. Res. Commun.* **46**, 1623.

Shyamala, G., and Gorski, J. (1969). *J. Biol. Chem.* **244**, 1097.

Shyamala, G., and Nandi, S. (1972). *Endocrinology* **91**, 861.

Sinha, D., Cooper, D., and Dao, T. L. (1973). *Cancer Res.* **33**, 411.

Spelsberg, T. C., Steggles, A. W., and O'Malley, B. W. (1971). *J. Biol. Chem.* **246**, 4188.

Steggles, A. W., Spelsberg, T. C., Glasser, S. R., and O'Malley, B. W. (1971). *Proc. Nat. Acad. Sci. U.S.* **68**, 1479.

Sterental, A., Dominguez, J. M., Weissman, C., and Pearson, O. H. (1963). *Cancer Res.* **23**, 481.

Terenius, L. (1968). *Cancer Res.* **28**, 328.

Terenius, L. (1971). *Eur. J. Cancer* **7**, 57.

Terenius, L. (1972). *Eur. J. Cancer* **8**, 55.

Williams, D., and Gorski, J. (1971). *Biochem. Biophys. Res. Commun.* **45**, 258.

Williams, D., and Gorski, J. (1972). *Proc. Nat. Acad. Sci. U.S.* **69**, 3464.

Wittliff, J. L., Gardner, D. G., Battema, W. L., and Gilbert, P. J. (1972a). *Biochem. Biophys. Res. Commun.* **48**, 119.

Wittliff, J. L., Hilf, R., Brooks, W. F., Savlov, E. D., Hall, T. C., and Orlando, R. A. (1972b). *Cancer Res.* **32**, 1983.

Chapter IV

CHARACTERIZATION OF HUMAN BREAST CANCER BY EXAMINATION OF CYTOPLASMIC ENZYME ACTIVITIES AND ESTROGEN RECEPTORS

RUSSELL HILF AND JAMES L. WITTLIFF

I.   Introduction

Although it has been known since Beatson's report (1896) that growth of breast cancer may be dependent on the secretions from the ovaries (estrogens), the ability to correctly classify the individual breast cancer as hormone-dependent or hormone-independent* has only recently reached a degree of certainty to be useful as a predictor of response to known therapeutic manipulations. From clinical observations of women with breast cancer, a proportion of women with this disease (20 to 30%, or perhaps higher in the premenopausal patient) possesses lesions that are affected by altering the hormonal milieu of the host. Thus, ablation of steroid-producing glands, e.g,. ovaries and adrenals, or administration of pharmacological levels of estrogens or androgens results in objective regression of

---

* The terminology found in the literature on breast cancer may create some confusion. Strictly defined, hormone-dependent breast tumors are those that regress after endocrine organ ablation or those tumors that do not grow in the absence of certain hormones. These tumors can also be defined as hormone-responsive. Another class of tumor exists, which is not dependent but hormone-responsive; recurrent or metastatic breast cancer that regresses after administration of pharmacological doses of estrogens or androgens are such examples. These sometimes occur in patients who had undergone oophorectomy or adrenalectomy at a prior time in the course of the disease. There are numerous experimental tumor models that are inhibited in growth by hormonal therapy but are not dependent on the presence of the host's ovaries or adrenals for growth; these are termed autonomous-responsive. We shall use the terms dependent and responsive in the more general sense in this paper; the term hormone-independent needs no further qualification.

neoplastic lesions, relief of pain, and prolongation of survival of women with advanced metastatic breast cancer (Stoll, 1972). If one can identify those women who possess hormone-responsive cancers, the clinician may approach a plan of therapy on a sound basis, avoiding the use of agents which have little likelihood of success.

One of the first approaches toward a diagnostic test for hormone responsiveness of mammary tumors was initiated by Bulbrook and his colleagues (see review, Bulbrook, 1970). Analyses of urinary specimens demonstrated that higher levels of 17-hydroxysteroids relative to 17-oxosteroids (17-ketosteroids) were found in women who showed a poorer response to adrenalectomy or hypophysectomy than in those who demonstrated a higher amount of 17-ketosteroids relative to 17-hydroxycorticosteroids. From the data obtained in a retrospective study, they constructed a discriminant function, such that a positive discriminant (more etiocholanolone relative to 17-hydroxycorticosteroids) correlated with a good response to hypophysectomy; patients with a negative discriminant generally failed to respond to endocrine organ ablation. As these studies were expanded, additional factors were recognized to play a role in identifying those women with the poorest chance to respond to ablative procedures. Thus, women with negative discriminants, who were within 6 years of menopause and who showed a free period (time from mastectomy to recurrence) of less than two years were essentially unresponsive and such patients are no longer treated by endocrine ablation (Hayward and Bulbrook, 1968). Projecting these approaches in a forward prognostic study, Bulbrook and his colleagues examined urine from 5000 disease-free women living on Guernsey to ascertain if a particular pattern of urinary steroids might predict for eventual appearance of breast cancer (Bulbrook and Hayward, 1967; Bulbrook, 1970). The results obtained to date suggest that tumors may arise in women of low fertility who excrete subnormal amounts of androgen and estrogen metabolites (etiocholanolone); their neoplasms would be predicted to be rapidly growing and hormone-independent (negative discriminant). Obviously, additional data will be forthcoming and the results will be awaited with great interest. Although reservations have been expressed concerning the physiological significance of these urinary steroids, the advantages of this approach are obvious; the ease of collecting samples is enviable and the ability to perform analyses on repetitive samples adds greatly to the validity of the data.

We have utilized a somewhat different approach by examining the biochemical properties of the tumor itself. This approach is an outgrowth of studies of experimental rodent mammary tumors and attempts to relate data obtained from the animal models to human breast cancer (Hilf et al., 1967; Hilf, 1968, 1970, 1971, 1973). Information on the responsiveness of experimental tumors to endocrine manipulations was utilized as a basis for tumor classification. At the same time, studies were initiated with human breast carcinomas (1) to establish and identify characteristics of human malignancies that were unique to neoplasia and (2) to seek correlations of these parameters with the clinical course of the disease. Inherent in such studies is the gathering of data on the clinical course of the disease in the patient and the response, or lack of it, to the therapeutic maneuvers employed by the clinician.

The initial studies, which began in 1967, dealt with measuring the activities of several selected enzymes in infiltrating ductal carcinoma of the breast, chosen because it is the most common malignant breast lesion in women (McDivitt *et al.*, 1968; Hilf *et al.*, 1969b, 1970a,b). In addition to the tumors, samples of "normal" breast (normal defined as breast tissue free of abnormalities by light microscopic criteria) were obtained and analyzed. It was desirable to examine other lesions of the breast, enabling one to compare the biochemical characteristics of nonmaligant diseases with both normal and carcinomatous tissue; alterations unique to frank carcinoma might be found and would not reflect proliferative capacity of the tissue studied. To this end, we obtained samples of fibrocystic disease of the breast and of fibroadenomas, both representing proliferative but benign diseases (McDivitt *et al.*, 1968).

The other biochemical parameter measured was specific estrogen-binding capacity of the cytoplasmic receptor in normal and neoplastic breast tissues. Much of our present understanding of the mechanism of steroid hormone action on tumor cells has been derived from investigations of the effects of estrogens on normal target tissues such as the uterus and mammary gland (Mueller, 1965; Gorski *et al.*, 1968; Williams-Ashman and Reddi, 1971; Jensen and DeSombre, 1972a,b). It is now well accepted that an estrogen target organ, such as the breast and uterus, has the capacity to bind labeled estradiol-17β specifically with high affinity due to the presence of protein macromolecules termed "estrogen-binding proteins" or "estrogen receptors." Since the binding of the steroid preceded changes in synthesis of nucleic acids and proteins in target tissues such as the uterus, and since prevention of the uterotrophic response to estrogen by anti-estrogenic agents, e.g., MER-25, U-11100A, and CI-628, was correlated with the decreased binding of estradiol-17β to receptor, it was logical to conclude that the interaction of steroid with receptor was an early and necessary step in the action of the hormone. The demonstration by Folca *et al.*, (1961) of a higher uptake of labeled hexestrol by breast tumors of patients showing a response to ablation and the many more recent reports that certain primary and metastatic mammary tumors possess estrogen-binding capacity (Jensen *et al.*, 1967; Sander, 1968; Johansson *et al.*, 1970;

Korenman and Dukes, 1970; Feherty *et al.*, 1971; Hahnel *et al.*, 1971; Wittliff *et al.*, 1972b; McGuire, 1973) suggest that such properties of neoplasms might provide a basis for prediction of response. Jensen *et al.*, (1971b, 1972) have now shown that those patients whose breast tumors lack estrogen receptors have little chance of demonstrating remission of their disease following adrenalectomy. Thus, as part of our long-term investigations of breast cancer, we initiated studies of specific estrogen-binding capacity in normal and neoplastic human breast tissues (Wittliff *et al.*, 1972b; Savlov *et al.*, 1974).

The data presented here represent a summary of our findings over the past few years. Correlations of the biochemical studies with the clinical course of the disease are still quite preliminary but will become apparent as the time after surgery progresses. The utility of these assays as predictive indices for therapy remains to be demonstrated in a prospective study; the data accumulated here in a retrospective study will surely form a firm basis for future studies.

II. Methodology

The methods employed for these studies have been published in detail earlier (Hilf *et al.*, 1969a,b, 1970a,b, 1973; Wittliff *et al.*, 1972b). However, it should be noted that we have used two somewhat different approaches for obtaining human samples. In conjunction with Drs. R. A. Orlando, F. L. Archer, H. Fanger, and J. Ree, samples were collected by them, trimmed of necrotic and hemorrhagic areas, and frozen until shipped by air in dry ice to our laboratory. Upon receipt, the samples were placed in our deep freeze ($-80°C$) until assayed. The second approach used was with fresh material obtained by the Division of Oncology nurses from the Pathology Departments at various local hospitals. In these latter cases, tissues were kept on ice until delivered to our laboratory, at which time they were trimmed, weighed, put into plastic vials, and quick frozen in liquid nitrogen prior to storage. Although less time elapsed prior to freezing in the former case, we have noted no alteration in enzyme activities or estrogen-binding capacity attributable to either of the methods used to obtain samples. Studies have also indicated little or no significant changes in biochemical parameters in human tissues stored at $-80°C$ for 1–2 months.

It is essential in studies of human tumors that a careful microscopic surveillance of the tissues be an integral part of the program. As biochemists, we have relied on the microscopic evaluation of sections made from a random selection of tissue immediately adjacent to the tissues used for biochemical assays. Diagnoses from these slides were used to classify these tissues (McDivitt *et al.*, 1968). In addition, semiquantitative estimation of various cellular components have been made of these tissues to estimate the percentage represented by each cell type, i.e., carcinoma, fibrous tissue, adipose cells, epithelial cells, inflammation, etc. These data are used to seek correlations between biochemical parameters and morphology. Thus, while the pathology of the tissues represents adjacent areas to those actually assayed, the need for such morphological monitoring is particularly relevant to breast tissues and breast diseases.

III.   Enzyme Activities in Human Breast Tissues

In an earlier publication, it was pointed out that the human tissues examined had an acceptable degree of variability; studies on replicate samples from the same lesion provided us with an estimate of homogeneity (Hilf *et al.*, 1970b). Data on infiltrating ductal carcinoma indicated a good degree of biochemical uniformity such that the standard error did not exceed 10% of the mean value. This was also the case with samples of fibrocystic disease and fibroadenomas but a somewhat greater variability was observed with samples of "normal" breast. This latter variability in normal breast tissue may be due in part to the relatively low levels of enzyme activity (a small variation in activity from sample to sample would create a substantial percent error), to the greater variability in cell population, to the possible influences of hormonal milieu, and to the fact that such samples may not be "normal" in the true sense of the word. Regardless of the greater variability (standard error of the mean may be 20 to 25% of the mean), the results obtained comparing nondiseased breast tissue with the abnormal breast tissue clearly demonstrate many highly significant alterations in enzyme activities in diseased tissue.

The results of examination of human tissues are presented in Table I, where enzyme activity was expressed per unit of tissue weight. With the exception of α-glycerolphosphate dehydrogenase, the activities of the enzymes examined were significantly higher in carcinoma samples compared to either normal breast tissue, to fibrocystic disease, or to fibroadenoma. These changes in carcinomas were in the order of a 5-fold increase for lactate dehydrogenase to as high as 14-fold increase for pyruvate kinase when compared to normal breast. It is also of interest that the enzyme activities in fibroadenomas were generally higher than those seen in normal breast or fibrocystic disease, indicating the elevated metabolic potential of the benign neoplasm. Fibrocystic disease, however, was not strikingly different in the activities of these enzymes from normal breast tissue, although fibrocystic disease samples demonstrated elevated activities of isocitrate dehydrogenase and phosphoglucomutase. In most instances, one could ob-

TABLE I Biochemical Characteristics of Human Breast Tissues[a,b]

Enzyme (µmoles/min/100 mg tissue)	Normal breast	Fibrocystic disease	Fibroadenoma	Infiltrating ductal carcinoma
G6PD	0.018 ± 0.008 (58)	0.019 ± 0.003 (33)	0.030 ± 0.005 (19)	0.121 ± 0.014[c,d,e] (135)
ICD	0.022 ± 0.003 (58)	0.047 ± 0.008[c] (33)	0.086 ± 0.017[c,d] (19)	0.209 ± 0.014[c,d,e] (131)
GPI	0.59 ± 0.05 (57)	0.82 ± 0.10 (32)	1.47 ± 0.19[c,d] (19)	3.06 ± 0.18[c,d,e] (130)
PGM	0.003 ± 0.001 (50)	0.009 ± 0.002[c] (29)	0.017 ± 0.003[c,d] (18)	0.030 ± 0.003[c,d,e] (119)
αGPD	0.082 ± 0.010 (58)	0.076 ± 0.013 (33)	0.049 ± 0.030 (19)	0.063 ± 0.005 (134)
GDH	0.008 ± 0.003 (56)	0.004 ± 0.001 (29)	0.009 ± 0.002 (18)	0.036 ± 0.009[c,d,e] (120)
AAT	0.069 ± 0.008 (57)	0.109 ± 0.019 (28)	0.182 ± 0.024[c,d] (20)	0.343 ± 0.020[c,d,e] (126)
PYK	0.250 ± 0.044 (53)	0.569 ± 0.181 (28)	1.255 ± 0.279[c] (20)	3.480 ± 0.274[c,d,e] (117)
HK	0.005 ± 0.001 (56)	0.004 ± 0.001 (25)	0.014 ± 0.003[c,d] (17)	0.038 ± 0.005[c,d,e] (120)
LDH	0.444 ± 0.047 (38)	0.540 ± 0.125 (17)	0.876 ± 0.144[c] (11)	2.069 ± 0.143[c,d,e] (86)

[a] Abbreviations used are G6PD, glucose-6-phosphate dehydrogenase; ICD, NADP-isocitrate dehydrogenase, decarboxylating; GPI, glucose phosphate isomerase; PGM, phosphoglucomutase; αGPD, α-glycerolphosphate dehydrogenase; GDH, glutamate dehydrogenase; AAT, aspartate aminotransferase; PYK, pyruvate kinase; HK, hexokinase; and LDH, lactate dehydrogenase.

[b] Mean ± S.E.M. Numbers in parentheses, number of samples assayed.

[c] Significantly different ($P < 0.01$) compared with normal breast.

[d] Significantly different ($P < 0.01$) compared with fibrocystic disease.

[e] Significantly different ($P < 0.01$) compared with fibroadenoma.

serve a graded elevation in enzyme activities, such that one might rank the tissues on the following basis: normal breast < fibrocystic disease < fibroadenoma < carcinoma.

An important aspect of enzyme activity measurements relates to the manner of expressing data. One classic method expresses enzyme activity per unit of protein, often considered to represent specific activity. As can be seen from the data in Table II, there was essentially no difference in protein content among the tissues examined and, thus, the expression of enzyme activity per milligram protein provided data that were quite similar to that seen when expressing enzyme activity on a wet tissue weight basis (Table I). However, the values for DNA content were significantly different between normal and abnormal tissues. If one assumes that DNA content reflects overall cellularity, then it is obvious that a neoplasm presents with a greater number of cells per unit volume than normal breast. Therefore, we have used a more conservative approach by expressing enzyme activity per milligram DNA, which would normalize any differences in enzyme activity that would be due to differences in cell number. These data are shown in Figs. 1–4. The glycolytic enzymes (Fig. 1) demonstrate an elevated activity in carcinomas, with both LDH and GPI demonstrating a significant increase only in the malignant neoplasms. Pyruvate kinase, while markedly elevated in carcinomas (approximately 5-fold that found in normal breast tissue), was slightly increased in fibroadenomas compared to normal breast. Both G6PD and ICD, enzymes that produce NADPH as a result of the reactions that they catalyze, were found to be uniquely elevated in carcinomas (Fig. 2), suggesting that these enzymes play an important role in the metabolism of malignant tissues. We also found that hexokinase, phosphoglucomutase (Fig. 3), and aspartate aminotransferase (Fig. 4) were increased in activity in the carcinomas, whereas the activities of the enzymes were similar in normal breast, in fibrocystic disease, and in fibroadenomas. In contrast, the activity of glutamate dehydrogenase (Fig. 3) was unchanged in any of the tissues examined. Although most of the changes observed demonstrated an increase in enzyme activity in neoplastic tissues, the opposite pattern was seen for α-glycerolphosphate dehydrogenase. In the case of α-GPD (Fig. 4), the highest level of activity was seen in normal breast tissue and the activity of this enzyme was markedly reduced in both fibroadenomas and infiltrating ductal carcinomas, probably reflecting the decreased content of adipose tissue in the benign and malignant tumors.

Thus, the data clearly show that there exist significant biochemical differences between malignant tumors and either normal or nonmalignant disease of the breast in women. These data indicate that the infiltrating ductal carcinomas possess a distinctive metabolic capacity, which is not due only to an increase in cellularity; expression of enzyme activity per milli-

TABLE II

Protein and Nucleic Acid Content of Human Breast Tissues[a]

End point	Normal breast	Fibrocystic disease	Fibroadenoma	Infiltrating ductal carcinoma
Protein (mg/100 mg)	3.10 ± 0.18 (38)	2.93 ± 0.22 (17)	3.99 ± 0.53 (10)	3.65 ± 0.12 (82)[c]
RNA (μg/mg)	1.21 ± 0.13 (56)	1.29 ± 0.15 (33)	2.93 ± 0.37 (20)[b,c]	3.43 ± 0.15 (133)[b,c]
DNA (μg/mg)	1.26 ± 0.15 (56)	1.53 ± 0.22 (33)	2.99 ± 0.41 (20)[b,c]	4.24 ± 0.22 (134)[b,c,d]

[a] Data presented as mean ± SEM. Numbers in parentheses represent the number of samples assayed.
[b] Significantly different ($P < 0.01$) compared to normal breast.
[c] Significantly different ($P < 0.01$) compared to fibrocystic disease.
[d] Significantly different ($P < 0.01$) compared to fibroadenoma.

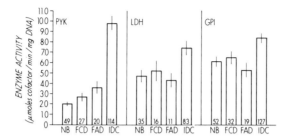

Fig. 1. Activities of pyruvate kinase (PYK), lactate dehydrogenase (LDH), and glucosephosphate isomerase (GPI) in samples of normal breast (NB), fibrocystic disease (FCD), fibroadenoma (FAD), and infiltrating ductal carcinoma (IDC). Each bar represents the mean for the number of samples shown in each bar; vertical lines represent the standard error of the mean.

gram DNA indicated that carcinomas possess unique elevations in the activities of LDH, GPI, G6PD, ICD, HK, and AAT. These data also suggest that fibrocystic disease may not be a preneoplastic lesion, since there appear to be few fundamental biochemical alterations in samples of fibrocystic disease compared with normal breast.

Recently, we have initiated studies on the isoenzyme patterns for lactate dehydrogenase and glucose-6-phosphate dehydrogenase in these human tissues. Several studies of LDH isoenzymes in malignant tissues have demonstrated that the tumors contain predominantly LDH-3, LDH-4, and LDH-5 (muscle-type isoenzymes) irrespective of the tissue from which the tumor arose (see review by Criss, 1971). In constrast, no reports of G6PD isoenzymes in human tumors were found, although some data on normal and neoplastic rodent tissues have been published (Hershey *et al.,* 1966;

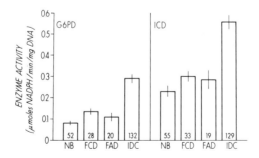

Fig. 2. Activities of glucose-6-phosphate dehydrogenase (G6PD) and NADP-isocitrate dehydrogenase (ICD) in samples of normal breast (NB), fibrocystic disease (FCD), fibroadenoma (FAD), and infiltrating ductal carcinoma (IDC). Each bar represents the mean for the number of samples shown in each bar; vertical lines represent the standard error of the mean.

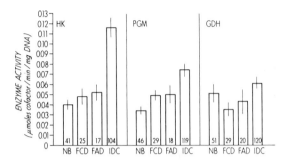

Fig. 3. Activities of hexokinase (HK), phosphoglucomutase (PGM), and glutamate dehydrogenase (GDH) in samples of normal breast (NB), fibrocystic disease (FCD), fibroadenoma (FAD), and infiltrating ductal carcinoma (IDC). Each bar represents the mean for the number of samples shown in each bar; vertical lines represent the standard error of the mean.

Richards and Hilf, 1971, 1972). Thus, it seemed logical to examine normal breast tissue for isoenzymes and determine if any alterations in these patterns occurred in human breast carcinomas and in benign diseases of the breast. The results of these initial studies are summarized in Table III. The data demonstrate an elevated level of LDH-5 in the infiltrating ductal carcinomas compared with normal breast or with benign lesions of the breast, results in agreement with earlier reports (Goldman *et al.*, 1964).

The data in Table III indicate that there are 3 discrete bands for G6PD in the human breast tissues examined. The fastest migrating species,

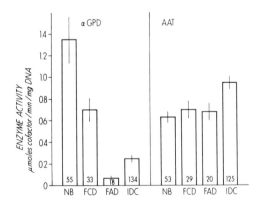

Fig. 4. Activities of α-glycerolphosphate dehydrogenase (αGPD) and aspartate aminotransferase (AAT) in samples of normal breast (NB), fibrocystic disease (FCD), fibroadenoma (FAD), and infiltrating ductal carcinoma (IDC). Each bar represents the mean for the number of samples shown in each bar; vertical lines represent the standard error of the mean.

TABLE III

G6PD and LDH Isoenzymes in Normal and Abnormal Human Breast Tissues[a]

Tissue	No. Samples	% G6PD Isoenzyme			No. Samples	% LDH Isoenzyme				
		G6PD-3	G6PD-2	G6PD-1		LDH-5	LDH-4	LDH-3	LDH-2	LDH-1
Carcinoma	8	5 ± 1	44 ± 6	51 ± 6	12	16 ± 3	27 ± 3	30 ± 1	20 ± 2	7 ± 2
Normal breast	2	21 ± 2	24 ± 1	55 ± 1	7	4 ± 1	24 ± 1	38 ± 2	25 ± 1	9 ± 1
Fibrocystic disease	5	16 ± 4	32 ± 4	51 ± 7	9	3 ± 1	20 ± 2	40 ± 2	27 ± 1	10 ± 1
Fibroadenoma	2	6 ± 2	45 ± 10	49 ± 10	2	< 1	13 ± 2	42 ± 2	31 ± 3	14 ± 1

[a] Data presented as mean ± S.E.M.

designated G6PD-1, represents about 50% of the total G6PD enzyme and appeared to be unchanged in normal or abnormal breast specimens. The species demonstrating an intermediate mobility, G6PD-2, was lowest in the normal breast and slightly higher in samples of fibroadenoma and carcinoma. The slowest migrating species, G6PD-3, showed a contrasting pattern, i.e., greatest levels in normal tissue and least amount in tumors. Thus, there appear to be distinctive G6PD isoenzyme patterns found in tumors compared to normal breast or fibrocystic disease, although the patterns were similar between malignant and nonmalignant tumors. These preliminary results are being extended.

IV. Estrogen-Binding Proteins in Human Breast Tissues

Currently it is accepted that an essential characteristic of an estrogen target cell, such as those in the uterus or mammary gland, is the capacity to bind estradiol specifically and with high affinity. Binding of female sex hormones (E) to entities termed "estrogen-binding proteins" or "estrogen-receptors" (designated R_c in Fig. 5) precedes alterations in the rates of transcription and translation in a target cell. Investigations from many laboratories (Mueller, 1965; Gorski et al., 1968; Hamilton, 1968; Williams-Ashman and Reddi, 1971; Jensen and DeSombre, 1972a,b,) have established that estradiol-17β interacts with these receptors by the sequential process illustrated in this figure. The steroid enters the target cell, apparently by passive diffusion, and combines with the cytoplasmic form of the receptor protein (R_c). The receptor hormone complex of the mammary gland sediments at 8–9 Svedbergs (S) on sucrose gradients containing low salt (Gardner and Wittliff, 1973c). If the hormone–receptor complex is extracted with salt solutions of greater then physiological ionic strength, a

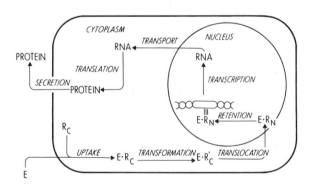

Fig. 5. Proposed steps in the interaction of estradiol-17β with a target cell.

binding protein sedimenting at 4–5 S is seen. These entities represent the two forms of the estrogen receptor isolated *in vitro* from the cytoplasm of the mammary gland. The true molecular size of the cytoplasmic form of the receptor, R_c, in a target cell is not known presently, although recent evidence (Stancel *et al.*, 1973) suggests the 4–5 S form may predominate. In the presence of estradiol-17β, the receptor (R_c) apparently undergoes a temperature-dependent transformation to the new species (designated E · R_c') which sediments at about 5 S (Jensen *et al.*, 1971a). The transformed complex (E · R_c') migrates to the nucleus where it binds to an acceptor site presumably in the chromatin of the target cell. This 5 S form of the receptor may be extracted from target cell nuclei by 0.4 M KCl (Jensen *et al.*, 1968; Shyamala and Gorski, 1969). Only the transformed complex, E · R_c', has the ability to translocate to the nucleus and stimulate RNA polymerase activity, resulting in an elevation of the synthesis of nucleic acids (Mohla *et al.*, 1972). An example of the target cell response would be the increase in growth of the uterus after estrogen stimulation.

Since specific estrogen-binding proteins presumably are found only in estrogen-responsive or -dependent cells, a knowledge of their presence and perhaps properties may serve as a molecular basis for the distinction between breast carcinomas in patients that are responsive to endocrine ablative surgery and/or hormone therapy and those that are not.

Of the multitude of hormones interacting with the mammary gland, the principal steroid hormones are the estrogens, progestagens, and glucocorticoids. Estrogens and progestagens apparently stimulate the differentiation of breast epithelial cells in readiness for milk protein synthesis and secretion (Juergens *et al.*, 1965; Cowie and Tindal, 1971). Glucocorticoids, on the other hand, apparently play a role in the formation and stabilization of rough endoplasmic reticulum, the principal site of milk protein synthesis (Oka and Topper, 1971, 1972). Receptors which bind glucocorticoids in a special fashion and with high affinity have been reported in the normal mammary gland (Tucker *et al.*, 1971; Gardner and Wittliff, 1973b; Shyamala, 1973) and in a hormone-responsive mammary adenocarcinoma (Gardner and Wittliff, 1973a).

Following the pioneering work of Jensen and Jacobson in the late 1950's and early 1960's (Jensen, 1960; Jensen and Jacobson, 1960, 1962), Talwar and colleagues (1964) provided the first evidence that estradiol-17β was associated with a particular macromolecule using Sephadex column chromatography. The use of centrifugation in sucrose gradients of labeled estradiol–receptor complex from the cytoplasm of target cells was first reported by Toft and Gorski (1966). This important finding provided an easy method for the separation of the specific forms of the receptor from nonspecifically bound steroid. In addition to the separation of specific estrogen receptors by centrifugation on sucrose gradients (Jensen et al., 1971b; Wittliff et al., 1971, 1972b), estrogen-binding capacity of human breast carcinoma has been studied by tissue slice procedure (Sander, 1968; Johansson et al., 1970; Hahnel and Twaddle, 1971; Maass et al., 1972) as well as the dextran-coated charcoal technique (Korenman and Dukes, 1970; Feherty et al., 1971; Gorlich and Heise, 1971; Leung et al., 1973). With each of the assays it is important that estrogen-binding capacity be measured in the presence and in the absence of unlabeled estradiol-17β or a competitive inhibitor of binding such as CI-628 (CN-55,945-27) or nafoxidine (U-11100) to assure measurements of specific estrogen-binding capacity. Both the dextran-coated charcoal procedure and sucrose gradient analyses have the added advantage that they separate the unreacted tritiated-ligand from protein-bound hormone by either adsorption of the unbound steroid to the surface of the dextran-coated charcoal or by its inability to penetrate the gradient of sucrose. Although sucrose gradient centrifugation as a means of measuring specific estrogen-binding capacity is one of the most time-consuming and expensive procedures, it is one of the most satisfactory in terms of visualization of specific estrogen receptors.

Presently in our laboratories data (as cpm) from either sucrose gradient or charcoal adsorption assays of estrogen-binding proteins are handled as previously described (Wittliff et al., 1972b), using specific programs (Brooks and Wittliff, 1973). Specific estrogen-binding proteins sedimenting at 8–9 S as well as 4–5 S are easily identified by their isotopic profiles from the sucrose gradient analyses. Specific estrogen binding is estimated as the differences in radioactivity found in either the 8–9 S region or the 4–5 S region of the gradient, since each cytosol is measured in the presence and in the absence of a competitive ligand (usually unlabeled estradiol-17β). Specific estrogen-binding capacity is expressed as femtomoles (10^{-15} moles) estradiol bound per milligram cytosol protein or femtomoles per microgram DNA.

Using sucrose gradient analysis, we have shown that certain infiltrating ductal carcinomas of the human breast contain specific estrogen-binding proteins (Wittliff et al., 1972b). The majority of these receptors sediment at 8–9 S when extracted from the tissue in buffers containing low salt (Fig. 6). The ligand specificity of these binding proteins was determined in each tissue by simultaneous incubation of an aliquot of cytosol with a competitive inhibitor such as CI-628 or unlabeled estradiol-17β prior to sucrose gradient centrifugation. In a small number of tumors from breast cancer patients separation of estrogen-binding proteins from the cytosol revealed only 4–5 S receptors (Fig. 6). Although these proteins sediment with approximately the same sedimentation velocity as human serum

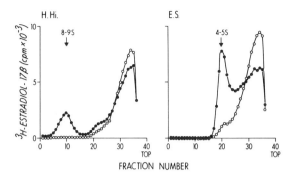

Fig. 6. Sedimentation of specific estrogen receptors in the cytosols of patients with breast carcinoma. Cytosols of tumors were reacted with [³H]estradiol-17β, layered onto linear gradients of sucrose, and centrifuged overnight at 308,000 g. Fractions were collected into scintillation vials and the radioactivity measured. The profiles presented using the closed circles represent binding in the presence of [³H]estradiol alone, those using the open circles represent nonspecific binding of [³H]estradiol. The difference between the two types of profiles represents specific binding at either 8–9 S or 4–5 S.

albumin, i.e., 4.6 S, which binds estradiol nonspecifically, these receptors were apparently specific since, in the presence of unlabeled estradiol, binding of [³H]estradiol was inhibited. Another group of human breast carcinomas exhibited both the 8–9 S receptor and the 4–5 S receptor when these tissues were extracted with low salt buffers and sedimented on sucrose gradients (Fig. 7). Although we cannot determine the specific nature of 4–5 S binding species by current procedures *in vitro*, these receptors may represent either the initial estrogen–receptor complex, $E \cdot R_c'$, or the transformed complex, $E \cdot R'_c$, both of which are found in the cytosol of tumor cells.

Jensen *et al.* (1971b) reported earlier that the majority of human breast carcinomas which were examined in their study contained only the specific estrogen receptors sedimenting at 8–9 S. However, several of the tissues which they examined also contained the receptors which sedimented at 4–5 S similar to the profile shown in Fig. 7. A recent report by McGuire and DeLaGarza (1973) confirmed these data.

The specificity of estrogen binding by the 8–9 S and 4–5 S forms of the receptors was also checked (Fig. 7). The gradient profiles indicate that hydrocortisone, progesterone, and dihydrotestosterone had little inhibitory effect although estrone inhibited binding significantly. In one case we have also found that triamcinolone acetonide, a synthetic glucocorticoid, does not inhibit specific binding. Table IV summarizes several determinations of the specificity of [³H]estradiol-17β binding to the receptors in the cytosol of infiltrating ductal carcinomas of the human breast. These data and those of

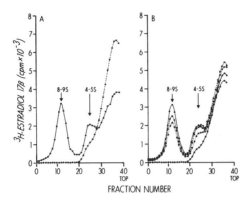

Fig. 7. Steroid-binding specificity of the estrogen receptors in the cytosol of a human breast carcinoma. Isotopic profiles following sucrose gradient centrifugation of cytosol from infiltrating ductal carcinoma incubated *in vitro* with 2 nM [³H]estradiol-17β (solid line, panel A). The dashed line (panel A) represents a reaction preincubated 10 minutes with 1 mM unlabeled estradiol-17β which serves as a measure of *nonspecific* binding. Notice that specific binding of [³H]estradiol-17β is indicated in both 8–9 S and 4–5 S peaks. The solid line (panel B) represents a reaction preincubated 10 minutes with 1 mM hydrocortisone; the dashed line (panel B), with 1 mM progesterone; the dotted line (panel B), with 1 mM dihydrotestosterone. The profile (indicated by the solid line which shows *no* binding by the 8–9 S peak, panel B) was preincubated with 1 mM estrone for 10 minutes. Notice that the binding of [³H]estradiol-17β to the 8–9 S and 4–5 S peaks is reduced significantly by estrone, indicating further the specificity of the receptor sites.

other investigators (Korenman and Dukes, 1970; Hahnel and Twaddle, 1971; Jensen *et al.*, 1971b; McGuire and DeLaGarza, 1973) indicate the ligand-binding characteristics of receptors in human breast tumors are similar to those of receptors from the normal mammary gland (Wittliff *et al.*, 1972a; Gardner and Wittliff, 1973c) as well as the uterus (Jensen and DeSombre, 1972b).

Both the 8–9 S and 4–5 S forms of the receptors are apparently protein in nature since they are sensitive to digestion by pronase. However, they are not sensitive to the presence of ribonuclease or deoxyribonuclease (J. L. Wittliff, R. Hilf, and B. W. Beatty, unpublished results). The sensitivity of these receptors to pronase digestion is similar to that exhibited by specific estrogen-binding proteins in other target cells such as the uterus (Jensen and DeSombre, 1972b) and the mammary gland (Gardner and Wittliff, 1973c). Titration of these specific estrogen-binding proteins with increasing concentrations of [³H]estradiol-17β indicated a single type of binding site exhibiting high affinity ($K_d \sim 10^{-10}$ M) for the ligand (Feherty *et al.*, 1971; Hahnel and Twaddle, 1971; Wittliff *et al.*, 1972b; McGuire, 1973). Other properties of estrogen-binding proteins in human breast tumors such as the temperature dependence of the binding reaction (Hahnel and Twaddle, 1971; Feherty et al., 1971) and effects of ionic strength and polyanions on the sedimentation properties of the receptors (McGuire and DeLaGarza, 1973) have been studied.

Table V summarizes some of the properties of specific estrogen-binding proteins from the cytosol of normal and neoplastic mammary cells. The estrogen receptor found in infiltrating ductal carcinoma of the human breast has many properties which are similar to those of specific estrogen-binding proteins in the lactating mammary gland of the rat.

Specific estrogen receptors have not been demonstrated in nonmalignant lesions of the breast such as fibrocystic disease or fibroadenoma (Wittliff et al., 1972b) (Fig. 8). However, significant binding of labeled estradiol has been reported for a few nonmalignant diseases of the breast when measured by the tissue slice (Johansson et al., 1970) or dextran-coated charcoal (Feherty et al., 1971) procedure. Although normal breast tissue from women is known to concentrate [³H]estradiol in vivo (Demetriou et al., 1964; Braunsberg et al., 1967; Deshpande et al., 1967; Pearlman et al., 1969) the levels of steroid retained are considerably lower than those found in tumor tissue. One explanation for this reduced binding is that normal breast tissue during states other than pregnancy and lactation contains few epithelial cells and a predominance of adipose cells when compared to most

TABLE IV

Specificity of [³H]Estradiol-17β Binding to the Receptors in the Cytosol
of Infiltrating Ductal Carcinomas of the Human Breast

| | | [³H]Estradiol-17β bound (%) | |
Competitive substance	Concentration (μM)	8–9 S Receptors	4–5 S Receptors
None	—	100	100
Estradiol-17β	1	3 ± 1[a]	62 ± 8[b]
Estrone	1	4 ± 1	61 ± 9
Dihydrotestosterone	1	82 ± 4	82 ± 3
Progesterone	1	82 ± 10	97 ± 1
Hydrocortisone	1	90 ± 6	98 ± 1
Triamcinolone	1	98[c]	98[c]

[a] Mean ± S.E.M., 4 tumor specimens.

[b] Mean ± S.E.M., 3 tumor specimens.

[c] Single sample.

TABLE V

Properties of Specific Estrogen-Binding Proteins from the Cytosol of Normal and
Neoplastic Mammary Cells

	Lactating rat	Infiltrating ductal carcinoma—human
Dissociation constant	10^{-9}–10^{-10} M	10^{-9}–10^{-10} M
Sedimentation velocity	8–9 Svedbergs	8–9 Svedbergs
Subunits (0.4 M KCl)	4–5 Svedbergs	4–5 Svedbergs
Ligand specificity	Estrogens	Estrogens
Pronase sensitivity	+	+
DNase sensitivity	−	−
RNase sensitivity	−	−
pCMB sensitivity	+	+
Temperature stability (*in vitro*)	Stable at 0°C Unstable at 37°C	Stable at 0°C Unstable at 37°C
Ligand stability (*in vitro*)	Estrogens	Estrogens

malignant breast cancers. To date, normal breast tissue from only one
patient has exhibited specific estrogen receptors sedimenting at 8 S (Wittliff
et al., 1972b). Recent results from our group suggest that the simple explanation of a lack of cellularity may not be the answer. Examination of the
estrogen-binding capacity of mammary gland from virgin, pregnant, and
lactating rats revealed that levels of specific estrogen receptors were low in

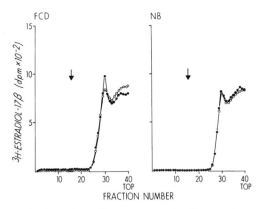

Fig. 8. Representative isotopic profiles of estrogen-binding proteins separated by sucrose
gradient centrifugation of cytosols of fibrocystic disease (FCD) of the breast and normal
breast (NB). Assay conditions were similar to those described in the legend of Fig. 6. Arrows
indicate the position of sedimentation of the 8–9 S receptor.

glands of virgin and pregnant animals but increased throughout lactation reaching a maximum which was comparable to that of infiltrating ductal carcinoma of the human breast (Beers and Wittliff, 1973). We have not examined normal breast tissue from pregnant or lactating women, however, because of the unavailability of specimens.

The distribution of specific receptors in malignant breast cancers examined in our study is shown in Table VI. Eighty-one of 175 primary breast tumors (approximately 46%) contained significant estrogen-binding capacity (Table VI). Of the 81 tumors exhibiting the capacity to bind estradiol specifically, 64 contained the 8–9 S receptors. The specific binding capacity of these carcinomas demonstrated a range from 5 to 224 fmoles estradiol bound/mg of protein, with an overall mean of 67 fmoles/mg of protein. Twenty-one of these 64 tumors also contained the 4–5 S receptors. The specific binding capacity of the receptors sedimenting at 4–5 S was 47 fmoles estradiol bound/mg of cytosol protein with a range of 10 to 213. Seventeen specimens of infiltrating ductal carcinoma contained only the 4–5 S receptors; binding capacity of this receptor was 73 fmoles/mg cytosol protein with a range of 10 to 262. The remaining 94 tumor tissues did not exhibit specific estrogen-binding capacity. The significance of this distribution of receptor species is not known presently.

Distribution of estrogen-binding capacity in human breast cancers appears to be similar whether measured by the sucrose gradient or the dextran-coated charcoal procedure, i.e., approximately 50% contain receptors, even though measurements were made in different laboratories (Table VII). By all assays, i.e., the tissue slice procedure, dextran-coated charcoal, and sucrose gradient analyses, approximately 44% of the primary breast carcinomas examined contain specific estrogen receptors although the absolute amount of receptor varies considerably from tumor to tumor (Table VII).

No histological feature has been found which might explain the variation in levels of estrogen receptors in human breast tumors. In *our* experience, the proportion of tumor cells to surrounding connective tissue and adipose cells does not appear to be correlated with the variation in estrogen-binding capacity. It has been reported that adipose cells of rodent mammary glands do not contain the specific estrogen receptors (Puca and Bresciani, 1969; Shyamala and Nandi, 1972), although these cells will take up a considerable amount of the steroid because of its lipid solubility. Presently we are not able to determine if the level of estrogen-binding proteins in a breast tumor is a reflection of a heterogenous cell population in which a variable number of tumor cells demonstrates estrogen sensitivity or a more homogeneous cell population in which individual cells exhibit variable estrogen-binding capacity.

TABLE VI

Summary of Specific Binding of Estradiol-17β by Malignant and Nonmalignant Breast Tissues from Humans

Breast tissue examined	Rating	No. with 8–9 S receptor	Estrogen-binding capacity: 8–9 S (fmol/mg protein)	No. with 8–9 and 4–5 S receptor	Estrogen-binding capacity: 4–5 S (fmol/mg protein)
Infiltrating ductal carcinoma	+	64/64	67 ± 7 (5–224)[a]	21/64	47 ± 12 (10–213)[a]
Infiltrating ductal carcinoma	+	0/17	<1	17/17[b]	73 ± 17 (10–262)[a]
Infiltrating ductal carcinoma	–	0/94	<2	0/94	<1
Total with receptors		81/175 (46%)			
Fibrocystic disease	–	0/9	<1	0/9	<1
Normal breast	–	1/20	<1	0/20	<1

[a] Number refers to range of values.
[b] Only 4–5 S.

TABLE VII

Distribution of Estrogen-Binding Capacity in Human Breast Carcinoma

Investigator	No. of tumors examined	No. of tumors exhibiting estrogen-binding capacity	Assay procedure
Sander (1968)	25	9	Tissue slice
Johansson et al. (1970)	31	14	Tissue slice
Gorlich and Heise (1971)	38	8	Tissue slice
Hahnel et al. (1971)[a]	71	13	Tissue slice
Maass et al. (1972)[b]	164	67	Tissue slice
	329	111 (34%)	
Korenman and Dukes (1970)	15	7	Charcoal adsorption
Feherty et al. (1971)	53	37	Charcoal adsorption
McGuire (1973)[c]	43	14	Charcoal adsorption
Leung et al. (1973)	58	34	Charcoal adsorption
	169	92 (54%)	
Jensen et al. (1971b)	84	46	Sucrose gradient
Wittliff et al. (1972b, 1974)[a]	175	81	Sucrose gradient
	259	127 (49%)	
Total (by all assays)	757	330 (44%)	

[a] Also used charcoal adsorption assay.

[b] Also used gel electrophoresis assay.

[c] Also used sucrose gradient procedure.

Another important consideration is the endogenous concentration of estrogens in the plasma and tumor of the patient. Estrogen levels are known to influence the number of specific binding sites on receptor proteins occupied *in vivo* by the steroid hormone (Gorski *et al.*, 1968; Baulieu *et al.*, 1971; Jensen and DeSombre, 1972a,b). For example, Maass and his colleagues (1972) have found that estrogen-binding capacity in the human uterus varies during the menstrual cycle; it is low in midcycle and is reduced further in the second phase. They have also shown that there is no binding of [^{3}H]estradiol-17β to receptors in breast tumors from patients with plasma estradiol-17β levels exceeding 300 pg/ml. Furthermore, the report of Willcox and Thomas (1972) that human tumors maintained in organ culture can convert estrone to estradiol-17β is of particular interest since the concentration of estrone is significant in the plasma (Baird *et al.*,

1969) of postmenopausal women and in certain breast tumors (James *et al.*, 1970; Korenman and Dukes, 1970).

Breast cancer becomes clinically evident more often in postmenopausal women, whose circulating estrogen levels are low. However, data on tumors which lack estrogen-binding capacity and which were removed from women with high plasma levels of estrogens (premenopausal) should be excluded in order to avoid false negative results. In our study it was shown that a small number (approximately 30%) of tumors from premenopausal women contained measurable levels of specific estrogen-binding proteins (Fig. 9). Therefore, data on these tumors may be of predictive value for selection of appropriate therapies for certain breast cancer patients who are premenopausal. A greater number (approximately 65%) of tumors from women who were postmenopausal exhibited specific estrogen capacity (Fig. 9). Fifty-five was chosen as an age at which virtually every woman was postmenopausal. Data such as these suggest that there may be a relationship between the level of estrogen receptors in breast carcinomas and the age (or endocrine state) of the patient at the time of surgery. Whether these

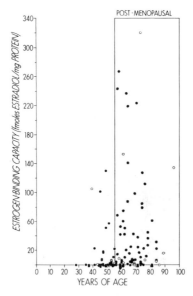

Fig. 9. Relationship of specific estrogen-binding capacity of cytosols from primary malignant tumors and the age of the patient at the time of surgery. Fifty-five years of age was chosen as a time at which virtually every woman had undergone the menopause. The closed circles represent patients with infiltrating ductal carcinoma of the breast; open circles represent patients with other types of malignant breast disease such as medullary carcinoma and colloid carcinoma.

results reflect endogenous levels of estrogen will have to await additional analyses. Figure 9 also illustrates the considerable variation in the binding capacity in tumors from women of the same age. The estrogen-binding capacity of certain tumors reaches such a magnitude that the carcinoma may be competitive with other body tissues for available estradiol. Although there is a considerable variation in the binding capacity of tumors from women who are postmenopausal, a considerable number of tumors from this age group do not demonstrate significant estrogen-binding capacity (Fig. 9). Therefore, it is plausible that the presence of specific estrogen-receptor proteins in a breast tumor may be the expression of a phenotype characteristic of a hormonally responsive cell. However, consideration of the absence of a patient's response to endocrine therapy in whose tumor estrogen receptors were demonstrated will be discussed.

V. Preliminary Clinical Correlations

Preliminary evidence from our study (Savlov *et al.,* 1974) and of other investigators (Jensen *et al.,* 1971b; Maass *et al.,* 1972; Braunsberg *et al.,* 1973; Leung *et al.,* 1973) indicates that remission of breast cancer after adrenalectomy, and in some cases after additive hormone therapy, occurred more often in women with breast tumors containing estrogen receptors than in those patients whose carcinomas did not exhibit measurable quantities of estrogen-binding proteins (Table VIII). The study of Jensen and co-workers (1971b) provided the first evidence that the lack of specific estrogen-binding protein in breast tumors may be correlated with the absence of an objective clinical remission of disease following adrenalectomy. The data in Table VIII on the lack of responsiveness of patients with breast cancer containing specific estrogen receptors, 6 of 36, may be explained from the following considerations. First since breast carcinomas are heterogeneous with regard to cellular composition, it is reasonable to suggest that although hormonally dependent cells "die" as a result of ablation of endocrine organs, hormonally independent cells continue to proliferate. Second, the lack of responsiveness of these patients to ablative therapy may be that events beyond the initial interaction of the steroid with a tumor cell are defective. Some obvious events to consider as possible sites of defectiveness are (1) at the level of transformation of the receptor, (2) at the level of translocation, or (3) in the final binding of the receptor–hormone complex to the chromatin prior to the initiation of transcription (Fig. 5).

Although these data (Table VIII) support the original observation of Folca and co-workers (Folca *et al.,* 1961), it is necessary that we increase the number of patients whose tumors are examined for specific estrogen-binding capacity and to correlate these data with the patient's response. In

TABLE VIII

Relationship between Estrogen-Binding Capacity of Breast
Tumors and the Patient's Response to Therapy

	No. of patients exhibiting objective remission following additive or ablative hormone therapy	
Investigator	Tumors containing estrogen receptors	Tumors lacking estrogen receptors
Jensen *et al.* (1971b)	10/13	1/29
Maass *et al.* (1972)	6/7	0/14
Leung *et al.* (1973)	12/12	2/10
Savlov *et al.* (1974)	2/4	0/7
Total	30/36	3/60

that way, we may determine the relevance of the receptor mechanism to the selection of therapeutic regimens.

Since we had reported earlier that, in a spectrum of rodent mammary tumors, there appeared to be a relationship beween certain enzyme activities and hormone responsiveness (Hilf *et al.*, 1969a, 1970a; Hilf, 1970, 1971) and since Smith and King (1970) had also shown a relationship between glycolytic enzymes and hormonal dependence of a mammary tumor in BR6 mice, we examined enzyme activities of human carcinomas possessing estrogen receptors and enzyme activities of human tumors that lacked specific estrogen receptors. These results are summarized in Fig. 10. The data indicate that the activities of the glycolytic enzymes, GPI, PYK, and LDH, were significantly higher in carcinomas that lack specific estrogen receptors. Further, G6PD and ICD, two enzymes that catalyze reactions that result in production of NADPH, were also significantly elevated in carcinomas that lack estrogen receptors. The ratio of $G6PD/\alpha GPD$ activities appeared to be higher in tumors lacking estrogen-binding capacity. Thus, human tumors which may be considered as hormonally independent (lack estrogen receptors) demonstrate higher glycolytic capacity, a result that could be predicted from the data reported for hormone-responsive and hormone-independent animal tumors.

It is certainly pertinent that 4 of the patients in our series, whose tumors did not possess significant levels of estrogen receptors, did demonstrate objective responses to chemotherapy, using agents such as 5-fluorouracil, prednisone, cytoxan, and methotrexate (Savlov *et al.*, 1974). Three of those patients had carcinomas that contained an elevated G6PD/αGPD ratio, suggesting a hormonally independent tumor on the basis of earlier studies with rodent tumors (Hilf, 1971). In the fourth patient, although the G6PD/αGPD ratio was < 1, the activity of the glycolytic enzymes GPI and PYK was strikingly elevated. It would appear that either an increased G6PD/αGPD ratio and/or elevated activities of glycolytic enzymes may predict for response to chemotherapy. Studies are currently underway to seek confirmation of the above proposals.

VI. Conclusion

Direct examination of breast tumors for specific biochemical parameters is useful in the characterization of the neoplasm as to its response to alterations of the endocrine status of the host. It would appear from preliminary data that the lack of specific estrogen-binding capacity, often accompanied by elevated activities in glycolytic enzymes, would predict for a lack of response to endocrine organ ablation, i.e., adrenalectomy; a chemotherapeutic regimen may be warranted. In those patients whose tumors possess significant levels of specific estrogen receptors, ablative procedures and/or administration of steroids should result in an objective clinical response. A

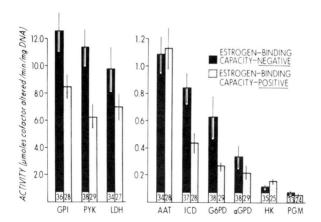

Fig. 10. Enzyme activities in infiltrating ductal carcinomas that lack estrogen receptors (solid bars) compared with carcinomas that possess specific estrogen receptors (stippled bars). Values presented as mean ± standard error of the mean (vertical line in each bar); number of samples examined is shown at the base of each bar. Enzymes measured were GPI, glucosephosphate isomerase; PYK, pyruvate kinase; LDH, lactate dehydrogenase; AAT, aspartate amino transferase; ICD, isocitrate dehydrogenase; G6PD, glucose-6-phosphate dehydrogenase; αGPD, α-glycerolphosphate dehydrogenase; HK, hexokinase; and PGM, phosphoglucomutase.

further discrimination of the response may arise from a consideration of the concentration and, perhaps, properties of the receptors as well as the profile of enzymes selected to reflect the metabolic status of the carcinoma. Assuming that the present clinical correlations are confirmed, it is not unreasonable that this approach, i.e., direct biochemical characterization of the tumor, may become a routine procedure for the oncologist to employ in defining the breast cancer patient.

ACKNOWLEDGMENTS

The authors wish to acknowledge the competent technical assistance of W. D. Rector, W. F. Brooks, Jr., C. Littrell, and B. Beatty, the efforts of our Oncology nurses, D. O'Hagan, J. Evra, and S. Kinsella, in obtaining and transporting human tissues to our laboratories, and the interest by the many physicians whose cooperation make such studies possible to be performed. We thank M. Palmer for her secretarial assistance. The continued encouragement and provocative discussions with T. C. Hall and W. B. Patterson should be noted. The investigations presented here were made possible through the financial support of USPHS Grants CA-12836 and CA-11198 from the National Cancer Institute, and by a grant, CI-6, from the American Cancer Society.

REFERENCES

Baird, D. T., Horton, R., Longcope, C., and Tait, J. F. (1969). *Recent Progr. Horm. Res.* **25,** 611.

Baulieu, E. E., Alberga, A., Jung, I., LeBeau, M. C., Mercier-Bodard, C., Milgrom, E., Raynaud, J. P., Raynaud-Jammet, C., Rochefort, H., Truong, H., and Robel, P. (1971). *Recent Progr. Horm. Res.* **27,** 351.

Beatson, G. T. (1896). *Lancet* **2,** 104.

Beers, P. C., and Wittliff, J. L. (1973). *Fed. Proc., Fed. Amer. Soc. Exp. Biol.* **32,** 651.

Braunsberg, H., Irvine, W. T., and James, V. H. T. (1967). *Brit. J. Cancer* **21,** 714.

Braunsberg, H., James, V. H. T., Irvine, W. T., James, F., Jamieson, C. W., Sellwood, R. A., Carter, A. E., and Hulbert, M. (1973). *Lancet* **1,** 163.

Brooks, W. F., Jr., and Wittliff, J. L. (1973). *Anal. Biochem.* **54,** 464.

Bulbrook, R. D. (1970). *Advan. Steroid Biochem. Pharmacol.* **1,** 387–417.

Bulbrook, R. D., and Hayward, J. L. (1967). *Lancet,* **1,** 519.

Cowie, A. T., and Tindal, J. S. (1971)."The Physiology of Lactation," pp. 151–168. Williams & Wilkins, Baltimore, Maryland.

Criss, W. E. (1971). *Cancer Res.* **31,** 1523.

Demetriou, J. A., Crowley, L. G., Kushinski, S., Donovan, A. J., Kotin, B., and MacDonald, I. (1964). *Cancer Res* **24,** 926.

Deshpande, N., Jensen, V., Bulbrook, R. D., Berne, T., and Ellis, F. (1967). *Steroids* **10,** 219.

Feherty, P., Ferrer-Brown, G., and Kellie, A. E. (1971). *Brit. J. Cancer* **25,** 697.

Folca, P. J., Glascock, R. F., and Irvine, W. T. (1961). *Lancet* **2,** 796.

Gardner, D. G., and Wittliff, J. L. (1973a). *Brit. J. Cancer* **27,** 441.

Gardner, D. G., and Wittliff, J. L. (1973b). *Biochem. Biophys. Acta* **320,** 617.

Gardner, D. G., and Wittliff, J. L. (1973c). *Biochemistry* **12,** 3090.

Goldman, R. D., Kaplan, N. D., and Hall, T. C. (1964). *Cancer Res.* **24,** 389.

Gorlich, M., and Heise, E. (1971). *Arch. Geschwulstforsch.* **38,** 139.

Gorski, J., Toft, D., Shyamala, G., Smith, D., and Notides, A. (1968). *Recent Progr. Horm. Res.* **24,** 45.

Hahnel, R., and Twaddle, E. (1971). *Steroids* **18**, 653.

Hahnel, R., Twaddle, E., and Vivian, A. B. (1971). *Steroids* **18**, 681.

Hamilton, T. H. (1968) *Science* **161**, 649.

Hayward, J. L., and Bulbrook, R. D. (1968). *In* "Prognostic Factors in Breast Cancer" (A. P. M. Forrest and P. B. Kunkler, eds.), pp. 383–392. Livingstone, Edinburgh.

Hershey, F. B., Johnston, G., Murphey, S. M., and Schmitt, M. (1966). *Cancer Res.* **26**, 265.

Hilf, R. (1968). *Cancer Res.* **28**, 1888.

Hilf, R. (1970). *In* "Protein Metabolism and Biological Function" (C. P. Bianchi and R. Hilf, eds.), pp. 251–261. Rutgers Univ. Press, New Brunswick, New Jersey.

Hilf, R. (1971). *Nat. Cancer Inst., Monogr.* **34**, 43.

Hilf, R. (1973). *Methods Cancer Res.* **7**, 55–114.

Hilf, R., Michel, I., and Bell, C. (1967). *Recent Progr. Horm. Res.* **23**, 229.

Hilf, R., Goldenberg, H., Michel, I., Carrington, M. J., Bell, C., Gruenstein, M., Meranze, D. R., and Shimkin, M. B. (1969a). *Cancer Res.* **29**, 977.

Hilf, R., Goldenberg, H., Orlando, R. A., and Archer, F. L. (1969b). *Proc. Soc. Exp. Biol. Med.* **132**, 613.

Hilf, R., Goldenberg, H., Bell, C., Michel, I., Orlando, R. A., and Archer, F. L. (1970a). *Enzymol. Biol. Clin.* **11**, 162.

Hilf, R., Goldenberg, H., Michel, I., Orlando, R. A., and Archer, F. L. (1970b). *Cancer Res.* **30**, 1874.

Hilf, R., Wittliff, J. L., Rector, W. D., Savlov, E. D., Hall, T. C., and Orlando, R. A. (1973). *Cancer Res.* **33**, 2054.

James, F., Braunsberg, H., Irvine, W. T., and James, V. H. T. (1970). *Steroids* **15**, 669.

Jensen, E. V. (1960). *Proc. Int. Congr. Biochem. 4th, 1958* Vol. 15, 119.

Jensen, E. V., and DeSombre, E. R. (1972a). *In* "Biochemical Actions of Hormones" (G. Litwack, ed.), Vol. 2, pp. 215–255. Academic Press, New York.

Jensen, E. V., and DeSombre, E. R. (1972b). *Annu. Rev. Biochem.* **41**, 203.

Jensen, E. V., and Jacobson, H. I. (1960). *In* "Biological Activities of Steroids in Relation to Cancer" (G. Pincus and E. P. Vollmer, eds.), pp. 161–178. Academic Press, New York.

Jensen, E. V., and Jacobson, H. I. (1962). *Recent Progr. Horm. Res.* **18**, 387.

Jensen, E. V., DeSombre, E. R. and Jungblut, P. W. (1967). *In* "Endogenous Factors Influencing Host-Tumor Balance" (R. W. Wissler, T. L. Dao, and S. Wood, eds.), pp. 15–30. Univ. of Chicago Press, Chicago, Illinois.

Jensen, E. V., Suzuki, T., Kawashima, T., Stumph, W. E., Jungblut, P. W., and DeSombre, E. R. (1968). *Proc. Nat. Acad. Sci. U.S.* **59**, 632.

Jensen, E. V., Numata, M., Brecher, P. I., and DeSombre, E. R. (1971a). *In* "The Biochemistry of Steroid Hormone Action" (R. M. S. Smellie, ed.), p. 133. Academic Press, New York.

Jensen, E. V., Block, G. E., Smith, S., Kyser, K., and DeSombre, E. R. (1971b). *Nat. Cancer Inst., Monogr.* **34**, 55.

Jensen, E. V., Block, G. E., Smith, S., Kyser, K., and DeSombre, E. R. (1972). *In* "Estrogen Target Tissues and Neoplasia" (T. L. Dao, ed.), pp. 23–57. Univ. of Chicago Press, Chicago, Illinois.

Johansson, H., Terenius, L., and Thoren, L. (1970). *Cancer Res.* **30**, 692.

Juergens, W. G., Stockdale, F. E., Topper, Y. J., and Elias, J. J. (1965). *Proc. Nat. Acad. Sci. U.S.* **54**, 631.

Korenman, S. G., and Dukes, B. A. (1970). *J. Clin. Endocrinol. Metab.* **30**, 639.

Leung, B. S., Fletcher, W. S., Lindell, T. D., Wood, D. C., and Krippaehne, W. W. (1973). *Arch. Surg. (Chicago)* **106**, 515.

Maass, H., Engel, B., Hohmeister, H., Lehmann, F., and Trams, G. (1972). *Amer. J. Obstet. Gynecol.* **113,** 377.

McDivitt, R. W., Stewart, F. W., and Berg, J. W. (1968). *In* "Atlas of Tumor Pathology," No. 34, p. 000. Armed Forces Inst. Pathol. Washington, D.C.

McGuire, W. L. (1973). *J. Clin. Invest.* **52,** 73.

McGuire, W. L., and DeLaGarza, M. (1973). *J. Clin. Endocrinol. Metab.* **36,** 548.

Mohla, S., DeSombre, E. R., and Jensen, E. V. (1972). *Biochem. Biophys. Res. Commun.* **46,** 661.

Mueller, G. C. (1965). *In* "Mechanisms of Hormone Action" (P. Karlson, ed.), pp. 228–239. Academic Press, New York.

Oka, T., and Topper, Y. J. (1971). *J. Biol. Chem.* **246,** 7701.

Oka, T,. and Topper, Y. J. (1972). *J. Nat. Cancer Inst.* **48,** 1225.

Pearlman, W. H., DeHertogh, R., Laumas, K. R., and Pearlman, M. R. J. (1969). *J. Clin. Endocrinol. Metab.* **29,** 707.

Puca, G. A., and Bresciani, F. (1969). *Endocrinology* **85,** 1.

Richards, A. H., and Hilf, R. (1971). *Biochim. Biophys Acta* **232,** 753.

Richards, A. H., and Hilf, R. (1972). *Cancer Res.* **32,** 611.

Sander, S. (1968). *Acta Pathol. Microbiol. Scand.* **74,** 301.

Savlov, E. D., Wittliff, J. L., Hilf, R., and Hall, T. C. (1974). *Cancer* **33,** 303.

Shyamala, G. (1973). *Fed. Proc., Fed. Amer. Soc. Exp. Biol.* **32,** 453.

Shyamala, G., and Gorski, J. (1969). *J. Biol. Chem.* **244,** 1097.

Shyamala, G., and Nandi, S. (1972). *Endocrinology,* **91,** 861.

Smith, J. A., and King, R. J. B. (1970). *Cancer Res.* **30,** 2055.

Stancel, G. M., Leung, K. M. T., and Gorski, J. (1973). *Biochemistry* **12,** 2130.

Stoll, B. A. (1972). "Endocrine Therapy in Malignant Disease." Saunders, Philadelphia, Pennsylvania.

Talwar, G. P., Segal, S. J., Evans, A., and Davidson, O. W. (1964). *Proc. Nat. Acad. Sci. U.S.* **52,** 1059.

Toft, D., and Gorski, J. (1966). *Proc. Nat. Acad. Sci. U.S.* **55,** 1574.

Tucker, H., Larson, B., and Gorski, J. (1971). *Endocrinology* **89,** 152.

Willcox, P. A., and Thomas, G. H. (1972). *Brit. J. Cancer* **26,** 453.

Williams-Ashman, H. G., and Reddi, A. H. (1971). *Ann. Rev. Physiol.* **33,** 31.

Wittliff, J. L., (1974). Seminars in Onocology (in press).

Wittliff, J. L., Hilf, R., and Brooks, W. F., Jr. (1971). *Proc. Amer. Ass. Cancer Res.* **12,** 47.

Wittliff, J. L., Gardner, D. G., Battema, W. L., and Gilbert, P. J. (1972a). *Biochem. Biophys. Res. Commun.* **48,** 119.

Wittliff, J. L., Hilf, R., Brooks, W. F., Jr., Savlov, E. D., Hall, T. C., and Orlando, R. A. (1972b). *Cancer Res.* **32,** 1983.

CHAPTER V

DEFECTS OF ANION AND ELECTRON TRANSPORT IN MORRIS HEPATOMA MITOCHONDRIA

KATHRYN F. LANOUE, JOHN G. HEMINGTON, TOMOKO OHNISHI, HAROLD P. MORRIS, and JOHN R. WILLIAMSON

I. Introduction and Background

By far the most remarkable and consistent metabolic abnormality of neoplastic tissue is the high glycolytic rate observed under aerobic conditions. Since the glycolytic rate apparently exceeds the capacity of the tissue to oxidize the reducing equivalents formed during glycolysis, lactic acid accumulates. Different tumors vary enormously in their rates of formation of lactic acid under aerobic and anaerobic conditions (Aisenberg, 1961a). An overlap is seen in fact between the normal and the neoplastic tissue in this regard. It has been stated that the fastest growing, most malignant tumors have the highest rates of aerobic glycolysis (i.e., aerobic production of lactic acid) (Weber, 1972). However, the cause and functional significance of this finding have remained obscure. On a purely logical basis, the production of excess lactate could be due to (a) glycolytic rates exceeding the oxidative capacity of the mitochondria for pyruvate or to (b) ineffective mechanisms for reoxidation of NADH generated during glycolysis by the mitochondrial electron transport chain.

We have chosen to examine this problem by comparing a series of Morris hepatomas of different growth rates with normal liver. The normoxic or resting rate of oxygen utilization in a perfused rat liver is 250 μatoms/gm wet wt/hour (Scholz and Bücher, 1965). Rat liver slices give about the same rate of oxygen utilization (i.e., Q_{O_2} = 6–12 μl/mg dry weight/hour) (Burk, 1939). If all the oxygen consumption of the liver was utilized for glucose oxidation, the normal rat liver could oxidize a maximum of 20 μmoles of glucose or 40 μmoles of lactate/gm wet weight/hour. Data are available from studies of the utilization of glucose in hepatoma slices (Sweeney *et al.*, 1963), indicating that that rate of aerobic lactate production varies from 14 to 66 μmoles/gm wet weight/hour, apparently depending on the growth rate of the tumor, while the aerobic production of lactate in normal liver slices varies from 2 to 18 μmoles/gm wet weight hour (Ashmore *et al.*, 1958; Sweeney *et al.*, 1963), depending on the composition of the incubation media and the nutritional state of the rats. When [6-^{14}C]glucose was used as the substrate for slices, Ashmore *et al.* (1958) found that the glucose oxidation rates (rate of production of $^{14}CO_2$) were similar but low in liver and heptaoma (1–3 μmoles lactate equivalents/gm wet weight/hour), by no means straining the oxidative capacity of either tissue. The oxidation rate (3.3 μmoles lactate equivalents/gm wet weight/hour) of the liver slice compared well with its production of [^{14}C]lactate (6.0 μmoles/gm wet weight/hour). However, the production of [^{14}C]lactate in Novikoff hepatomas was 31.8 μmoles/gm wet weight/hour, and the oxidation rate was only 1.14 μmole lactate/gm wet weight/hour. This work was confirmed and expanded to a series of Morris hepatomas in a later paper (Sweeney *et al.*, 1963). Thus, in some instances the glycolytic rates observed in tumor slices exceed the oxidative capacity of normally functioning mitochondria, but even in the face of high glycolytic rates, only a very small proportion of the oxidized substrate comes from glucose. Glycolytic rates are low in the liver because of the presence of gluconeogenic enzymes. When reducing equivalents are generated in the liver cytosol via other pathways [*e.g.*, the oxidation of alcohol (Williamson *et al.*, 1969b), xylitol (Williamson *et al.*, 1971), glycerol, or sorbitol (Berry *et al.*, 1973)], rates of utilization of the generated NADH are high, approaching 108 μmoles/gm wet weight/hour (Berry *et al.*, 1973). Hepatomas lack the gluconeogenic enzymes and, therefore, are rather more like heart or skeletal muscle tissue in their enzyme pattern. Perfused rat hearts have high glycolytic rates and about 80% of the glucose utilized goes to CO_2 (Safer and Williamson, 1973).

The apparent inability of tumor tissue to respond to the high levels of cytosol-generated reducing equivalents may be due to ineffective mechanisms for the removal of cytoplasmic-reducing equivalents related to abnormalities of anion transport across the mitochondrial membrane or deficiencies of mitochondrial content and electron transport. Since NADH produced in the cytoplasm does not penetrate liver (Lehninger, 1951; Purvis and Lowenstein, 1961) or hepatoma (Boxer and Devlin, 1961) mitochondria directly, reducing equivalents must be carried from extramitochondrial NADH to the intramitochondrial electron transport chain by indirect routes, or "shuttle mechanisms." Two such mechanisms which have been studied extensively are the malate–aspartate cycle (Borst, 1963) and the α-glycerophosphate cycle (Bücher and Klingenberg, 1958). These are illustrated in Fig. 1. The α-glycerophosphate cycle requires the presence in the cytoplasm of an NAD-linked α-glycerophosphate dehydrogenase and the presence of a flavin-linked α-glycerophosphate dehydrogenase in the mitochondria. The malate–aspartate cycle requires the activity of cytoplasmic and mitochondrial malate dehydrogenase and glutamate oxalacetate transaminase and the operation of specific transport mechanisms (Chappell, 1968) across the mitochondrial membrane allowing

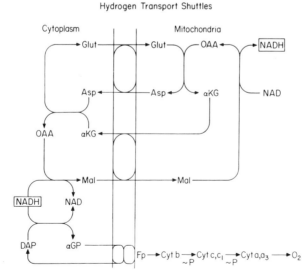

Fig. 1. Shuttle mechanisms for the transport of reducing equivalents across the mitochondrial membrane. Abbreviation used: Glut, glutamate; OAA, oxalacetate; Asp, aspartate; NAD and NADH, nicotinamide adenine dinucleotide (oxidized and reduced forms, respectively); αKG, α-ketoglutarate; Mal, malate; DAP, dihydroxyacetone phosphate; αGP, $_a$-glycerophosphate; Fp, flavoprotein; $\sim$P, high energy phosphate bond.

influx of glutamate and malate and efflux of α-ketoglutarate and aspartate. In recent years emphasis has been placed on the dominant role of the malate–aspartate cycle in transporting cytoplasmic reducing equivalents to the mitochondrial electron transport chain in liver (Anderson *et al.*, 1971; Ylikahri *et al.*, 1971), heart (Safer *et al.*, 1971), and kidney (Rognstad and Katz, 1970).

Studies carried out several years ago which attempted to evaluate the capacity of neoplastic tissue to carry out these "shuttle mechanisms" (Boxer Devlin, 1961) did not include the functioning of the malate–aspartate cycle. A report by Gordon *et al.*, (1967), however, indicates that by using menadione (vitamin K_3) to provide an artificial transfer of electrons from the cytoplasm directly to the mitochondrial respiratory chain, oxidation rates of ascites cells could be increased, and aerobic lactic acid accumulation substantially reduced. The inference is that the endogenous "H-shuttle" is rate-limiting. However, since menadione enters the electron transport chain at a point beyond the first phosphorylation site, any limitation in the ascites cells of electron transport in the region of the first phosphorylation site might be rate-limiting rather than the "H-shuttle" mechanism itself.

Most studies of tumor mitochondria have indicated that they are similar in many respects, although not identical to the mitochondria of the tissue of origin (Aisenberg, 1961b; Mehard *et al.*, 1971; Pedersen *et al.*, 1970). One recent series of papers has indicated a possible abnormality of glutamate metabolism which correlated with the growth rate of the tumors (Kovacevic, 1971, 1972; Kovacevic and Morris, 1972). Thus, it is appropriate to study the energy metabolism of a series of hepatomas of different growth rates with special emphasis placed on possible differences between hepatoma and liver mitochondria in the functioning of the malate–aspartate cycle and the electron transport chain.

II. Methods

A. *Source of Hepatomas*

Buffalo strain rats either with (host) or without (control) tumors implanted subcutaneously and intramuscularly in the hind limb were shipped by Dr. H. P. Morris to Philadelphia by air. The animals were maintained on food and water *ad libitum* and housed in the university vivarium. Rats bearing tumors 7777 (fast growth rate), 7800 and 7794A (intermediate growth rate), and 16 (slow growth rate) were sacrificed at an average of 25, 35, 40, and 135 days, respectively, from the time of implantation of the hepatomas. At these times the tumors were usually 2–3 cm in diameter and relatively free of hemorrhagic areas. The biology and growth characteristics of these and other Morris hepatomas have been described previously (Morris and Wagner, 1968; Nowell *et al.*, 1967).

B. Preparation of Mitochondria

Livers and tumors were removed and disected free of fat and extraneous tissue. Hemorrhagic and necrotic areas in the tumors were carefully removed. All tumor, host liver, and control liver mitochondria were isolated by a modification of the method of Pedersen *et al.* (1970). The isolation medium contained 2 mM morpholinopropane sulfonic acid (MOPS), EDTA (0.5–5 mM) and fraction V bovine serum albumin (0.5 gm/liter) defatted by the method of Chen (1967). The minced tissue was homogenized in 2–3 volumes of the isolation medium with a Polytron PT 10, rather than a Potter-Elvehjem tissue grinder.

C. Incubation Conditions

Incubations were carried out at 28°C in a buffer media containing 150 mM KCl, 20 mM Tris-Cl, 10 mM phosphate-Tris, 0.1 mM EDTA, 5 mM MgCl$_2$, and 30 mM glucose (pH 7.2). When intramitochondrial concentrations of metabolites were required, the silicone oil method for rapid separation of mitochondria from the incubation medium was used and dextran (MW 40,000) was included in the buffer mixture (LaNoue *et al.*, 1972). Various metabolic states are specified in the text. They are defined as follows: *State 4*, no additions to buffer other than substrate and 1–4 mg mitochondrial protein; *state 3*, additions to the basic buffer system include substrate, 100 μM ADP, 8 units of hexokinase (Type F-300, Sigma Chemical Company), and 1–4 mg of mitochondrial protein; *Uncoupled*, additions to the buffer system include substrate, 0.2–0.3 nmoles/mg protein of *p*-trifluoromethoxyphenylhydrazone of carbonylcyanide (FCCP), and 1–4 mg of mitochondrial protein. Measurements of oxygen utilization in these metabolic states were made polarographically using a Clark oxygen electrode.

D. Metabolite and Enzyme Assays

Citric acid cycle intermediates, glutamate, aspartate, NADH, and NADPH were assayed as described by Williamson and Corkey (1969). Phosphate levels were measured by the method of Wahler and Wollenberger (1958). Malate dehydrogenase (MDH), glutamate oxalacetate transaminase (GOT), and glutamate dehydrogenase (GDH) were assayed according to Pette (1965). Cytochrome a + a$_3$ was assayed in

50 mM phosphate buffer (pH 7.0) containing 50 mM reduced cytochrome c. The rate of oxidation of cytochrome c upon addition of mitochondrial protein (0.1 to 1.0 mg) was monitored at 550 nm with a Zeiss spectrophotometer.

E. Additional Methods

Electron paramagnetic resonance spectra were performed on a Varian model E-4 spectrophotometer. After addition of 20 mM glutamate plus 1 mM malate, samples of mitochondria were transferred to 3 mm inner diameter quartz EPR tubes, incubated for 5 minutes at room temperature, and rapidly frozen by immersion in liquid isopentane at 113°K. Sample temperatures below 77°K were obtained by cooling in a stream of helium gas. Temperatures were monitored with an Au/Co versus Pt thermocouple (Ohnishi *et al.,* 1971).

Mitochondrial levels of Ca^{2+} and Mg^{2+} were measured according to the method of Pybus (1968). The "reconstituted shuttle" used to evaluate the malate–aspartate cycle in mitochondria was adapted from previously published methods (LaNoue and Williamson, 1971; Robinson and Halperin, 1970). The techniques and interpretation of mitochondrial swelling studies essentially follow those of Chappell (1968).

III.   Results

A. Measurement of Respiration Rates of Hepatoma Mitochondria

Rates of oxygen utilization by Morris hepatoma mitochondria were measured using a variety of substrates, and these were compared with the rates obtained with host liver mitochondria. Since respiratory rates of mitochondrial preparations from livers of host rats with different tumors showed no significant differences, these values were pooled and compared with values obtained from liver mitochondria of normal rats. Again, no significant differences were observed as reported in Table I. It can be seen from Table I that rates of ascorbate plus tetramethylphenylenediamine (TMPD) oxidation by tumor mitochondria appeared normal except for hepatoma 7777. This indicates that the electron transport chain is normal in the region from cytochrome c to cytochrome oxidase, and that no large errors have been incurred due to the inclusion of oxidatively inert protein with the possible exception of tumor 7777. State 3 (Chance and Williams, 1955) is the metabolic state which includes buffer, substrate, phosphate, and phosphate acceptor (ADP). Mitochondria normally respire actively in this state and produce ATP. State 4 (Chance and Williams, 1955) lacks phosphate ac-

TABLE I

Respiration Rates of Morris Hepatoma and Host Liver Mitochondria[a]

Preparation	Glutamate-malate			Succinate-rotenone			Ascorbate–TMPD uncoupled
	State 3	State 4	Uncoupled	State 3	State 4	Uncoupled	
Control liver	(4) 78.7 ± 4.6	10.2 ± 0.6	124.3 ± 7.1	(4) 102.5 ± 5.4	16.5 ± 1.5	149.3 ± 7.0	(4) 164.5 ± 3.4
Host liver	(41) 88.4 ± 2.6	12.9 ± 0.8	123.4 ± 4.1	(25) 117.4 ± 3.6	24.5 ± 1.4	164.7 ± 4.1	(25) 166.2 ± 3.1
Tumor 7777	(12) 47.9 ± 7.1	11.1 ± 1.7	76.9 ± 7.6	(7) 38.5 ± 6.0	14.3 ± 1.6	58.0 ± 9.2	(5) 83.5 ± 10.4
Tumor 7800	(13) 78.3 ± 4.2	11.4 ± 0.9	109.3 ± 6.0	(7) 99.1 ± 7.0	26.2 ± 3.4	119.0 ± 9.2	(5) 180.7 ± 9.0
Tumor 7794A	(7) 41.7 ± 3.0	12.9 ± 1.9	73.9 ± 4.5	(4) 67.8 ± 4.0	23.0 ± 4.1	112.5 ± 8.4	—
Tumor 16	(12) 38.3 ± 1.8	8.6 ± 0.4	51.9 ± 2.5	(10) 83.0 ± 2.1	23.3 ± 1.8	108.4 ± 4.4	(8) 144.1 ± 13.5

[a] Reaction conditions are described in Section II. Mitochondrial protein was 1 to 2 mg/ml reaction media. Substrate concentrations were 12.5 mM glutamate, 5 mM malate, 10 mM succinate plus 5 μM rotenone, and 2 mM ascorbate plus 0.9 mM tetramethylphenylene diamine (TMPD). Values are means ± standard error, and number of determinations are shown in parentheses. Values are expressed in nanoatoms O/min·mg.

ceptor and is normally associated with very low respiratory rates. The ratio of the respiratory rate in state 3 to that in state 4 (respiratory control ratio) is frequently used as a measure of the integrity and intactness of the mitochondrial membranes. When mitochondrial membranes are damaged or the mitochondria are uncoupled, state 4 rates are increased. The data in Table I indicate that state 4 rates are not increased in the hepatoma mitochondria. This would imply that the mechanisms of energy coupling are unaffected although state 3 rates are somewhat low, particularly with glutamate–malate as substrate.

The different tumors exhibit several patterns of inhibited respiration. Electrons from the three substrates used to test the mitochondria enter the electron transport chain at the sites indicated in Fig. 2. Figure 2 is a diagram of the electron transport chain as currently conceived (Ohnishi, 1973), including the many different iron–sulfur proteins which can be identified by modern techniques of electron paramagnetic resonance spectroscopy. Table I shows that mitochondria from tumor 7777 respire rather slowly in state 3 and in the uncoupled state irrespective of the site of entry of electrons along the electron chain. Much lower rates with NAD-linked substrates were obtained if the mitochondria from tumor 7777 were not prepared in the presence of high (2 mM) concentrations of EDTA. Addition of NAD to tumor 7777 mitochondria increased respiratory rates of NAD-linked

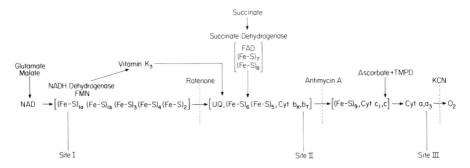

Fig. 2. Scheme for sequence of respiratory chain components, energy coupling sites, reaction sites of respiratory inhibitors, and points of entry of various substrates. Iron–sulfur centers (Fe–S) are numbered for identification. The $(Fe–S)_{1 \leftleftarrows 4}$ and $(Fe–S)_{1a,1b,5}$ in the NADH dehydrogenase region are designated according to Orme-Johnson *et al.* (1971) and Ohnishi *et al.* (1972), respectively. $(Fe–S)_7$ and $(Fe–S)_8$ are iron–sulfur centers associated with the succinate dehydrogenase; the $(Fe–S)_7$ signals are detectable at 77°K (Beinert *et al.*, 1962), while the $(Fe–S)_8$ signals are detectable only below 30°K (Ohnishi, 1973). $(Fe–S)_6$ is a newly identified iron–sulfur center with the half-reduction potential around 0 mV (Ohnishi, 1973), and $(Fe–S)_9$ is that originally reported by Rieske *et al.* (1964).

substrates only if the mitochondria were prepared with low (0.1 mM) concentrations of EDTA.

Tumor 7800, also a rather rapidly growing tumor, oxidized all the substrates tested at normal rates. On the other hand, tumors 7794A and 16 oxidized glutamate relatively poorly. Succinate respiration was also inhibited, but to a smaller extent. Although not shown in Table I, rates of respiration with 2 mM pyruvate plus 1 mM malate or 2 mM α-ketoglutarate in tumor 16 were 80% of the rates obtained with host liver mitochondria. However, although the degree of respiratory inhibition was less with these substrates, the rates of oxygen uptake (35 to 39 natoms/min · mg) in state 3 were no greater than the rates obtained with glutamate–malate as substrate.

The apparently greater degree of inhibition of glutamate respiration is of particular interest in the study of tumor metabolism since transport of glutamate across the mitochondrial membrane and transamination to aspartate are involved in the transport of reducing equivalents from the cytosol to the intramitochondrial electron transport chain. For this reason the inhibition of glutamate respiration was examined in more detail. Since the apparent K_m of glutamate for respiration by rat liver mitochondria (Kovacevic and Morris, 1972), i.e. 1 mM is of the same order of magnitude as the tissue glutamate concentration (Weber *et al.,* 1971; Williamson *et al.,* 1969a) it seemed appropriate to examine the rates of respiration of the tumor mitochondria as a function of the concentration of glutamate. The results of these studies are shown in Table II. A typical set of titration data comparing tumor 7777 and 7794A with host liver are shown in Fig. 3. The results of this study show that the apparent K_m for glutamate was increased 3-fold in tumor 7777 but was unchanged in the other tumors. On the other hand, the V_{max} of respiration was low in all tumors studied except tumor 7800. The V_{max}'s reported in Table II are lower than the corresponding respiration rates reported in Table I because the kinetic data were obtained in the presence of glutamate without malate and endogenous respiration was subtracted from the observed rates. The discrepancies are smaller in the case of the tumors because malate did not stimulate the respiration of tumor mitochondria in the presence of glutamate.

B. Pyridine Nucleotide Redox Ratios

In order to gain some insight into the cause of the slow rates of glutamate respiration, the state of reduction of the pyridine nucleotides was estimated by measuring enzymatically the levels of the reduced pyridine nucleotides in state 3, state 4, and the rotenone inhibited or fully reduced state. The level of NADH in the rotenone inhibited state is approximately

TABLE II

Kinetic Parameters of Glutamate Oxidation in a
Series of Hepatomas[a]

Preparation	K_m	V_{max}
	(mM)	(natoms O/min·mg)
Host liver	0.49 ± 0.06	50.3 ± 4.6
Tumor 7777	1.50 ± 0.17	38.5 ± 8.0
Tumor 7800	0.57 ± 0.04	56.8 ± 9.9
Tumor 7794A	0.27 ± 0.05	37.2 ± 5.0
Tumor 16	0.47 ± 0.05	35.1 ± 8.5

[a] State 3 conditions were used and are described in Section II. A mitochondrial protein of 1 to 2 mg/ml of incubation media was used. Glutamate concentrations were varied and no malate was added. Values are means ± standard error of at least 4 determinations.

equal to the level of the total reducible pyridine nucleotide pool of the mitochondria so that NADH/NAD ratios can readily be calculated. Values for the NADH levels and the calculated NADH/NAD ratios are given in Table III. The total pyridine nucleotide content of tumor 7777 was low in comparison with other mitochondrial preparations, while all other tumors had a higher content than the host liver mitochondria. The NADH/NAD ratio is state 3 was higher with mitochondria from tumors 7794A and 16 than the host liver mitochondria despite an inhibited respiratory rate, suggesting that the rate-limiting step cannot be glutamate entry into the

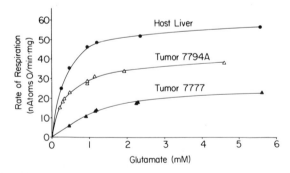

Fig. 3. The effect of glutamate concentration on respiration of hepatoma mitochondria and host liver mitochondria. Reaction conditions are described in the footnote to Table II.

mitochondria. The data imply an inhibition of the electron transport chain or possibly of some step in the entry or utilization of ADP and phosphate to produce state 3 respiration.

C. Adenosine Triphosphatase Activity

Low activity of uncoupler-stimulated mitochondrial adenosine triphosphatase (ATPase) in tumor mitochondria has been observed in several laboratories (Pedersen *et al.,* 1971). If this ATPase were inhibited in the direction of ATP synthesis, a reduced state of the pyridine nucleotides would be expected. Likewise, a positive correlation among the activity of the ATPase, rates of respiration, and the degree of oxidation of the nucleotide pool might be expected. Consequently, ATPase activity was measured by the release of phosphate from ATP in the presence of high concentrations of FCCP. Tumor mitochondria were compared with the host mitochondria. The results are shown in Fig. 4. Simultaneous measurements (not shown) of intramitochondrial phosphate levels indicated that there was no inhibition per se of phosphate transport out of the mitochondria in the tumors. Since uncoupler stimulated ATPase activity was virtually absent in mitochondria from tumor 7800, which exhibit normal respiration rates and low state 3 NADH levels, it was concluded that the phosphate transferring function of the ATPase in the direction of ATP synthesis was unlikely to be responsible for the inhibition of state 3 respiration in tumors 16 and 7794A.

TABLE III

Redox State of Host Liver and Tumor Mitochondria in State 3 and State 4 with Glutamate and Malate as Substrates[a]

	State 3		State 4		
Preparation	NADH (nmoles/mg)	$\dfrac{\text{NADH}}{\text{NAD}^+}$	NADH (nmoles/mg)	$\dfrac{\text{NADH}}{\text{NAD}^+}$	Rotenone NADH (nmoles/mg)
Host liver	0.81 ± 0.05	0.68	1.85 ± 0.08	11.6	2.01 ± 0.13
Tumor 7777	0.36 ± 0.06	0.49	0.78 ± 0.05	2.52	1.09 ± 0.02
Tumor 7800	0.64 ± 0.04	0.28	2.11 ± 0.04	2.57	2.93 ± 0.03
Tumor 7794A	2.01 ± 0.05	1.02	3.17 ± 0.04	3.87	3.99 ± 0.05
Tumor 16	1.83 ± 0.06	0.99	2.70 ± 0.03	2.76	3.68 ± 0.06

[a] State 3 and state 4 conditions are described in Section II. A mitochondrial protein of 2 mg/ml of incubation media was used. Glutamate (12.5 mM) and malate (1.0 mM) were used as substrates. Rotenone when added was 2.5 μM. Incubation times were 1 minute.

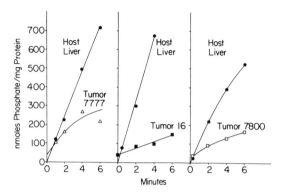

Fig. 4. Activity of uncoupler(FCCP)-stimulated ATPase in hepatoma mitochondria and host liver mitochondria. Mitochondria (5–6 mg/ml) were incubated in phosphate-free buffer mixture (cf. Methods, Section II) containing 8% dextran, 10 mM ATP, and 0.67 μM FCCP in a total volume of 3 ml. Samples (0.5 ml) were taken for phosphate determination at 0, 1, 2, 4, and 6 minutes.

D. Iron–Sulfur Proteins in Tumor Mitochondria

Although several studies have shown that the cytochrome contents of tumor mitochondria are in the normal range (Chance and Hess, 1959; Mehard *et al.,* 1971; Pedersen, 1972), we know of no previous attempts to measure iron–sulfur proteins in tumor mitochondria. Many iron–sulfur proteins are involved in the transport of electrons from substrates to oxygen. A large number of these iron–sulfur centers have recently been detected in mammalian, avian, and yeast mitochondria by Orme-Johnson *et al.* (1971) and Ohnishi and co-workers (1972; Ohnishi, 1973), using electron paramagnetic resonance (EPR) techniques at temperatures between that of liquid nitrogen (77°K) and liquid helium (4.2°K). This low temperature EPR technique offers a specific and sensitive tool for the study of individual iron–sulfur centers in the respiratory chain. As shown in Fig. 2, five iron–sulfur centers (one iron–sulfur center is probably composed of two or four atoms of iron and acid labile sulfide) have been shown on the substrate side of the rotenone inhibition site and five on the oxygen side (Ohnishi *et al.,* 1972). In spite of many overlapped EPR signals appearing in a narrow range of magnetic field, different species of EPR signals can be measured separately in mitochondrial preparations because of their different temperature and power dependence and half-reduction potentials. The role of these iron-sulfur centers as the electron carries in the respiratory chain has been suggested from kinetic studies of their redox reactions (Beinert and Palmer, 1965) and from an observed close relationship between the maximum rate of electron transfer and relative intensities of EPR signals arising from iron–sulfur proteins in the different dehydrogenases, using various yeast systems (Ohnishi *et al.,* 1971). Peak positions and line shape of these signals from liver and tumor mitochondria and their temperature and power dependence were very similar to those previously obtained with corresponding iron–sulfur centers in pigeon heart or *Candida utilis* mitochondria.

Figure 5 shows typical EPR spectra of reduced iron–sulfur centers in

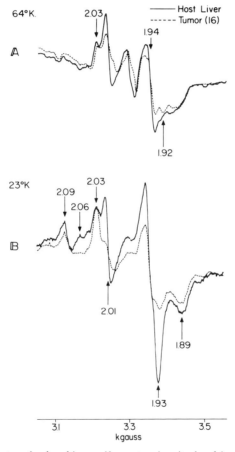

Fig. 5. EPR spectra of reduced iron–sulfur centers in mitochondria prepared from Morris hepatoma 16 and from host liver, measured at 64° and 23°K. Mitochondrial suspensions were brought to anaerobiosis in EPR tubes by incubation with 8.3 m*M* glutamate plus 8.3 m*M* malate for 10 minutes at room temperature. Protein concentration of both preparations was 60 mg/ml. EPR operating conditions were modulation frequency, 100 kHz; modulation amplitude, 12.5 G; microwave power, 50 mW; microwave frequency, 9.113 GHz; time constant, 0.3 seconds; scan time, 500 G/minute.

mitochondria prepared from the slow growing tumor 16 and its host liver. As seen in spectra A (taken at 64°K) iron–sulfur center 1 (g = 2.03 and 1.94), center 7 (g = 2.03, 1.94 and 1.92), and center 9 (g = 1.90; described by Rieske *et al.,* 1964) are all clearly visible in the host liver mitochondria. As seen also in spectrum A, the "g = 1.94" peak to peak amplitude of mitochondria from tumor 16 showed a 30% decrease with respect to host liver mitochondria which was considered largely due to the decrease of center 1 because the "g = 1.92" peak, which is mostly from center 7 at this temperature, showed only a very slight decrease.

At a lower temperature (23°K) signals from iron–sulfur center 2 (g = 2.06 and 1.93) and center 5 (g = 2.09 and 1.89) were obtained as shown in spectrum B of Fig. 5. The center 2 signals of tumor 16 are diminished drastically with respect to the host liver. Although spectra are not presented here, EPR signals arising from iron–sulfur centers 3 and 4 also showed a diminished intensity in the tumor mitochondria.

In contrast to iron–sulfur centers 1, 2, 3, and 4, EPR signals due to centers 7, 9, and 5 showed a relatively smaller decrease of intensity in the tumor mitochondria. These results show that the centers associated with the NADH dehydrogenase region of the respiratory chain are specifically diminished. This was reflected in the decreased respiratory rate of NAD-linked substrate oxidation in hepatoma 16 mitochondria, while little decrease occurred in the succinate or ascorbate plus TMPD oxidation rate.

Spectra A and B in Fig. 6 show that the intensity of all the EPR signals from tumor 7800 are very similar to those of the host liver. This result correlates well with the observation that respiratory rates of tumor 7800 mitochondria were normal.

In Fig. 7 typical EPR spectra of the iron–sulfur centers in mitochondria from the rapidly growing tumor 7777 are presented. In spectrum A, EPR signals from center 6 (g = 2.11 and 1.90), center 5 (g = 1.50), and center 9 (g = 1.90) in addition to "g = 1.94 signals" from centers 1 and 7 are apparent in host liver mitochondria. All these signals show diminished intensity in the fast growing tumor 7777 mitochondria. At a lower temperature, center 1, 2, and 5 signals were obtained as in spectrum B, Fig. 7. All the observed EPR signals showed similarly decreased intensity in rapidly growing tumor 7777 mitochondria.

The decrease of the parmagnetic signals from iron–sulfur centers in the tumor mitochondria correlates very well with the observed respiratory deficiencies and also with reduced state of the pyridine nucleotides in the case of tumor 16. The situation with tumor 7777 is obviously different. These mitochondria had a very different appearance from normal liver mitochondria. They formed a much less tightly packed pellet than mitochondria from normal liver and were also lighter in color.

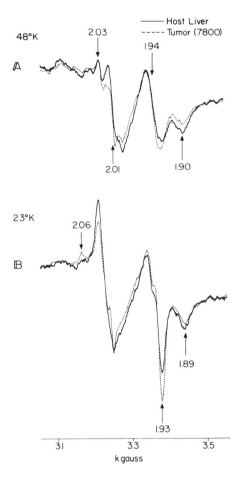

Fig. 6. EPR spectra of reduced iron–sulfur centers in mitochondria prepared from Morris hepatoma 7800 and host liver, measured at 48° and 23°K. Mitochondria used in this experiment were stored frozen in liquid nitrogen and thawed prior to the preparation of samples for EPR measurement. Anaerobiosis was obtained by incubating frozen and thawed mitochondrial suspensions with 8.3 mM glutamate plus 8.3 mM malate and 3.3 mM NADH. The protein concentration of both hepatoma 7800 and host liver mitochondria was 50.0 mg/ml. EPR operating conditions were the same as described in the legend of Fig. 5.

E. Endogenous Ca^{2+} and Mg^{2+} Levels

Previous studies (van Rossum *et al.*, 1971) have shown that Ca^{2+} levels in tumor tissue are abnormally high compared to the tissues from which the tumors are derived. The reason for the high levels of intracellular Ca^{2+} is not known, but is presumably related to a deficiency of energy-linked Ca^{2+}

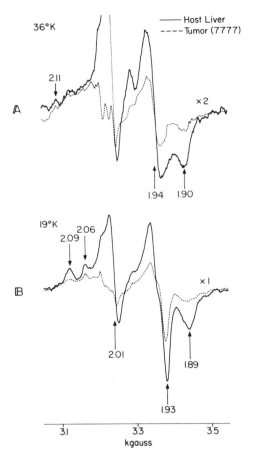

Fig. 7. EPR spectra of reduced iron–sulfur centers in mitochondria prepared from Morris hepatoma 7777 and host liver, measured at 36° and 19°K. Protein concentrations of tumor and host liver mitochondria were 62.5 mg/ml and 65 mg/ml, respectively. EPR operating conditions are the same as in Fig. 5.

efflux from the cell. This in turn may be related to abnormal functioning of the Na^+–K^+ ATPase of the cell membrane. An energy deficiency for ion pumping may be involved since ATP levels of Morris hepatomas freeze-clamped *in situ* (Weber *et al.*, 1971) have been found to be considerably lower than those of normal, freeze-clamped liver.

Table IV shows the measured levels of Ca^{2+} and Mg^{2+} in the mitochondria as isolated. Tumor 7777 was isolated in 2 mM EDTA. All other mitochondria were isolated in 100 μM EDTA. The table clearly shows that although all tumor mitochondria had abnormally high Ca^{2+} levels, these levels were an order of magnitude higher in tumor 7777. The Mg^{2+} content, on the other hand, was relatively constant.

Previous studies have indicated that mitochondria isolated from neoplastic tissue are low in pyridine nucleotide and required supplementation with added NAD (Aisenberg, 1961a). Interactions between Ca^{2+} and pyridine nucleotides in the mitochondrial membrane have been explored in a recent paper (Vinogradov et al., 1972). It was found that the accumulation of large amounts of Ca^+ in mitochondria caused a depression of respiration with NAD^+-linked substrates. The inhibition of respiration was accompanied by a depletion of endogenous pyridine nucleotides. The effects were not related to mitochondrial swelling and were attributable in part to the formation of a Ca^{2+}–NADH complex in the membrane. It is possible, therefore, that the abnormally low total pyridine nucleotide content and possibly other altered functions of mitochondria isolated from tumor 7777 are not intrinsic properties of the mitochondria in situ, but reflect damage to the mitochondria during isolation as a result of the abnormally high Ca^{2+} content of the tumor. Isolation of the mitochondria in medium containing high EDTA concentrations certainly provided some protection and yielded mitochondria with coupled respiration, but the high Ca^{2+} content of these mitochondria suggests that the protection by EDTA was not complete.

F. Measurements of NADH Utilization in a "Reconstituted Shuttle" System

The studies outlined above, which were designed to characterize and evaluate the basic properties of the tumor mitochondria, revealed abnor-

TABLE IV

Calcium and Magnesium Content of Tumor Mitochondria[a]

Preparation	No. of determinations	Ca^{2+}	Mg^{2+}
Host Liver	27	4.45 ± 0.26	26.8 ± 0.77
Tumor 7777	6	99.8 ± 23.6	21.5 ± 3.1
Tumor 7800	5	15.3 ± 2.4	28.7 ± 3.0
Tumor 16	9	14.8 ± 2.3	28.6 ± 2.0

[a] Ca^{2+} and Mg^{2+} Levels were measured with a Varian Techtron atomic absorption spectrophotometer. Strontium Cl (15 mM) was included in all Ca^{2+} samples to prevent interference from phosphate. Values expressed in nanomoles per milligram.

malities in their rates of glutamate respiration, contents of iron–sulfur proteins, ATPase activities, and Ca^{2+} content. These abnormalities do not appear to be related in a very strict way to growth rates. In order to evaluate whether a defect also exists in the pathway of NADH transfer to the mitochondria via the malate–aspartate cycle, use was made of a "reconstituted shuttle" system (LaNoue and Williamson, 1971).

The rate of oxidation of NADH was observed directly by disappearance of NADH fluorescence from a reaction mixture containing buffer (cf. Methods, Section II), isolated mitochondria, malate dehydrogenase, glutamate oxalacetate transaminase, ADP, NADH, aspartate, glutamate, and malate. Both glutamate and malate were varied to obtain operational apparent Michaelis constants. Figure 8 is an illustration of the traces obtained using rat liver mitochondria. The complete shuttle system (trace A) is defined in the legend. As shown in the figure, the reaction is initiated by the addition of mitochondria to the cuvette containing the other shuttle components. Trace C shows that the rate of NADH oxidation without added malate dehydrogenase and glutamate oxalacetate transaminase is very slow. Trace B, the rate without glutamate, is greater than trace C because of the production of α-ketoglutarate from endogenous substrates. Data of this type were obtained for all tumors studied and for their host livers. Mitochondria from livers of control rats of the Buffalo strain were indistinguishable in this system from host liver mitochondria.

Figure 9 illustrates in representative titrations the effect of glutamate concentration on the rate of oxidation of exogenous NADH. It is apparent

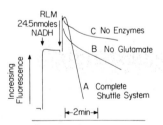

Fig. 8. Fluorometric traces of oxidation of exogenous NADH by liver mitochondria via a reconstituted malate–aspartate shuttle. Trace A: incubation media (2.0 ml) included the standard buffer mixture (cf. Methods, Section II), dialyzed glutamate oxalacetate transaminase (6 units/ml), dialyzed malate dehydrogenase (6 units/ml), 2 mM ADP, 2 mM aspartate, 5 mM glutamate, and 1 mM malate. At the times indicated, 24.5 nmoles of NADH was added followed by liver mitochondria (0.69 mg protein). Trace B: glutamate was omitted from the reaction media. Trace C: glutamate oxalacetate transaminase and malate dehydrogenase were omitted from the reaction media.

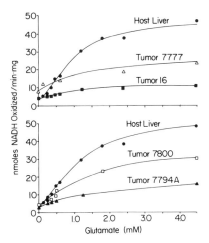

Fig. 9. The effect of glutamate concentration on the rate of oxidation of exogenous NADH via a reconstituted malate–aspartate shuttle. Conditions were the same as described in Fig. 8, trace A, with the exception that glutamate concentrations were varied as shown. Mitochondrial protein varied from 0.5 to 1.0 mg/ml.

that maximal shuttle flux is much lower in the tumors. As one would expect, the tumors 16 and 7794A with the slowest rates of oxidation of glutamate were the ones with the slowest shuttle fluxes. However, tumor 7800 which had a normal respiratory rate with glutamate and malate as substrate was less active than host liver mitochondria in oxidizing NADH by the reconstituted shuttle. Double reciprocal plots of the data showed that the K_m for glutamate was similar for host and tumor mitochondrial preparations (0.5 to 1 mM) except for tumor 7777 which was 3- to 4-fold higher (Table V). The major difference between the tumor and host liver mitochondria resides in the maximal rates attainable at high concentrations of glutamate.

The effect of malate concentration was studied in a similar manner. The results are shown in Fig. 10. As in Fig. 9, there is a significant flux when no substrate is added. This is due to the endogenous malate in the mitochondrial preparations. The Michaelis constants and V_{max}'s for the malate titration are listed in Table V. Again, the apparent K_m's for malate were similar in all preparations studied except for tumor 7777. The apparent maximum velocities were lower for all the tumor mitochondria compared with the host liver mitochondria. These studies suggest that there is probably a defect of anion transport in the tumor mitochondria in addition to a defect of electron transport.

TABLE V

Kinetic Parameters of the Oxidation of Exogenous NADH via a
Reconstituted Malate–Aspartate Shuttle[a]

Preparation	Glutamate varied		Malate varied	
	K_m	V_{max}	K_m	V_{max}
Host liver	(6) 1.65	68.7	(4) 0.125	54
Tumor 7777	(3) 4.0	25	(2) 0.48	26.0
Tumor 7800	(3) 1.34	43	(2) 0.12	32.0
Tumor 7794A	(2) 0.91	11.0	(2) 0.08	12.8
Tumor 16	(2) 0.8	12.1	(2) 0.05	13.0

[a] Conditions used are the same as those described in Fig. 8 with
the exception that glutamate and malate concentrations were
varied. The number of determinations is shown in parentheses.

G. Measurements of Metabolite Accumulations during Glutamate Oxidation

Direct enzymatic assays were made of the production of aspartate and α-ketoglutarate with glutamate and malate as substrates in order to confirm and extend the studies with the reconstituted shuttles. These measurements were made in the absence of external NADH, malate dehydrogenase, and glutamate oxalacetate transaminase. In order to obtain maximal rates, state 3 conditions were employed with 5 mM glutamate and 1mM malate. Figure 11 shows the rates of aspartate production for the various tumors and their host livers, while Fig. 12 shows the kinetics of the accumulation of α-ketoglutarate. Aspartate production was always greater than α-ketoglutarate production because it is the end product of glutamate transamination and is transported irreversibly out of the mitochondria to the incubation medium, which contains no extramitochondrial enzymes. Thus, the rate of aspartate production is a measure of the rate of glutamate transamination. Although α-ketoglutarate is formed both by glutamate transamination and deamination, it is also oxidized in the mitochondria via α-ketoglutarate dehydrogenase. Furthermore, unlike aspartate transport, the α-ketoglutarate:malate exchange across the mitochondrial membrane is reversible and reaches a steady state. Figures 11 and 12 show that all tumor mitochondria exhibited a smaller accumulation of both aspartate and α-ketoglutarate than the respective host liver mitochondria.

Measurements of oxygen utilization were also carried out during the course of these experiments. If one assumes a negligible accumulation of succinate in the medium, which was verified with studies on normal rat liver mitochondria, flux through glutamate dehydrogenase may be roughly estimated from the difference between oxygen utilization calculated from glutamate transamination and oxidation of α-ketoglutarate to oxalacetate and the measured oxygen consumption. Since oxidation of glutamate to malate *via* glutamate dehydrogenase requires 3 atoms of oxygen per mole of glutamate, one-third of the difference will be equal to the flux through glutamate dehydrogenase. Likewise, oxygen utilization due to productivity of α-ketoglutarate from glutamate transamination will be equal to three times the aspartate accumulation minus twice the α-ketoglutarate accumulation. Table VI gives the calculated fluxes through glutamate oxalacetate transaminase and glutamate dehydrogenase and the measured oxygen utilization for three of the tumors together with their host livers. It is apparent from the table that transamination is more severely inhibited than oxygen utilization. Glutamate dehydrogenase accounts for a small percentage of the flux in the liver mitochondria and a somewhat larger percentage in tumor mitochondria. This is a significant finding since the transaminase pathway will support flux through the malate–aspartate shuttle, whereas the dehydrogenase pathway will not.

Vitamin K_3, 2-methyl-1,4-napthoquinone, can accept electrons directly from NADH and donate them to the electron transport chain in the region

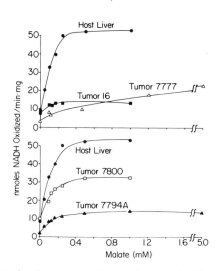

Fig. 10. The effect of malate concentration on the rate of oxidation of exogenous NADH via a reconstituted malate–aspartate shuttle. Conditions were the same as described in Fig. 8, trace A, with the exception that malate concentrations were varied as shown. Mitochondrial protein varied from 0.5 to 1.0 mg/ml.

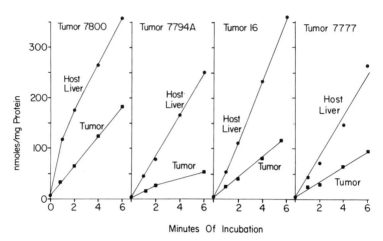

Fig. 11. Comparison of the rates of aspartate production by hepatoma mitochondria and host liver mitochondria. Mitochondria (1mg/ml) were incubated under state 3 conditions (cf. Methods, Section II). Glutamate (5 mM) and malate (1 mM) were used as substrates. Total volume of the incubation mixture was 3 ml, and 0.5 ml samples were taken for analysis at the times shown.

of cytochrome b, thus bypassing the iron–sulfur protein deficiency of the tumor 16 mitochondria in the NADH dehydrogenase region. For this reason we included vitamin K_3 in an experiment using tumor 16 mitochondria and mitochondria from its host liver. Oxygen utilization, aspartate production, and α-ketoglutarate accumulation were measured as previously, and the results are presented in Table VII. The data shown that vitamin K_3 stimulates metabolism in both control and tumor mitochondria. A more dramatic stimulation of both oxygen uptake and transamination is observed in the case of the tumor. However, even in the presence of the vitamin K_3 bypass, flux through the transaminase pathway is only 38% of the control, indicating that although the deficiency of the iron–sulfur proteins undoubtedly plays a role in the observed inhibition of glutamate oxidation, it does not account for it entirely. However, further work along these lines is needed since in other experiments, which included 2 mM arsenite to inhibit α-ketoglutarate dehydrogenase and rotenone to inhibit at the first phosphorylation site, addition of vitamin K_3 stimulated the rates of respiration and aspartate and α-ketoglutarate production of tumor 16 mitochondria to a similar extent as in the host liver mitochondria. Under these conditions, α-ketoglutarate production was 10 to 20% greater than aspartate production, illustrating the small activity of glutamate dehydrogenase.

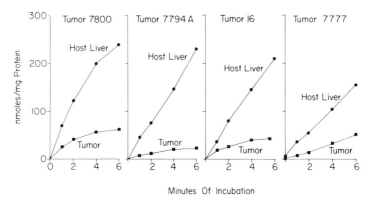

Fig. 12. Comparison of the rates of α-ketoglutarate production by hepatoma mitochondria and host liver mitochondria. Reaction conditions are described in Fig. 11.

The mitochondrial enzyme content of certain of the critical enzymes involved in glutamate metabolism (i.e., malate dehydrogenase, glutamate oxalacetate transaminase, and glutamate dehydrogenase) in tumor mitochondria compared with the host liver mitochondria are shown in Fig. 13. Mitochondria were sonicated and assayed by spectrophotometric methods based on the disappearance of NADH (Pette, 1965).As one would

TABLE VI

Parameters of Glutamate Metabolism in Liver and Tumor Mitochondria[a]

Preparations	O₂ uptake		Glutamic–oxalacetic transaminase		Glutamate dehydrogenase	
	Flux (natoms O/min·mg)	Percent control	Flux (nmoles/ min·mg)	Percent control	(nmoles/ min·mg)	Percent control
Host 16	74.0		49.7		0.0	
Tumor 16	43.1	58	15.0	30	4.1	∞
Host 7794A	80.4		43.5		1.0	
Tumor 7794A	50.4	62	13.1	30	6.4	640
Host 7800	110		58		13.3	
Tumor 7800	91.5	83	30	52	11.2	84

[a] Reaction conditions are described in Fig. 11.

TABLE VII

Effect of Vitamin K_3 on Glutamate Metabolism in Liver and Tumor Mitochondria[a]

Preparation	O_2 Uptake		Glutamic–oxalacetic transaminase		Glutamate dehydrogenase	
	Flux (natoms O/min·mg)	Percent control	Flux (nmoles/ min·mg)	Percent control	Flux (nmoles/ min·mg)	Percent control
Host 16	99	100	42	100	11	100
Tumor 16	42	42	9	22	10	90
K_3 + host 16	122	100	53	100	20	100
K_3 + tumor 16	81	65	20	38	16	82

[a] Reaction conditions are described in Fig. 11. 30 μM of 2-methyl-1,4-naphthoquinone (vitamin K_3) was included in the reaction media as shown.

expect, the enzyme contents cannot be used to account for the results observed. Glutamate dehydrogenase activity was decreased more than that of the transaminase in the tumors, and the activity of the transaminase was in all cases well above that which could cause any limitation of the flux observed in these experiments, suggesting that regulation was mediated by substrate availability to the enzymes.

H. Measurements of Anion Transport

1. Swelling Experiments

Transport of glutamate and malate across the membrane into the mitochondrial matrix and efflux of aspartate and α-ketoglutarate are required for operation of the malate–aspartate shuttle. The capacity of tumor mitochondria to catalyze operation of the shuttle is low compared to host liver mitochondria. Since the low rates observed appeared not to be explained entirely on the basis of deficiencies of iron–sulfur proteins or of low enzyme contents, it seemed most reasonable to examine the properties of the anion transport systems involved.

One relatively simple, straightforward method of obtaining information about transport phenomenon takes advantage of mitochondrial swelling in concentrated ammonium salts (Chappell, 1968). Buffered solutions of 100 mM ammonium salts of the anions to be studied containing EDTA together with rotenone to prevent metabolism were used to produce large volume swelling. Light scattering at 550 nm was observed after addition of mitochondria to the buffered salts. Several reviews are available which outline results obtained with this method (Chappell, 1968; Klingenberg, 1970). Mitochondria will not swell in K^+ salts because this cation is nonpermeant, and they do not swell in NH_4Cl because Cl^- is nonpermeant. Mitochondria placed directly in 100 mM ammonium phosphate, acetate, or glutamate swell readily, while the transport systems which allow swelling in ammonium malate and ammonium succinate require a small amount of phosphate for activation. Control experiments (not shown) indicated that tumors 16, 7800, and 7777 swell normally in ammonium acetate. Acetate, however, requires no specific membrane carrier (Klingenberg, 1970). These same tumors showed no impairment of phosphate transport. The swelling of tumors 7800 and 7777 in ammonium salts of phosphate, glutamate, malate, and succinate are compared with swelling of host liver mitochondria (host 7800) in Fig. 14. Tumor 16 is compared with its host in Fig. 15. Swelling in ammonium glutamate does not occur in tumor 16 and is very slow or absent in tumor 7777, while tumor 7800 appears to be similar to host liver in this respect. All tumors show impairment of malate and succinate swelling. It is not surprising that transport of both these anions is similarly inhibited because studies have shown that the same carrier system is involved (Klingenberg, 1970).

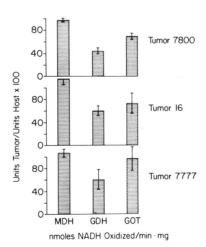

Fig. 13. Enzyme activities of mitochondria isolated from host rat livers and from hepatomas 7800, 16, and 7777. Mitochondria were sonicated and spun at 12,000 g to remove unbroken mitochondria. The supernatant material was assayed for enzymes as described by Pette (1965).

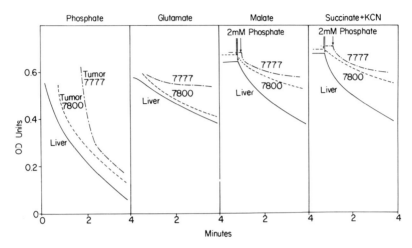

Fig. 14. Light-scattering changes induced by mitochondrial swelling in concentrated ammonium salts. Light-scattering changes were observed at 550 mμ using 1.6 mg mitochondrial protein (host liver, hepatoma 7777 or 7800) in 2 ml of reaction media. The incubation mixture included 100 m*M* ammonium salts of the anions listed at the top of the figure panels; 5 μ*M* rotenone, 0.1 m*M* EDTA, and in the case of succinate, 1 m*M* KCN. Swelling was initiated by the addition of mitochondria to buffer containing 100 m*M* phosphate or glutamate. Phosphate was used to initiate swelling in buffer containing mitochondria and 100 m*M* malate or succinate.

2. Measurement of Anion Gradients across the Mitochondrial Membrane

There are a great many limitations inherent in swelling studies. For example, in the present studies, differences in initial degree of swelling of tumor and liver mitochondria cannot be excluded. Likewise, it is impossible to evaluate the capacity for anion efflux by swelling. This becomes especially necessary in the case of aspartate because transport of aspartate is largely unidirectional in the outward direction (LaNoue and Williamson, 1971; Palmieri *et al.*, 1971). Also, the relevance of glutamate swelling to our specific problem is open to question. Glutamate entry occurs via two carrier systems. One seems to involve an exchange across the membrane with OH⁻ ions and is inhibited by *N*-ethylmaleimide (Meijer *et al.*, 1972). The other, which is active in the malate–aspartate cycle, involves an exchange of glutamate with aspartate and is not inhibited by *N*-ethylmaleimide (LaNoue and Hemington, 1973). Since mitochondrial swelling with ammonium glutamate is completely inhibited by *N*-ethylmaleimide exchange of glutamate with an hydroxyl ion is responsible for this swelling. Consequently, the more difficult task of measuring intramitochondrial concentrations of anions during active metabolism was undertaken. The techniques for doing this are described in Methods, Section II and in more detail elsewhere (LaNoue *et al.*, 1972).

Intramitochondrial concentrations of glutamate, malate, α-ketoglutarate, and aspartate were measured during state 3 metabolism of tumors 16 and 7800. The results are shown in Figs. 16 to 19. Measurement of intramitochondrial levels of anions in the presence of very high extramitochondrial levels is difficult because of the necessity for making large corrections for the amount of extramitochondrial fluid carried down through the silicone oil layer. Thus, when intramitochondrial glutamate contents were required, the initial concentration of glutamate in the medium was 0.5mM. Similarly, when malate was measured in the matrix phase, its initial external concentration was 0.1 mM. Figure 16 shows the results of an experiment using mitochondria prepared from tumor 7800 and its host liver in state 3 with 5 mM glutamate and 0.1 mM malate. The top half of the figure shows the disappearance of malate from the external

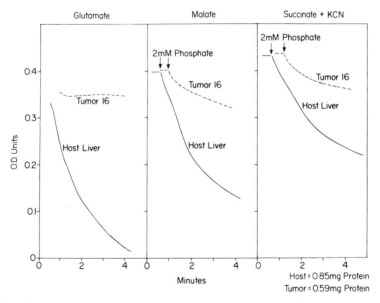

Fig. 15. Light-scattering changes induced by mitochondrial swelling. Light scattering changes were observed at 550 mμ using 0.8 mg of host liver mitochondria protein and 0.6 mg of hepatoma 16 mitochondrial protein in 2 ml of reaction media. The mixture included 100 mM ammonium salts of the anions listed at the top of the figure panels, 5 μM rotenone, 0.1 mM EDTA and in the case of succinate, 1 mM KCN. Swelling was initiated by the addition of mitochondria to buffer containing 100 mM glutamate. Phosphate was used to initiate swelling in buffer containing mitochondria and 100 mM malate or succinate.

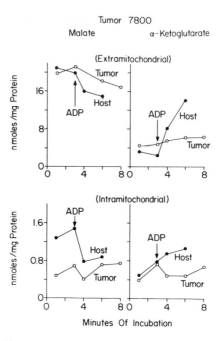

Fig. 16. Intra- and extramitochondrial levels of α-ketoglutarate and malate during oxidation of glutamate and malate by hepatoma 7800 and rat liver mitochondria. The initial incubation mixture included the standard buffer mixture (cf. Methods, Section II), 8% dextran, 5 mM glutamate, 0.1 mM malate, and 0.1 μC/ml [^{14}C]sucrose. The reaction was started with 30 mg of mitochondrial protein added to a total volume of 6 ml. At 3 minutes, 100 μM ADP and 5 units of hexokinase were added. Duplicate 0.5 ml samples were taken at 1, 3, 4, 5, and 6 minutes. Mitochondria and media were separated by rapid centrifugation through silicone oil (LaNoue *et al.,* 1972).

media and the appearance of α-ketoglutarate. The intramitochondrial concentration of malate was lower in the tumor than in the liver mitochondria, although the extramitochondrial concentration of malate was higher due to the diminished rate of glutamate metabolism. Thus the influx of malate may be rate limiting under these conditions. On the other hand, no specific inhibition of α-ketoglutarate transport is suggested by the data. Figure 17 illustrates similar results from an identical experiment using tumor 16.

Figures 18 and 19 give the results of experiments using tumors 7800 and 16, in which 0.5 mM glutamate and 1.0 mM malate were the substrates. Glutamate disappearance and aspartate appearance were measured. High levels of intramitochondrial glutamate measured in the tumor mitochondria indicate that transport of glutamate does not limit metabolism. Rates of efflux of aspartate were slow in the tumor, while measured intramitochondrial aspartate levels were high, suggesting a specific inhibition of the transport of aspartate. Both aspartate efflux and malate entry cannot be rate-limiting under the same situations, although both functions may be impaired.

In order to evaluate the importance of the aspartate transport impairment, flux of aspartate was measured, as well as intramitochondrial aspartate levels under three different conditions shown in Table VIII. When the malate concentration in the medium is high, aspartate efflux would appear to be rate limiting; whereas when the malate concentration is low (0.1 mM), the data suggest (by the very low levels of intramitochondrial aspartate measured) that flux through transaminase is rate limiting, probably due to a deficiency of intramitochondrial malate.

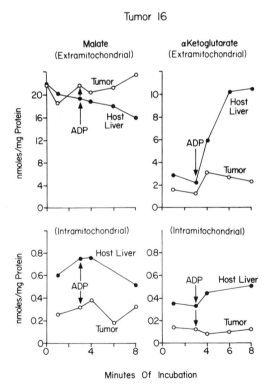

Fig. 17. Intra- and extramitochondrial levels of α-ketoglutarate and malate during oxidation of glutamate and malate by hepatoma 16 and rat liver mitochondria. Reaction conditions are identical to those described in Fig. 16.

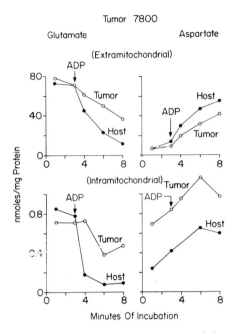

Fig. 18. Intra- and extramitochondrial levels of aspartate and glutamate during oxidation of glutamate and malate by hepatoma 7800 and host liver mitochondria. Incubation conditions are identical to those described in Fig. 16, with the exception that the initial glutamate concentration was 0.5 m*M* and the malate concentration was 1 m*M*.

I. Relationship between Glycolysis and Oxidation in Morris Hepatomas

A few preliminary experiments have been carried out in an attempt to relate our studies with isolated mitochondria to the metobolism of the intact tumor. Initially, an estimate was made of the mitochondrial content of tumor 16 and liver. This was accomplished by assaying cytochrome oxidase enzymatically from its rate of reduction of cytochrome c in preparations of sonicated mitochondria and sonicated tissue homogenates. The results of these measurements are shown in Table IX. The data may be used to estimate the mitochondrial content of the tissue, assuming only that all the cytochrome a + a_3 content is contained in the mitochondria. The finding that the mitochondrial content of the tumor is very similar to the host is in agreement with Pedersen who finds that the intermediate growing tumor 7800 has normal mitochondrial cytochrome oxidase content (Pedersen, 1972), while the rapidly growing tumor 3924A has a diminished mitochondrial content (Schreiber *et al.*, 1970).

Several experiments have been carried out using the tissue slice technique, measuring respiration rates and lactate production. Standard Warburg respirometers were used in this experiment. The medium contained Krebs Ringer phosphate, pH 7.2, together with 20 mM glucose. Slices were equilibrated with O_2 at 0°C and then incubated at 37°C for 70 minutes. Oxygen utilization was measured during the course of the experiment. At the end of 10, 20, 40, or 70 minutes, perchloric acid (0.1 ml of a 10%, w/v, solution) was tipped into each flask. Lactate was measured in the neutralized perchloric acid extracts of the media. Respiration of the host liver slices was 150 μatoms oxygen/gm wet weight/hour compared with 94 μatoms/gm wet weight/hour for slices of tumor 16. Lactate production, on the other hand, was 9.6 and 20.1 μmoles/gm wet weight/hour for the host liver and tumor 16, respectively, when measured over the time interval from 20 to 70 minutes of incubation. The respiration

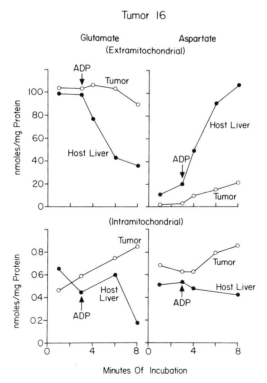

Fig. 19. Intra- and extramitochondrial levels of aspartate and glutamate during oxidation of glutamate and malate by hepatoma 16 and host liver mitochondria. Reaction conditions are identical to those described in Fig. 16.

TABLE VIII

Relationship of Intramitochondrial Aspartate Levels and Aspartate Flux across the Mitochondrial Membrane in Hepatoma 16 and Host Liver Mitochondria[a]

Substrate concentrations	Tumor 16		Host liver	
	Flux (nmoles/ min·mg)	Intramito- chondrial aspartate (nmoles/mg)	Flux min·mg	Intramito- chondrial aspartate (nmoles/mg)
5 mM Glutamate 1 mM Malate	12.7	1.31	69.8	2.17
5 mM Glutamate 0.1 mM Malate	13.5	0.29	26.2	0.53
0.5 mM Glutamate 1.0 mM Malate	4.0	0.76	22.3	0.45

[a] Reaction conditions were identical to those described in Fig. 16 with the exception that the substrate concentrations were varied as shown.

rates can be converted to rates per milligram of mitochondria since the mitochondrial content is known. It appears that these are about twice the state 4 rates recorded in Table I. These data illustrate that defective respiration and possible diminished transfer of reducing equivalents to the mitochondria, relative to the host liver, are exhibited by the whole tumor as well as by mitochondria isolated from the tumor.

IV. Discussion

Mitochondria isolated from the variety of Morris hepatomas covered in this study exhibit a diminished capacity for transporting reducing equivalents from cytosol to mitochondria via the malate–aspartate shuttle. The extent of the defect varies between tumors and does not appear to be a function of growth rate. Three factors may be involved in the inhibition. Low levels of iron–sulfur proteins are indicated by the very low EPR signals obtained in certain specific regions of the magnetic field. In addition, at least three of the tumors have defects in their capacity to transport two specific anions. Swelling studies and measurements of intramitochondrial contents show that the dicarboxylate carrier, which may transport malate into the mitochondrial matrix, does not function as well in the tumor as in the liver. In addition, the transport of aspartate out of the mitochondria may be defective.

Recent studies by Kovacevic and co-workers (Kovacevic, 1971, 1972; Kovacevic and Morris, 1972) have indicated that some tumor mitochondria show a decreased capacity for the oxidation of glutamate and an increased capacity for oxidation of glutamine. This was related to changes in transport properties of the respective substrates. The K_m for glutamate was reported to be increased, whereas the K_m for glutamine was decreased. We cannot confirm these results except with respect to the increased K_m for glutamate oxidation by mitochondria from tumor 7777. Glutamine was not found to be oxidized at appreciable rates by any of the tumor mitochondria studied.

Kinetic studies of the reconstituted malate aspartate shuttle indicate that the Michaelis constants for glutamate and malate are in a normal range, whereas maximal rates obtainable at high substrate levels are low in the tumor. This result does not eliminate the possibility that anion transport is rate limiting since it could be produced by lack of carrier proteins. However, the reduced state of the pyridine nucleotides measured in state 3 indicates that in tumors 16 and 7794A substrate entry is not rate limiting. The high NADH/NAD ratio in these tumors suggests that the metabolic lesion causing the slow fluxes is on the oxygen side of the dehydrogenases rather than on the substrate side. However, addition of vitamin K_3 which presumably bridges the iron–sulfur protein-deficient area in the tumor mitochondria produces only partial stimulation of glutamate metabolism. Thus, it would appear that there may be at least three separate defects in the tumors, which under different conditions may lead to slow transport of reducing equivalents from cytosol to mitochondrial matrix. The extra abnormalities noted in the mitochondria from tumor 7777 are probably arti-

TABLE IX

Mitochondrial Content of Tumor 16 and Host Liver Tissue[a]

Preparation	Tissue content of cytochrome a + a₃ $\left(\dfrac{\mu\text{moles cyto. c oxidized}}{\text{min} \cdot \text{gm wet weight}}\right)$	Mitochondrial content of cytochrome a + a₃ $\left(\dfrac{\mu\text{moles cyto. c oxidized}}{\text{min} \cdot \text{min protein}}\right)$	Tissue content of mitochondria $\left(\dfrac{\text{mg mito. protein}}{\text{gm wet weight tissue}}\right)$
Host liver	47.6	0.507	93.9
Tumor 16	42.3	0.495	85.5

[a] Homogenates and mitochondrial suspensions were extensively sonicated prior to assay. The assay procedure is described in the Section II. Values shown are means of three determinations.

factual, resulting from the high Ca^{2+} content of the isolated mitochondria. Whether this represents the situation *in situ* cannot be ascertained. Extrapolating from our very small sampling of hepatomas, we might postulate that not all of the defects appear in all tumors and that other lesions might appear if the sampling were larger. The explanation may be that optimal functioning of the pathways for cytosolic NADH oxidation via the respiratory chain has little survival value for the tumor. Thus, mistakes or changes in DNA material relative to the pathway would not be correctable.

The relevance of our studies using isolated mitochondria to the metabolism of the neoplastic cell requires further exploration. If the malate–aspartate shuttle is rate limiting for the oxidation of lactate, then tumors with relatively normal capacities for transport of reducing equivalents should have negligible rates of aerobic glycolysis and lactate production. Several reports (Aisenberg and Morris, 1963; Lin *et al.*, 1962) have appeared in the literature that indicate that Morris hepatoma 7800 has a normal rate of lactate accumulation. Since no information concerning tumors 7777, 7794A, and 16 was available, a preliminary examination of tumor 16 was undertaken, revealing that accumulation of lactate by tumor slices was considerably higher than that of host liver slices. However, measured lactate production was in a low range when compared to most hepatomas (i.e., 20 μmoles/gm wet weight/hour compared to 20–60 μmoles/gm wet weight/hour).

A recent study by Weber *et al.* (1971) of metabolite levels in freeze-clamped hepatomas of different growth rates is pertinent to this discussion. Tumors were freeze-clamped *in situ* and levels of lactate, pyruvate, β-hydroxybutyrate, and acetoacetate determined. Since lactate and pyruvate are in equilibrium via the cytosolic enzyme lactate dehydrogenase, the cytosolic ratio of $NAD^+/NADH$ can be estimated. From this, the oxidation–reduction potential of the cytosolic pyridine nucleotide pool can be calculated. Likewise, the β-hydroxybutyrate/acetoacetate ratio can be used to calculate the mitochondrial oxidation–reduction potential (Williamson *et al.*, 1967). Table X taken from the data of Weber *et al.* (1971) lists the results of these calculations. The potential difference between the mitochondria and the cytosol is mediated by an energy input at the level of the shuttle. It has been shown, in this laboratory, that aspartate efflux is energy driven (LaNoue and Hemington, 1973; LaNoue and Williamson, 1971; Williamson *et al.*, 1973). Any impairment of shuttle operation should act to diminish the potential differential. The last column of the table indicates that tumor 5123, a low glycolyzing tumor which is similar in growth rate to tumor 7800, has a fairly normal potential difference, whereas tumor 9618A, a very slow growing tumor, has a diminished potential. The results using tumor 3924A may not be valid since it has very low β-hydroxybutyrate dehydrogenase activity (Pedersen *et al.*, 1970).

TABLE X

Cytosolic and Mitochondiral NAD Redox Potentials of Rat Livers and Hepatomas[a,b]

Preparation	Ratio of lactate to pyruvate	Cytosol[b] NAD⁺ redox potential (mV)	Ratio of β-hydroxy-butyrate to aceto-acetate	Mito-chondrial matrix[c] NAD[b] redox potential (mV)	Potential difference (mV)
Buffalo rat liver	12.2	251	2.40	309	58
AC/N rat liver	21.9	258	1.78	305	47
Tumor 9618A (Buffalo rat)	43.3	269	0.96	297	28
Tumor 5123D (Buffalo rat)	55.0	271	3.73	315	44
Tumor 3924A (AC/N rat)	147.0	283	1.09	299	16

[a] Data are taken from Weber *et al.* (1971).

[b] The oxidation–reduction potential of the cytosolic NAD⁺ system is calculated using values of -337 mV for the midpotential of NAD⁺ and 1.11×10^{-4} for the equilibrium constant of lactate oxidation

$$\left[K = \frac{(\text{lact}) \, (\text{NAD}^+)}{(\text{pyr})(\text{NADH})} \right].$$

[c] The potential of the mitochondrial NAD⁺ system is calculated using values of -337 mV for the midpotential of NAD⁺ and 4.93×10^{-2} for the equilibrium constant of β-hydroxybutyrate oxidation

$$\left[K = \frac{(\beta\text{-OH-butyrate})(\text{NAD}^+)}{(\text{acetoacetate})(\text{NADH})} \right].$$

Thus, the data of Weber *et al.* (1971) when calculated in this way seem to indicate that the slowest growing tumor has the most impaired transport of reducing equivalents. This observation is in agreement with our studies with isolated mitochondria, indicating that impairment of H-transport shuttles need not be related directly with growth rate. Likewise, defects of iron–sulfur proteins do not appear to correspond with the growth rate of the tumors.

ACKNOWLEDGMENTS

This work was supported by grants from the American Cancer Society (P-585), the American Heart Association, and the United States Public Health Service (AM-15120 and CA-10729).

Kathryn F. LaNoue is a Dr. William Daniel Stroud Established Investigator of the American Heart Association.

REFERENCES

Aisenberg, A. C. (1961a). "The Glycolysis and Respiration of Tumors." Academic Press, New York.

Aisenberg, A. C. (1961b). *Cancer Res.* **21**, 295–303.

Aisenberg, A. C., and Morris, H. P. (1963). *Cancer Res.* **23**, 566–568.

Anderson, J. H., Nicklas, W. J., Blank, B., Refino, C., and Williamson, J. R. (1971). *In* "Regulation of Gluconeogenesis" (H.-D. Söling and B. Willms, eds.), pp. 293–315. Academic Press, New York.

Ashmore, J., Weber, G., and Landau, B. R. (1958). *Cancer Res.* **18**, 974–979.

Beinert, H., and Palmer, G. (1965). *In* "Oxidases and Related Redox Systems" (T. E. King, H. S. Mason, and M. Morrison, eds.), Vol. 2, pp. 567–590. Wiley, New York.

Beinert, H., Heinen, W., and Palmer, G. (1962). *Brookhaven Symp. Biol.* **15**, 229–265.

Berry, M. N., Kun, E., and Werner, H. V. (1973). *Eur. J. Biochem.* **33**, 407–417.

Borst, P. (1963). *In* "Funktionelle und morphologische Organisation der Zelle" (P. Karlson, ed.), pp. 137–158. Springer-Verlag, Berlin and New York.

Boxer, G. E., and Devlin, T. M. (1961). *Science* **134**, 1495–1501.

Bücher, T., and Klingenberg, M. (1958). *Angew. Chem.* **70**, 552–570.

Burk, D. A. (1939). *Cold Spring Harbor Symp. Quant. Biol.* **7**, 420–455.

Chance, B., and Hess, B. (1959). *Science* **129**, 700–708.

Chance, B., and Williams, G. R. (1955). *J. Biol. Chem.* **217**, 401–427.

Chappell, J. B. (1968). *Brit. Med. Bull.* **24**, 150–157.

Chen, R. F. (1967). *J. Biol. Chem.* **242**, 173–181.

Gordon, E. E., Ernster, L., and Dallner, G. (1967). *Cancer Res.* **27**, 1372–1377.

Klingenberg, M. (1970). *Essays Biochem.* **6**, 119–159.

Kovacevic, Z. (1971). *Biochem. J.* **125**, 757–763.

Kovacevic, Z. (1972). *Eur. J. Biochem.* **25**, 372–378.

Kovacevic, Z., and Morris, H. P. (1972). *Cancer Res.* **32**, 326–333.

LaNoue, K. F., and Hemington, J. G. (1973). *Fed. Proc., Fed. Amer. Soc. Exp. Biol.* **32**, 557 (abstr.).

LaNoue, K. F., and Williamson, J. R. (1971). *Metab., Clin. Exp.* **20**, 119–140.

LaNoue, K. F., Bryła, J., and Williamson, J. R. (1972). *J. Biol. Chem.* **247**, 667–679.

Lehninger, A. L. (1951). *J. Biol. Chem.* **190**, 345–359.

Lin, Y. C., Elwood, J. C., Rosado, A., Morris, H. P., and Weinhouse, S. (1962). *Nature (London)* **195**, 153–155.

Mehard, C. W., Packer, L., and Abraham, S. (1971). *Cancer Res.* **31**, 2148–2160.

Meijer, A. J., Brouwer, A., Reijngoud, D. J., Hoek, J. B., and Tager, J. M. (1972). *Biochim. Biophys. Acta* **283**, 421–429.

Morris, H. P., and Wagner, B. P. (1968). *Methods Cancer Res.* **4**, 125–152.

Nowell, P. C., Morris, H. P., and Potter, V. R. (1967). *Cancer Res.* **27**, 1565–1579.

Ohnishi, T. (1973). *Biochim. Biophys. Acta* **301**, 105–128.

Ohnishi, T., Katz, R., and Chance, B. (1971). *Abstr. Commun. Meet., Fed. Eur. Biochem. Soc., 7th, 1971* Abstract No. 655.

Ohnishi, T., Wilson, D. F., Asakura, T., and Chance, B. (1972). *Biochem. Biophys. Res. Commun.* **46**, 1631–1638.

Orme-Johnson, N. R., Orme-Johnson, W. H., Hansen, R. E., Beinert, H., and Hatefi, Y. (1971). *Biochem. Biophys. Res. Commun.* **44**, 446–452.

Palmieri, F., Senchi, G., and Quagliariello, E. (1971). *Experientia, Suppl.* **18**, 505–512.

Pedersen, P. L. (1972). *Gann Monogr. Cancer Res.* **13**, 251–265.

Pedersen, P. L., Greenawalt, J. W., Chan, T. L., and Morris, H. P. (1970). *Cancer Res.* **30**, 2620–2626.

Pedersen, P. L., Eska, T., Morris, H. P., and Catterall, W. A. (1971). *Proc. Nat. Acad. Sci. U.S.* **68**, 1079–1082.

Pette, D. (1965). *Naturwissenschaften* **52**, 597–616.

Purvis, J. L., and Lowenstein, J. M. (1961). *J. Biol. Chem.* **236**, 2794–2803.

Pybus, J. (1968). *Clin. Chim. Acta* **23**, 309–317.

Rieske, J. S., MacLennan, D. H., and Coleman, R. (1964). *Biochem. Biophys. Res. Commun.* **15**, 338–344.

Robinson, B. H., and Halperin, M. L. (1970). *Biochem. J.* **116**, 229–233.

Rognstad, R., and Katz, J. (1970). *Biochem. J.* **116**, 483–491.

Safer, B., and Williamson, J. R. (1973). *J. Biol. Chem.* **248**, 2570–2579.

Safer, B., Smith, C. M., and Williamson, J. R. (1971). *J. Mol. Cell. Cardiol.* **2**, 111–124.

Scholz, R., and Bücher, T. (1965). *In* "Control of Energy Metabolism" (B. Chance, R. W. Estabrook, and J. R. Williamson, eds.), pp. 393–414. Academic Press, New York.

Schreiber, J. R., Balcavage, W. X., Morris, H. P., and Pedersen, P. L. (1970). *Cancer Res.* **30**, 2497–2501.

Sweeney, M. J., Ashmore, J., Morris, H. P., and Weber, G. (1963). *Cancer Res.* **23**, 995–1002.

van Rossum, G. D. V., Gosalvez, M., Galeotti, T., and Morris, H. P. (1971). *Biochim. Biophys. Acta* **245**, 263–276.

Vinogradov, A., Scarpa, A., and Chance, B. (1972). *Arch. Biochem. Biophys.* **152**, 646–654.

Wahler, B. E., and Wollenberger, A. (1958). *Biochem. Z.* **329**, 508–520.

Weber, G. (1972). *Gann Monogr. Cancer Res.* **13**, 47–77.

Weber, G., Stubbs, M., and Morris, H. P. (1971). *Cancer Res.* **31**, 2177–2183.

Williamson, D. H., Lund, P., and Krebs, H. A. (1967). *Biochem. J.* **103**, 514–527.

Williamson, J. R., and Corkey, B. E. (1969). *In* "Methods in Enzymology" (J. M. Lowenstein, ed.), Vol. 13, pp. 434–513. Academic Press, New York.

Williamson, J. R., Scholz, R., and Browning, E. T. (1969a). *J. Biol. Chem.* **244**, 4617–4627.

Williamson, J. R., Scholz, R., Browning, E. T., Thurman, R. G., and Fukami, M. H. (1969b). *J. Biol. Chem.* **244**, 5044–5054.

Williamson, J. R., Jakob, A., and Refino, C. (1971). *J. Biol. Chem.* **246**, 7632–7641.

Williamson, J. R., Safer, B., LaNoue, K. F., Smith, C. M., and Wałajtys, E. (1973). *In* "Proceedings of the Society for Experimental Biology" (D. D. Davies, ed.), Symp. No. 27, pp. 241–281. Cambridge Univ. Press, London and New York.

Ylikahri, R. H., Hassinen, I., and Kähönen, M. T. (1970). *Biochem. Biophys. Res. Commun.* **44**, 150–156.

CHAPTER VI

METABOLITE AND HORMONAL CONTROL OF ENERGY METABOLISM IN EXPERIMENTAL HEPATOMAS

WAYNE E. CRISS

There have been numerous reports in the literature associating cancer with energy metabolism and hormones. A few of these reports indicated a relationship between diabetes and malignant growth. In experimental animals, reports as early as the 1950's showed a reduction in the incidence of chemically induced hepatomas in allozanized rats (Salzberg and Griffin, 1952), decreased growth of mammary carcinoma (Henson and Legros, 1972) and Novikoff ascites cells (Goranson and Tilser, 1955) in diabetic rats, and decreased growth of Ehrlich ascites cells in alloxanized mice (Vangerov and McKee, 1955). Recent reports indicate decreased mammary carcinoma growth in diabetic mice (Racker, 1965; Puckett and Shingleton, 1972), decreased incidence of DMBA-induced mammary tumors in rats without prolactin (Heuson *et al.*, 1972), and a correlated response of the growth of solid Ehrlich cells (Kodama and Kodama, 1970) to estrogens and androgens. For humans, one finds studies citing a decreased incidence of cancer in male diabetics (Kessler, 1970) and faulty carbohydrate metabolism in patients with metastatic carcinoma (Waterhouse and Kemperman, 1971). One recent report concerning rats even attributes death of the tumor bearer to the ability of a particular ascites tumor line to induce hypoglycemia in the tumor bearer (Killington *et al.,* 1971). Therefore, we have concerned ourselves, over the last 4–5 years, with investigations designed to probe potential changes in the metabolic and hormonal controls of energy metabolism in neoplastic tissues.

I.   Anaerobic and Aerobic Metabolism

A. Faulty Respiration?

There is no doubt but what the fully developed tumor cell has an almost unlimited capacity for the production of energy that may be used for macromolecular synthesis and growth. Most of the early observed metabolic characteristics of neoplastic tissues revolved around altered forms of energy metabolism: (a) high rates of anaerobic glycolysis; (b) presence of aerobic glycolysis; and (c) low rates of respiration (Warburg, 1930; Weinhouse, 1955; Boxer and Devlin, 1961 and, Aisenberg, 1961c; Racker, 1965; Wenner, 1967). In 1930, Warburg proposed the first substantial theory of carcinogenesis. He concluded that the cancer cell had faulty respiration and had to develop its fermentative metabolism to survive. However, this concept could not be vigorously challenged until a group of readily transplantable tumors were available for laboratory study. Thus, the development and study of the Morris "minimal deviation" hepatomas (Morris, 1963, 1965; Morris and Wagner, 1968) over the last 13 years have provided ample data to illustrate that all three of these original biochemical findings are not found in all tumors (e.g., certain limited number of highly differentiated hepatomas) and that these characteristics can be observed in certain normal tissues (e.g., leukocytes, intestinal mucosa, retina). But the common observation of altered energy metabolism in highly malignant tumor tissue is still predominant.

Poorly differentiated tumors have undergone numerous enzymatic shifts (Weber and Lea, 1966; Criss, 1971b). These changes may have resulted in altering the potential of metabolic pathways for the competition of common metabolites. Soon after Warburg's hypothesis on "faulty respiration," Johnson (1941) and Lynen (1941) suggested that the Pasteur effect (inhibition of glycolysis by molecular oxygen) was mediated by competition between metabolic pathways for common metabolites. They independently postulated a competition for substrates or metabolites between the transphorylating enzymes of glycolysis and the respiratory enzymes of mitochondrial oxidative phosphorylation. Recently, Weinhouse and his colleagues (Lo *et al.,* 1968) demonstrated a direct competition for metabolites between the enzymatic systems involved in nonoxidative (glycolyzing) and oxidative (respiratory) phosphorylation. These latter studies were interpreted to suggested that a powerful glycolytic system could carry out glycolytic phosphorylation at the expense of respiratory phosphorylation.

B. Increased Glycolytic Potential

In attempts to elucidate the specific intracellular sites of potential competition between glycolysis and respiration in normal and neoplastic tissues, we began a series of studies in Morris "minimal deviation" hepatomas which were designed to measure intracellular competition for the universal energy precursor, ADP (Criss, 1969, 1970, 1971a,b, 1973a,b,c; Criss *et al.,* 1970a,b; Sapico *et al.,* 1970; Filler and Criss, 1971). The activities of several substrate level phosphorylating enzymes from liver and hepatomas were determined: cytoplasmic adenylate kinase (EC 2.7.4.3), pyruvate kinase (EC 2.7.1.40), and phosphoglycerate kinase (EC 2.7.2.3), mitochondrial adenylate kinase (EC 2.7.4.3), and nucleoside diphosphokinase (EC 2.7.4.6). Tabulation of these enzymatic measurements were made by setting up a ratio of cytoplasmic to mitochondrial nonoxidative phosphorylation potential (Table I). The ratio was 0.44 in normal liver tissue, 0.50 in a group of highly differentiated hepatomas, 22.2 in a group of poorly differentiated hepatomas, (solid), and 71.2 in Novikoff ascites cells. The poorly differentiated tumor tissue seems to have acquired a 50 to 200 times greater potiential to produce ATP from its cytoplasmic systems versus its mitochondrial systems (anaerobically).

Even under aerobic conditions, it would appear that tumor respiration has developed specific "handicaps." All mitochondria require a constant supply of ADP and P_i, molecular oxygen, and reducing equivalents (NADH-NADPH) for normal ATP production. The reducing equivalents must be either produced cytoplasmically and transferred into the mitochondrion to a coupled electron transport chain or produced internally after transportation of specific reduced metabolites into the mitochondrial matrix. Therefore, we measured the enzymes from liver and hepatomas which are involved in the transportation of reducing equivalent into the mitochondria: (1) malate–aspartate shuttle systems by cytoplasmic and mitochondrial NAD^+-malate dehydrogenases (EC 1.1.1.37); (2) glycerophosphate shuttle system by cytoplasmic and mitochondrial NAD^+

TABLE I

Substrate-Level Phosphorylation in Liver and Hepatomas[a,b]

Tissue	Cytoplasmic enzymes			
	AK	PK	PGK	P.P.
Liver	47 ± 08	45 ± 11	34 ± 10	126
Highly dif. hepatomas				
9618A	45 ± 10	59 ± 14	39 ± 11 ⎫	
8999	40 ± 10	42 ± 09	43 ± 14 ⎬	133
7787	44 ± 11	53 ± 11	33 ± 13 ⎭	
Poorly dif. hepatomas				
3924A	42 ± 10	372 ± 48	203 ± 27 ⎫	
3683F	37 ± 09	395 ± 39	189 ± 29 ⎬	644
Novikoff hepatoma (solid)	44 ± 12	420 ± 46	231 ± 38 ⎭	
Novikoff ascites cells	45 ± 10	378 ± 35	218 ± 25	641

Tissue	Mitochondrial enzymes		
	AK	NDK	P.P.
Liver	252 ± 20	34 ± 05	286
Highly dif. hepatomas			
9618A	251 ± 27	36 ± 08 ⎫	
8999	210 ± 16	41 ± 11 ⎬	268
7787	226 ± 27	39 ± 10 ⎭	
Poorly dif. hepatomas			
3924A	21 ± 08	3 ± 01 ⎫	
3683F	13 ± 04	5 ± 03 ⎬	29
Novikoff hepatoma (solid)	37 ± 10	7 ± 03 ⎭	
Novikoff ascites cells	5 ± 02	4 ± 02	9

Cytoplasmic: mitochondrial phosphorylation
potential ratio

Liver	0.44
Highly dif. hepatomas	0.50
Poorly dif. hepatomas	22.20
Ascites hepatomas	71.22

[a] Reprinted with permission from Criss (1973a, b).

[b] Values for AK, PK, PGK, and NDK are given in $\mu m/gm$ tissue. AK, adenylate kinase; PK, pyruvate kinase; PGK, phosphoglycerate kinase; NDK, nucleoside diphospho-kinase; P.P., phosphorylation potential.

and FAD-glycerophosphate dehydrogenases (EC 1.1.1.8 and EC 1.1.99.5); (3) anaerobic metabolism by cytoplasmic lactate dehydrogenase (EC 1.1.1.27); (4) pentose phosphate pathway by cytoplasmic glucose-6-phosphate dehydrogenase (EC 1.1.1.49); and (5) glycolysis by cytoplasmic NAD^+-glyceraldehyde phosphate dehydrogenase (EC 1.2.1.12). Cytoplasmic NAD^+-malate dehydrogenase was decreased 5-fold in poorly differentiated hepatomas when compared to liver tissue. Cytoplasmic NAD^+-glycerophosphate dehydrogenase was decreased 6- to 10-fold in the poorly differentiated hepatomas (Table II). Glucose-6-phosphate dehydrogenase was increased 3-fold in the poorly differentiated tumors. Therefore, the fast growing hepatomas appear to have decreased ability to transfer cytoplasmically produced reducing equivalents into any coupled electron transport chain located within the mitochondria, but have potentially increased ability to synthesize nucleic acid precursors (ribose moieties via the pentose phosphate pathway).

Another indication of the shifts in metabolic pathway potential which would result in increased glycolysis in tumors can be observed from Table II. NAD^+-glycerophosphate dehydrogenase provides glycerol 3-phosphate for triglyceride and phospholipid synthesis; while NAD^+-lactate dehydrogenase is one of the key enzymes which allows recycling of NAD^+ during anaerobic glycolysis (Olson, 1951; Boxer and Devlin, 1961; White and Kaplan, 1969). There was a 5- to 8-fold increase in the ratio of lactate dehydrogenase to glycerophosphate dehydrogenase in the poorly differentiated hepatomas when compared to liver. A change of such magnitude could shift this bienzymatic competition for NADH in favor of glycolysis at the expense of lipid synthesis. Numerous other pathway eliminations or shifts have been observed in rapid growing tumors (Weber *et al.,* 1965; Weber and Lea, 1966; Criss, 1971b).

II.   Adenylate Energy Charge

A. How the Charge Works

Numerous postulates attempting to explain the alterations in the pathway shifts and modifications in intracellular control mechanisms which affect the production and utilization of ATP in tumor cells have been written over the years (Greenstein, 1956; Aisenberg, 1961a,b,c; Wenner, 1967). It has only been recently that Atkinson has developed and established a working mathematical relationship concerning the production and utilization or cellular energy (Atkinson, 1966, 1968a,b, 1969a; Liao and Atkinson, 1971a,b; Miller and Atkinson, 1972). Atkinson has defined an

TABLE II

Intracellular Hydrogen Transport Systems[a]

Tissue	Cytoplasmic enzymes[b]					
	NAD+-MDH	NAD+-GAPDH	*FAD-GPDH	NAD+-GPDH	NAD+-LDH	NADP-G6PDH
Liver	510 ± 43	134 ± 22	12 ± 04	123 ± 15	231 ± 32	10 ± 03
Highly dif. hep.						
9618A	497 ± 46	127 ± 18	16 ± 09	109 ± 10	204 ± 21	11 ± 04
8999	503 ± 53	146 ± 21	19 ± 06	116 ± 13	218 ± 14	15 ± 06
7787	478 ± 36	110 ± 09	10 ± 03	88 ± 11	236 ± 19	13 ± 05
Poorly dif. hep.						
3924A	87 ± 18	124 ± 24	17 ± 11	32 ± 09	198 ± 17	18 ± 05
3683F	116 ± 29	109 ± 16	12 ± 05	10 ± 04	222 ± 21	27 ± 10
Novikoff (solid)	106 ± 08	118 ± 18	14 ± 04	15 ± 04	209 ± 24	29 ± 09
Novikoff (ascites)	110 ± 11	111 ± 15	11 ± 05	11 ± 03	198 ± 22	24 ± 06

Tissue	Mitochondrial enzymes		
	NAD+-MDH	*FAD-GPDH	NAD+-GPDH
Liver	277 ± 19	499 ± 37	6 ± 3
Highly dif. hep.			
9618A	294 ± 28	487 ± 49	9 ± 3
8999	310 ± 19	399 ± 39	5 ± 2
7787	259 ± 33	541 ± 65	7 ± 3
Poorly dif. hep.			
3924A	288 ± 27	490 ± 36	5 ± 2
3683F	301 ± 39	508 ± 42	7 ± 3
Novikoff (solid)	354 ± 32	576 ± 44	7 ± 3
Novikoff (ascites)	380 ± 29	610 ± 43	6 ± 2

[a] Reprinted with permission from Criss (1973a, b).
[b] Values are given in μm/gm tissue.

adenylate energy charge as one-half the average number of anhydride bound phosphate groups per adenosine moiety, or:

$$\text{Adenylate energy charge} = \frac{[\text{ATP}] + 1/2\,[\text{ADP}]}{[\text{ATP}] + [\text{ADP}] + [\text{AMP}]}$$

When only AMP is present, there is a net charge of zero or complete discharge. When only ATP is present, there is a net charge of one or the cell is fully charged. Thus the adenylate system (adenylate kinase, ATP, ADP, and AMP) of a living cell can be compared to an electrochemical storage cell in its ability to accept, store, and supply energy. Atkinson and his colleagues have shown that certain key enzymes that participate in ATP-regenerating pathways show plots of enzyme activity against energy charge with negative slopes that increase with charge. Several enzymes of glycolysis and the citric acid cycle are inhibited by an energy charge of one (high ATP) and/or are stimulated by an energy charge of zero (high AMP). These include phosphofructokinase, pyruvate dehydrogenase, citrate synthetase, NAD$^+$-isocitrate dehydrogenase, and pyruvate kinase. Certain other key enzymes that participate in biosynthetic or other ATP-utilizing pathways show plots of enzyme activity against energy charge with positive slopes that increase with charge. Several biosynthetic enzymes are stimulated by an energy charge of one (high ATP) and/or are inhibited by an energy charge of zero (high AMP). These include citrate cleavage enzyme, phosphoribosyl-pyrophosphate synthetase, phosphoribosyl ATP synthetase, aspartokinase, and fructose-1, 6-diphosphatase. Thus, the adenylate energy system could provide the biological cell with a very sensitive intracellular regulatory control mechanism and also serve as a barometer for monitoring energy flow. Certainly, the adenine nucleotides are substrates or powerful modulators of enzymatic systems concerned with: glucose uptake; glycolysis; citrate acid cycle; activation, β-oxidation, and synthesis of fatty acids; glycogenesis and gluconeogenesis; oxidative phosphorylation; amino acid catabolism; and protein, RNA, and DNA synthesis.

Obviously, many enzymes and certain metabolites make varying contributions to the energy charge within a cell. Compartmentation could be an important factor in determining location and the quantity of the energy charge. It also raises the possibility of a distinct energy charge in distinct subcellular units. The energy charge in the cytoplasm would depend on the activity of several substrate level phosphorylating enzymes and transport of ATP out of the mitochondria. The energy charge within the mitochondria would depend on the efficiency of the malate–aspartate, oxalacetate (Haslam and Krebs, 1968), and glycerophosphate redox shuttle systems, coupling to the adenine nucleotides, and transport of ADP inward. It is thus apparent that there is a close link between the nicotinamide and adenine nucleotide systems (Williamson *et al.,* 1968; Veech *et al.,* 1970). If one considered the evidence which indicated that the adenine nucleotides contributed directly to the metabolic controlling elements involved in the Pasteur effect (Lo *et al.,* 1968; Atkinson, 1969b; Criss, 1969; Opie *et al.,* 1971; Clark *et al.,* 1973), and since one of the most notable and controversial features of the neoplastic cell was the inability of the Pasteur effect to completely inhibit the tumor cell's glycolysis (Warburg, 1930; Weinhouse, 1955; Boxer and Devlin, 1961; Aisenberg, 1961c; Racker, 1965), it became necessary to investigate the contribution of the adenylate energy charge to metabolic regulation (especially of glycolysis) in the neoplastic cell.

B. Levels of Charge in Tumors

We have already shown that several of the above-mentioned parameters, which are essential in establishing and maintaining an energy charge in the various subcellular compartments, are altered in neoplastic liver. Does this indicate a charge differential in neoplastic tissues? We have measured the levels of ATP, ADP, and AMP in normal and tumor tissues (Criss, 1973a,b) and calculated the overall adenylate energy charge. The charge was 0.87, 0.89, 0.90, and 0.91 in normal liver, a group of highly differentiated hepatomas, a group of poorly differentiated hepatomas, and Novikoff ascites cells, respectively (Table III). Novikoff ascites cells, under anaerobic conditions, were capable of maintaining a high charge when in-

TABLE III

Q and Adenylate Charge of Liver and Morris Hepatomas[a]

Tissue	ATP	ADP	AMP	Q	Adenylate charge
	(μm/gm tissue)				
Liver	2.47 ± .20	0.51 ± .03	0.15 ± .02	1.42	0.869
Highly dif. hepatomas					
9618A	2.63 ± .23	0.47 ± .04	0.14 ± .03	1.88	0.887
8999	2.78 ± .26	0.43 ± .06	0.14 ± .03		
Poorly dif. hepatomas					
3924A	2.90 ± .23	0.42 ± .05	0.13 ± .02		
3683F	2.72 ± .24	0.44 ± .06	0.14 ± .03	2.06	0.896
Novikoff (ascites)	2.91 ± .26	0.34 ± .04	0.15 ± .03		0.908

[a] Reprinted with permission from Criss (1973a, b).

cubated in the presence of glucose, but not in the presence of pyruvate, succinate, or 2-deoxyglucose (Figs. 1 and 2). Aerobically, in the presence of glyoxylate to inhibit aconitase and/or isocitrate dehydrogenase, Novikoff ascites cells maintained a high charge when incubated in the presence of glucose or glutamate, but not in the presence of pyruvate, citrate, or isocitrate (Tables IV and V). However, in the absence of glyoxylate, the adenylate energy charge was maintained (but not superenhanced) by any combination of the carbon sources. It would appear that Novikoff ascites cells can completely maintain a maximum adenylate energy charge utilizing only the cytoplasmic enzymatic phosphorylating systems or only the mitochondrial enzymatic phosphorylating systems [the latter is probably via the modified cycle as described by Borst (1962)]. However, when both systems are allowed to function, they do not raise the charge above that which each system is capable of maintaining on its own. Thus, the tumor cell has and maintains a very high (perhaps increased) adenylate energy charge. And it is likely that tumor mitochondria are functionally sound but may be unable to function at maximum capacity because they are unable to obtain adequate precursor metabolites. Therefore, it simply appears that the cancer cell has adapted itself for survival in an environment that is conducive to high cytoplasmic glycolysis regardless of the presence of oxygen

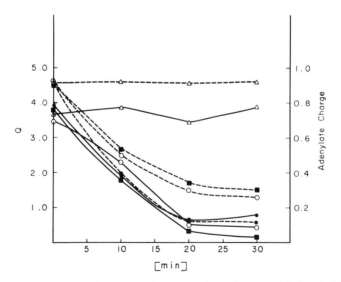

Fig. 1.   Response of Q and adenylate charge in ascites cells (anaerobically). Solid line, Q; dashed line, adenylate charge; closed circle, no additives; open triangle, +5 mM glucose; open hexagon, +5 mM pyruvate; closed square, +5 mM succinate. Reprinted with permission from Criss (1973b).

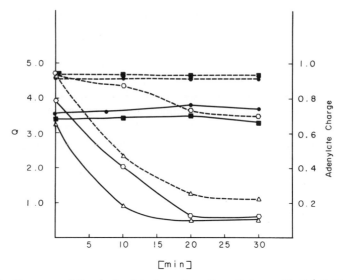

Fig. 2. Responses of Q and adenylate charge in ascites cells (anaerobically). Solid line, Q; dashed line, adenylate charge; closed circle, +5 mM glucose; open triangle, +5 mM 2-deoxy-glucose + 1 mM glucose; open hexagon, +5 mM 2-deoxyglucose + 5 mM glucose; +5mM 2-deoxyglucose + 15 mM glucose. Reprinted with permission from Criss (1973b).

or the availability of the necessary metabolites for oxidative phos-phorylation.

III.   Adenylate Kinase

Adenylate kinase (EC 2.7.4.3) is the enzymatic component of the adenylate energy charge system. Therefore, we investigated this enzymatic system in normal and neoplastic rat tissues. Summaries of our overall *in vivo* studies in Morris hepatomas and *in vitro* studies with homogenous preparations of adenylate kinase from liver and Morris hepatoma 3924A are given in Tables VI, VII, and VIII (Criss, 1971b, 1973a,b). Hepatoma 3924A is a poorly differentiated tumor.

A. In Vivo Comparisons

Liver adenylate kinase is located in the cytoplasm and in the outer com-partment of mitochondria. The overall reaction parameter (Q) of 1.3 is near the *in vitro* K_{eq} value for adenylate kinase indicating that this enzy-matic system may be near equilibrium in liver tissue and probably plays a

TABLE IV

Effect of Glyoxylate on the Production of ATP in Ascites Cells[a]

Preincubation additive	Incubation additive	ATP	ADP (μmoles/ml cells)	AMP	Q	Adenylate charge
		Experiment 1				
None	20 mM pyruvate	2.93 ± 0.21	0.34 ± 0.05	0.13 ± 0.02	3.31	0.91
10 mM glyoxylate	None	1.37 ± 0.19	1.16 ± 0.11	0.52 ± 0.09	0.53	0.64
10 mM glyoxylate	20 mM pyruvate	1.46 ± 0.22	1.11 ± 0.18	0.49 ± 0.11	0.58	0.66
		Experiment 2				
None	20 mM citrate	2.94 ± 0.18	0.34 ± 0.11	0.12 ± 0.06	3.04	0.91
10 mM glyoxylate	None	1.20 ± 0.22	1.37 ± 0.28	0.61 ± 0.10	0.39	0.59
10 mM glyoxylate	20 mM citrate	1.17 ± 0.16	1.42 ± 0.23	0.62 ± 0.17	0.36	0.59
		Experiment 3				
None	20 mM isocitrate	2.90 ± 0.21	0.33 ± 0.09	0.11 ± 0.04	2.93	0.92
10 mM glyoxylate	None	1.11 ± 0.26	1.32 ± 0.30	0.53 ± 0.14	0.34	0.60
10 mM glyoxylate	20 mM isocitrate	1.16 ± 0.17	1.41 ± 0.20	0.61 ± 0.19	0.37	0.58
		Experiment 4				
None	20 mM glutamate	2.88 ± 0.17	0.36 ± 0.08	0.15 ± 0.07	3.32	0.09
10 mM glyoxylate	None	1.50 ± 0.21	1.41 ± 0.26	0.41 ± 0.16	0.31	0.67
10 mM glyoxylate	20 mM glutamate	2.58 ± 0.24	0.51 ± 0.22	0.21 ± 0.13	2.08	0.86

[a] Reprinted with permission from Criss (1973b).

TABLE V

Effect of Glyoxylate on the Maintenance of the Adenylate Energy Charge in Ascites Cells[a]

Preincubation additive	Incubation additive	ATP	ADP (μmoles/ml cells)	AMP	Q	Adenylate charge
		Experiment 1				
None	Glucose	2.90 ± 0.22	0.32 ± 0.07	0.14 ± 0.04	3.94	0.91
None	Pyruvate	2.89 ± 0.26	0.33 ± 0.11	0.15 ± 0.05	3.97	0.91
None	Glutamate	2.92 ± 0.19	0.31 ± 0.08	0.13 ± 0.04	3.95	0.92
None	Glucose + pyruvate	3.02 ± 0.24	0.30 ± 0.09	0.17 ± 0.05	5.70	0.91
None	Glucose + glutamate	3.04 ± 0.27	0.29 ± 0.10	0.16 ± 0.06	6.07	0.91
None	Pyruvate + glutamate	2.97 ± 0.21	0.30 ± 0.12	0.16 ± 0.03	5.28	0.91
None	Glucose + pyruvate + glutamate	3.09 ± 0.25	0.38 ± 0.11	0.16 ± 0.04	6.33	0.92
		Experiment 2				
Glyoxylate	Glucose	2.93 ± 0.23	0.32 ± 0.07	0.14 ± 0.03	4.10	0.91
Glyoxylate	Pyruvate	0.40 ± 0.23	1.05 ± 0.30	1.50 ± 0.27	0.55	0.32
Glyoxylate	Glutamate	2.89 ± 0.19	0.32 ± 0.08	0.14 ± 0.03	3.97	0.91
Glyoxylate	Glucose + pyruvate	2.95 ± 0.27	0.32 ± 0.09	0.16 ± 0.06	4.62	0.91
Glyoxylate	Glucose + glutamate	2.93 ± 0.25	0.33 ± 0.11	0.15 ± 0.04	4.04	0.91
Glyoxylate	Pyruvate + glutamate	2.90 ± 0.25	0.32 ± 0.09	0.14 ± 0.03	3.98	0.91
Glyoxylate	Glucose + pyruvate + glutamate	2.97 ± 0.28	0.30 ± 0.09	0.15 ± 0.05	4.94	0.91

[a] Reprinted with permission from Criss (1973b).

TABLE VI

In Vivo Examination of Adenylate Kinase Activity[a]

	Liver	Hepatoma
Activity in cytosol	28[b]	9.8
Activity in ribosomes	2	0.1
Activity in mitochondria	133	0.5
Activity in nuclei	4	0.1
Location in mitochondria	Outer compartment	None
Reaction parameter Q^c	1.33	2.08
Response to fasting	+	+
Response to refeeding glucose	+	0[d]
Response to insulin	+	0
Relationship to respiration	+	0

[a] Composited from Criss (1970, 1971a) and Criss *et al.* (1970b).

[b] Activity is expressed as μmoles product per gram tissue wet weight at 25°C.

[c] $Q = [ATP][AMP]/[ADP]^2$; K_{eq} for the adenylate kinase catalyzed reaction *in vitro* would be equal to Q at equilibrium; $K_{eq} = 1.1 = Q$ at equilibrium.

[d] +, stimulatory; −, inhibitory; 0, no response.

major role in regulating energy levels. The liver enzyme is under direct control of the glucose–insulin axis and high levels of the mitochondrial form are correlated with high rates of tissue respiration. Tumor adenylate kinase is greatly decreased and found only in the cytoplasm. The lower activity is reflected in the overall reaction parameter which is four in the hepatoma. The tumor enzyme does not respond to dietary or hormonal manipulations like the liver enzyme. The latter type of studies will be reviewed in greater detail in a later section of this manuscript.

B. Kinetic Comparisons in Vitro

Both the liver and tumor enzyme use ATP, dATP, ADP, or AMP without added Mg^{2+} as substrates. However, Mg^{2+} does stimulate the liver enzyme 2- to 5-fold and the tumor enzyme 4- to 10-fold. Ca^{2+} stimulates both enzymes. Citrate (also isocitrate, fumarate, and malate) is stimulatory in the presence of Mg^{2+} and inhibitory in the absence of Mg^{2+}. Both enzymes are inhibited by free fatty acids, mercurial reagents, and detergent.

TABLE VII

Kinetic Studies with Liver and Tumor Adenylate Kinases[a]

	Liver[b]	Hepatoma[b]
Triphosphate substrate	ATP, dATP	ATP, dATP
Diphosphate substrate	ADP	ADP
Monophosphate substrate	AMP	AMP
Modulators[c]		
Mg^{2+}	+	++
Ca^{2+}	+	+
Citrate (in presence of Mg^{2+})	++	0
Citrate (in absence of Mg^{2+})	−	0
Mercurials	−	−
Detergents	−	−
Fatty acids	−	−

[a] Composited from manuscripts in press.
[b] +, stimulatory; −, inhibitory; 0, no response.
[c] Modulatory studies are from data in press.

C. Physical Protein Comparisons

The liver adenylate kinase has a molecular weight of 39,000 and is composed of three subunits. The hepatoma enzyme is 24,000 daltons and made up of two subunits. The liver enzyme shows changes in spectral absorbancies in the presence of Ca^{2+} or citrate; the tumor enzyme does not. Antibody to liver adenylate kinase cross reacts (Ouchterlong test) with liver, but not with tumor or purified rat skeletal muscle adenylate kinase. The muscle enzyme is found to have a molecular weight of 52,000, is composed of four subunits, and is not stimulated by citrate.

D. Possible Role of Liver Adenylate Kinase in Regulating Mitochondrial ATP Production

The production of mitochondrial ATP is dependent on several coordinated systems including: (1) efficiency of the redox shuttle systems; (2) tricarboxylic and dicarboxylic acid transport (Williamson et al., 1968); and (3) coupling to the adenine nucleotides.

Two of the redox shuttle systems (malate–aspartate and α-glycerophosphate) are greatly reduced in poorly differentiated hepatomas, as has been previously described.

Transportation of the tricarboxylic and dicarboxylic acids into the mitochondrion is dependent on the internal and external cation concentrations and pH (Chappell and Crofts, 1966; Palmieri et al., 1970). The inner membrane of the mitochondrion is appearently impermeable to most ions (Chappell and Crofts, 1966). And there probably exists an exchange diffusion mechanism for the entry of phosphate and an energy-dependent transportation system for the many multivalent ions, such as the mitochondrial substrates. The transportation of substrates (succinate, malate, etc.) was observed to be stimulated by a positive charge on the outer surface of the inner membrane. The charge being established by cation accumulation (Palmieri et al., 1970; Meisner et al., 1972). It is not unlikely that liver mitochondrial adenylate kinase which is localized in the outer compartment, which has been observed to undergo mitochonrial flux, which has a K_{eq} near unity, which is stimulated by citrate, and which has a substrate (ATP) that chelates cations ten times more readily than a product (ADP), may be involved not only in directly altering phosphorylated adenine nucleotide levels while leaving the concentration of PO_4^{3-} unchanged, but also in changing the surface charge on the inner mitochondrial membrane via chelation–nonchelation of cations. High ATP accumulation in the outer mitochondrial compartment could tend to decrease the positive charge in that compartment via Mg^{2+} chelation and would thereby decrease mitochondria substrate uptake. An accumulation of citrate acid cycle metabolites would stimulate adenylate kinase. Low ATP and high ADP in the outer compartment could allow for an increase in positive charge by decreased chelation of Mg^{2+} and would thereby enhance substrate uptake. Adenylate kinase could thus play a homeostatic role here by maintaining

TABLE VIII

Physical Studies with Liver and Tumor Adenylate Kinases[a]

	Liver	Hepatoma
Molecular weight	39,000	24,000
Number of subunits	3	2
Only amino acid differences[b]	11 Alanine	6 Alanine
Isoelectric point	8.1	9.2
Cross reaction with antibody to liver enzyme	Yes	No
Spectral changes with Ca^{2+}	Yes	No
Spectral changes with citrate	Yes	No

[a] Composited from manuscripts in press.

[b] Based on total amino acid analysis and given as residues per 13,000 daltons (smallest subunit).

an optimum level of phosphorylated adenine nucleotides and membrane charge to allow efficient mitochondrial functioning.

Translocation of ADP from outside the inner mitochondrial membrane to the phosphorylation sites within or inside the inner membrane appears to be a rate-limiting step in the oxidative phosphorylation of external (extramitochondrial) ADP (Bruni, 1966; Meisner and Klingenberg, 1968; Pfaff and Klingenberg, 1968; Duée and Vignais, 1969; Henderson and Lardy, 1970). The mitochondrial adenine nucleotide translocation system has the following characteristics: (1) It is specific for ATP, ADP, dATP, and dADP; (2) in a controlled state, the specificity of entrance is ten times greater for ADP than ATP; (3) in an uncontrolled state, the specificity of entrance is about the same for ATP and ADP; (4) the specificity of exit is about equal for ATP and ADP; (5) AMP inhibits the exchange of both ATP and ADP; and (6) Mg^{2+} causes preferential leakage of internal ATP. It is thought that the heterogenous exchange of ATP^{4-} and ADP^{3-} must be accompanied by the exchange of cations, such as H^+ or K^+, so that no resultant change in net charge results from the nucleotide exchange. Therefore, this system requires a very carefully regulated membrane potential to allow the preferred $ADP_{ex} \leftrightarrow ATP_{in}$ exchange.

High ATP accumulation in the outer compartment would decrease the positive charge (ATP chelation of Mg^{2+}) and thus not only decrease the inward transport of mitochondrial substrates (succinate, malate, etc.) but decrease the favorability of the $ADP_{ex} \leftrightarrow ATP_{in}$ exchange reaction. High levels of the other adenylate kinase substrate, AMP, could act as an inhibitor of the entire adenine nucleotide exchange reaction. In contradistinction, high levels of the adenylate kinase product, ADP, could allow for a higher positive charge in the outer compartment (via decreased chelation of Mg^{2+}) which would stimulate inward transport of mitochondrial substrates and would, of course, supply the translocase with transporter material. Adenylate kinase simultaneously decreases ATP and AMP and increases ADP. It could thus serve

$$ATP + AMP \underset{\text{kinase}}{\overset{\text{adenylate}}{\rightleftarrows}} 2ADP$$

as an excellent homogenous mechanism to maintain efficiently coupled liver mitochondria.

The postulated mechanism of the involvement adenylate kinase in the control of mitochondrial functioning would be as follows: Under conditions of adequate reduced precursors for mitochondrial oxidation, adenylate kinase would be stimulated. The stimulated enzyme could more readily maintain a coupled, oxidative phosphorylation of exogenous ADP by rapidly removing the buildup of ATP at the translocase exist while simultaneously supplying ADP to the translocase entrance. This would tend to present a decrease in the overall positive charge on the outside of the inner membrane which might result from ATP chelation of Mg^{2+}. The stimulated influx of the reduced metabolites which resulted from a high positive charge on the outside of the inner membrane would be maintained, and AMP, an inhibitor of the translocase system, would be kept low. Under conditions of a lack of reduced precursors for mitochondrial oxidation, adenylate kinase would not be stimulated. Therefore, a buildup of ATP at the translocase exit might occur. This could cause a possible decrease in the positive charge on the outside of the inner membrane. Thus, one result could be a reduction in the stimulation of metabolite and ADP translocation inward. If such a mechanism should prove to exist in liver tissue, it would not exist in poorly differentiated hepatoma tissue because of a lack of mitochondrial adenylate kinase in the latter.

IV.   Metabolic Patterns

Loss of a particular form of an enzyme (an isozyme) is not an unusual phenomena in neoplasia. Just as the process of differentiation results in the decoding of specific genes which results in specific adult tissue isozymes, so also does the process of dedifferentiation or neoplastic development result in the decoding of specific genes which results in specific noeplastic tissue isozymes. We have observed this phenomena in three isozymic systems (Table IX).

Rat tissue adenylate kinase was observed to exist as five different electrophoretic entities on isoelectrofocusing columns. The major isozyme in adult liver tissue was found to be the major isozyme in highly differentiated

TABLE IX

Comparison of Isozymes in Normal, Fetal, and Neoplastic Rat Tissues[a]

Enzyme	Adult liver	Adult muscle	Fetal liver[b]	Highly dif. hepatoma[c]	Poorly dif. hepatoma[d]
Adenylate kinase	III	II	IV	III	IV
Pyruvate kinase	I	II	III	I	III
Malate dehydrogenase	I	III	III	I	III

[a] Methods for identification of isozymes are described in Criss (1969) and Criss et al. (1970a).

[b] Liver from fetuses three days before birth.

[c] Highly differentiated Morris hepatoma 9618A.

[d] Poorly differentiated Morris hepatoma 3924A.

Morris hepatoma 9618A. Isozyme II was the major species in adult skeletal muscle; while isozyme IV was observed in both fetal liver and poorly differentiated hepatoma 3924A.

Pyruvate kinase existed as five electrophoretic forms upon isoelectrofocusing. Isozyme I was the major species in adult liver and a highly differentiated hepatoma. Isozyme II was the predominant form in skeletal muscle. While isozyme III was the pyruvate kinase in fetal liver and a poorly differentiated hepatoma.

Malate dehydrogenase was observed as three electrophoretic entities by isoelectrofucusing chromatography. Isozyme I was found in adult liver and a highly differentiated hepatoma. Isozyme III predominated in skeletal muscle, fetal liver, and a poorly differentiated hepatoma.

In all of the above systems, the major isozymic form which existed in adult liver was greatly diminished in the poorly differentiated heptoma. And the predominate enzymatic species in the poorly differentiated hepatoma was the same species of enzyme found in the fetal liver. This is the most significant aspect of studies of this type. These findings may be added to the large and ever growing body of evidence that tumors acquire fetal characteristics, both isozymes and antigens. So we must now become aware of the fact that neoplastic tissues do not have a large body of proteins (certainly not enzymatic machinery) which are unique to biology. But, rather, they have a group of proteins which are simply dissimilar to those of the parent (adult) differentiated tissue and may be similar to the embryonic or nondifferentiated tissue. Therefore, it is the derepression of otherwise repressed genes and/or the repression of otherwise derepressed genes that allows for the development of neoplastic characteristics.

Observations of the above type have led to two of the most recent cancer theories. The "concept of fetalism," as proposed by Knox (1972), explains the fetal-like patterns of tumors as a convergence of genetic expression which results in a common metabolic pattern. Just as different fetal tissues resemble each other more closely than do the adult tissues into which they develop, so also do different tumor tissues resemble each other more closely than do the adult tissues from which they may have developed. "Oncogeny as blocked ontogeny," which was proposed by Potter (Walker and Potter, 1972), is a theory based on observed changes in tissue isozymic composition. Many of the isozymic patterns observed in neoplastic tissues are similar to the isozymic patterns of the corresponding fetal tissue and dissimilar to the isozymic patterns of corresponding adult tissues. Both postulates would declare that the genetic readout in tumor tissues is very similar to the genetic readout in fetal tissues and not a unique form of genetic expression (Criss, 1971b).

V.   Control of Metabolic Patterns by Control of Genetic Expression

Much of the tumor cell's metabolic machinery and metabolic patterns conform to the machinery and patterns found in normal, immature, and rapidly growing cells. And one observes the same enzymatic and isozymic changes occurring during the differentiation from fetal to adult tissues that he observes during dedifferentiation from adult to neoplastic tissues (but opposite in direction). Therefore, one has hope that many of the "natural" controlling mechanisms are intact during the process of neoplastic development, but that they are either working in the opposite direction or result in a metabolic pattern which is opposite or nonadult-like in character. For example, enzymes which are not inducible in fetal liver at four days prior to birth are inducible in fetal liver at one to two days before birth (Greengard, 1969). So, if these controls are indeed functional but modified as in fetal liver four days prior to birth, it opens up a completely new area of specific chemical therapy. It would not be necessary to "eliminate" the tumor cell, but to simply redirect the controlling elements.

At present, we are working, at best, in a very dimly lit tunnel. Each of the known specific stimuli for genetic expression or even for differentiation acts strictly within the context of a definite stage of tissue and environmental milieu. At other tissue stages, in other tissues, or even in different stages of cell cycle, the same stimulus will not be effective. But perhaps this is precisely the problem in the differentiation of dedifferentiation of a tissue type. The controlling mechanisms, themselves, are very specific for a specific stage in a specific tissue. It is this specificity within the context of a specific tissue which must be critically examined for modification in neoplastic controls. One major "natural" controlling mechanism of tissue differentiation and development is certainly most specific; the action of trophic hormones on a target tissue.

A. Modified Controls in Poorly Differentiated Tumors

Control of genetic expression in malignant tissues is currently a very active area of tumor investigation (see Kaplan, 1963; Pitot and Cho, 1965; Pitot, 1966; Weber and Lea, 1966; Weinhouse 1966; Knox 1967; Criss, 1971b). There are many reports of modified controls of genetic expression in tumors. Most of these studies were performed by monitoring a final genomic product, e.g., enzymatic activity. Specific enzymes can be induced in specific differentiated tissues by treatment of the cell or tissue system with specific hormones and/or dietary metabolites. Most of these hormonal-dietary responses in normal adult tissues are found to be modified in complementary neoplastic tissues. Tables X–XIII illustrate three such systems where the responses of the genetic expression in the normal adult liver is different than the responses in poorly differentiated hepatomas. The results lead to obvious changes in metabolic patterns and control mechanisms. They are described below.

Liver and tumor adenylate kinase activity (AK) increased upon fasting of the animals for 36 hours. However, upon refeeding high glucose, the liver AK decreased while the tumor AK remained elevated. In the diabetic rat

TABLE X

Inductive Response of Adenylate Kinase in Normal and Neoplastic
Liver Tissues[a, b]

	Liver	Novikoff hepatoma	#3924A
Normal			
Fed	162 ± 11	33 ± 6	18 ± 4
Fasted	321 ± 19	59 ± 9	39 ± 9
Refed high glucose	116 ± 18	63 ± 10	33 ± 7
Fasted + actinomycin D	169 ± 16	39 ± 9	24 ± 4
Adrenalectomized			
Fed	122 ± 13	27 ± 6	13 ± 3
Fasted	208 ± 10	28 ± 7	14 ± 4
Refed high glucose	129 ± 15	24 ± 5	16 ± 4
Refed + hydrocortisone	133 ± 14	12 ± 4	16 ± 4
Diabetic			
Fed	390 ± 26	36 ± 7	21 ± 7
Fasted	381 ± 21	26 ± 5	25 ± 7
Refed high glucose	372 ± 17	33 ± 7	22 ± 5
Refed + insulin	180 ± 13	34 ± 6	19 ± 4
Ovariectomized			
Fed	172 ± 12	31 ± 7	17 ± 3
Fasted	193 ± 17	56 ± 12	31 ± 4
Refed high glucose	139 ± 14	52 ± 11	29 ± 6
Refed + estrogen	162 ± 13	20 ± 9	15 ± 3
Refed + progesterone	151 ± 12	18 ± 9	13 ± 4
Refed + testosterone	169 ± 14	26 ± 9	13 ± 4

[a] Reprinted with permission from Criss (1973d).

[b] Value are given in μm/gm tissue.

TABLE XI

Inductive Response of Pyruvate Kinase in Normal and Neoplastic
Liver Tissues[a,b]

	Liver	Novikoff hepatoma	#3924A
Normal			
Fed	30 ± 6	180 ± 17	165 ± 14
Fasted	9 ± 2	153 ± 14	149 ± 13
Refed high glucose	83 ± 9	192 ± 14	182 ± 14
Refed + actinomycin D	33 ± 7	151 ± 12	163 ± 14
Adrenalectomized			
Fed	37 ± 8	159 ± 14	149 ± 11
Fasted	21 ± 7	153 ± 10	156 ± 13
Refed high glucose	70 ± 11	164 ± 11	162 ± 14
Refed + hydrocortisone	55 ± 10	107 ± 10	154 ± 11
Diabetic			
Fed	12 ± 5	199 ± 19	149 ± 10
Fasted	8 ± 3	179 ± 16	146 ± 13
Refed high glucose	11 ± 3	163 ± 14	157 ± 16
Refed + insulin	27 ± 6	178 ± 14	155 ± 14
Ovariectomized			
Fed	22 ± 5	149 ± 11	179 ± 17
Fasted	19 ± 5	133 ± 11	161 ± 14
Refed high glucose	49 ± 7	162 ± 13	159 ± 14
Refed + estrogen	39 ± 7	156 ± 10	166 ± 14
Refed + progesterone	40 ± 8	162 ± 14	167 ± 16
Refed + testosterone	33 ± 6	138 ± 13	158 ± 13

[a] Reprinted with permission from Criss (1973d).
[b] Values are given in $\mu m/gm$ tissue.

liver AK was elevated and did not respond to dietary manipulation; however, tumor AK was elevated, decreased upon fasting, and increased upon refeeding high glucose. Liver AK was not affected but tumor AK was decreased in hydrocortisone-treated adrenalectomized animals. Responses of increase in enzymatic activity were inhibited by actinomycin D (Table X).

Liver pyruvate kinase activity (PK) decreased upon fasting and increased upon refeeding high glucose to normal and adrenalectomized animals.

TABLE XII

Inductive Response of Glucose-6-Phosphate Dehydrogenase in Normal and Neoplastic Liver Tissues[a,b]

	Liver	Novikoff hepatoma	#3924A
Normal			
Fed	8 ± 2	35 ± 5	27 ± 4
Fasted	4 ± 1	36 ± 5	27 ± 4
Refed high glucose	14 ± 2	41 ± 5	30 ± 5
Refed + actinomycin D	9 ± 2	33 ± 4	26 ± 3
Adrenalectomized			
Fed	7 ± 1	31 ± 3	25 ± 4
Fasted	5 ± 1	34 ± 4	29 ± 3
Refed high glucose	10 ± 2	35 ± 4	24 ± 3
Refed + hydrocortisone	8 ± 1	22 ± 2	15 ± 3
Diabetic			
Fed	3 ± 1	38 ± 6	30 ± 5
Fasted	4 ± 1	36 ± 5	27 ± 4
Refed high glucose	7 ± 2	32 ± 4	30 ± 4
Refed + insulin	8 ± 2	37 ± 5	29 ± 4
Ovariectomized			
Fed	6 ± 2	27 ± 4	21 ± 3
Fasted	5 ± 2	29 ± 4	24 ± 4
Refed high glucose	9 ± 2	32 ± 4	26 ± 4
Refed + estrogen	13 ± 4	39 ± 5	34 ± 5
Refed + progesterone	14 ± 4	36 ± 5	30 ± 5
Refed + testosterone	13 ± 3	40 ± 6	36 ± 6

[a] Reprinted with permission from Criss (1973d).

[b] Values are given in μm/gm tissue.

Liver PK was reduced in the fed diabetic animals and did not change upon alterations in the diet. Tumor PK was high and remained high during all dietary manipulations; except, it was repressed in the hydrocortisone-treated adrenalectomized animals. Responses of increase in enzymatic activity were inhibited by actinomycin D (Table XI).

Liver glucose-6-phosphate dehydrogenase (G6PD) decreased upon fasting, increased upon refeeding high glucose, and was decreased in the diabetic animals. Tumor G6PD did not change upon fasting and/or re-feeding high glucose, was not decreased in the diabetic animals, but was decreased by hydrocortisone treatment of the adrenalectomized animals. Responses of increases in enzymatic activity were inhibited by actinomycin D (Table XII).

It would appear that the enzymatic activities of adenylate kinase, and glucose-6-phosphate dehydrogenase, as extracted from tumor tissues, show

TABLE XIII

Modification of Genetic Expression in Tumors[a]

Enzymatic System	Type of Modification[b]	References
Aspartate aminotransferase	⊕ Hydrocortisone	Otani and Morris, 1968; Nisselbaum and Bodansky, 1969; Kopelovich et al., 1970
Serine dehydratase[c]	⊖ Dietary (multiple substrate)	Jost and Pitot, 1970
Arginase	⊕ Cortisol	Wee and Morris, 1970; Wee et al., 1971
Glutamine synthetase	⊕ Cortisol	Wee and Morris, 1970; Wee et al., 1971
Tryptophan pyrrolase[c]	⊖ Dietary (substrate)	Pitot and Pitot et al., 1965; Pitot and Jost, 1967; Pitot, 1968
Ornithine transaminase	⊖ Dietary (glucose)	Pitot, 1968
Hydroxymethylglutaryl-CoA reductase[c]	⊖ Dietary (substrate)	Pitot et al., 1965; Siperstein and Tagan, 1966; Pitot, 1968
Pyruvate carboxylase	⊖ Glucocorticoid	Weber, 1963
Phosphoenolpyruvate carboxylase	⊖ Glucocorticoid	Weber, 1963
Fructose-1,6-diphosphatase	⊖ Glucocorticoid	Weber, 1963
Glucose-6-phosphatase	⊖ Glucocorticoid	Weber, 1963
Glucose-6-phosphate dehydrogenase	⊕ ⊖ Insulin, cortisol, dietary	Wenner, 1960; Potter and Ono, 1961
Adenylate kinase	⊕ Hydrocortisone, ⊖ Insulin-dietary	d
Pyruvate kinase	⊕ Hydrocortisone ⊖ Insulin-dietary	d
Amino acid levels	⊖ Glucocorticoid	Weber et al., 1965
RNA levels	⊖ Glucocorticoid	Weber and Lea, 1966
Cyclic AMP levels	⊖ Glucagon	Butcher et al., 1972

[a] Data were summarized from the listed references.

[b] ⊕ = enhanced response; ⊖ = decreased response.

[c] Show differential sensitivity of enzyme induction to actinomycin D.

[d] Current manuscript.

a decreased overall response to dietary manipulations, decreased response to insulin, and increased response to hydrocortisone. These studies illustrate a "commonness" in the modified responses to hormones and/or dietary alterations of three enzymatic systems in rat liver tumors.

The modified responses of these three enzymatic systems (possibly three genetic units) in tumors are not unique. Table XIII is a tabulation of the modified responses of other enzymatic systems which have been observed in tumors. Most of these reports are from the Morris hepatoma lines. In many systems, the responses to glucocorticoids was diminished. In several systems, the response to glucocorticoid was increased. Genetic responses to the protein hormones (insulin or glucagon) were diminished. Therefore, not only has the neoplastic cell lost several of its adult enzymatic systems, but the overall response of many of the remaining enzymatic systems has undergone drastic modifications. Upon alterations in the environment, changes in hormonal or dietary milieu, the genetic unit, which would normally respond to such changes in the adult differentiated tissue in a specific manner, appears to be either not capable of responding or overresponds in the neoplastic tissue.

B. Modified Controls in Highly Differentiated Tumors

A modified response can even be observed in highly differentiated tumor tissues (Tables XIV and XV, Watanabe et al., 1969; Scott et al., 1972). All of these studies illustrate that the normal responses of a genetic system (to hormonal and/or dietary changes) in highly differentiated liver tissue have undergone some form of modification in highly differentiated hepatomas.

C. Heterogeneity of Modified Responses

However, we must keep in mind that the same modified responses have not been observed in all tumors. Tyrosine aminotransferase was inducible by insulin, hydrocortisone, and cAMP in H-35 cells, but it was induced only by insulin and hydrocortisone in HTC cells (Granner et al., 1968; Lee et al., 1970; Butcher et al., 1971). Examination of several enzymes in the slow growing and highly differentiated Morris hepatoma 9618A revealed that some enzymes respond to dietary manipulation and other enzymes do not respond; however, the response patterns in the hepatoma always differed from the response patterns in the host liver (Watanabe et al., 1969). The responses of α-aminoisobutyrate transport and tyrosine aminotransferase varied widely in a large group of highly differentiated Morris hepatomas (Scott et al., 1972). Thus, the genetic responses (using enzymatic activity to monitor gene expression) are modified but are not

TABLE XIV

Inductive Response of Adenylate Kinase in
Differentiated Liver Tissues[a]

	Activity of AK
Liver of fasted rat[b]	341 ± 23
Liver of refed rat[c]	111 ± 16
Tumor 9618A of fasted rat[d]	134 ± 19
Tumor 9618A of refed rat	110 ± 14
Tumor 7787 of fasted rat	132 ± 14
Tumor 7787 of refed rat	109 ± 11
Tumor 7794B of fasted rat	109 ± 10
Tumor 7794B of refed rat	138 ± 12
Tumor 8999 of fasted rat	140 ± 17
Tumor 8999 of refed rat	108 ± 15

[a] Methods are given in Criss (1969, 1973a).

[b] Assays made from hypotonic extracts of tissues taken from rats which were fasted 64 hours.

[c] Assays made from hypotonic extracts of tissues taken from rats which were fasted 64 hours and refed a 30% glucose-saline solution for 16 hours.

[d] All tumors are classified as highly differentiated Morris hepatomas.

identical in all neoplastic tissues. In general, the genetic responses in tumors are different from the complementary genetic responses in complementary adult differentiated tissues.

VI. Derepressive Interception

Modification in the responses of genetic units to protein hormones, catecholamines, and steroid hormones have been observed in many types of neoplastic tissue. One of the mechanisms by which the protein hormones and catecholamines function in adult differentiated tissues involves a cAMP system. One of the mechanisms by which the steroid hormones functions in adult differentiated tissues involves an intracellular binding protein.

A. Cyclic AMP System

Cyclic AMP has become of central importance as a second messenger of hormonal stimulation in tissues. In a large number of hormone-dependent

TABLE XV

Inductive Response of Pyruvate Kinase (PK)
in Differentiated Liver Tissues[a]

	Activity of PK
Liver of fasted rat	8 ± 3
Liver of refed rat	98 ± 14
Tumor 9618A of fasted rat	38 ± 9
Tumor 9618A of refed rat	45 ± 10
Tumor 7787 of fasted rat	34 ± 5
Tumor 7787 of refed rat	31 ± 7
Tumor 7794B of fasted rat	36 ± 8
Tumor 7794B of refed rat	34 ± 6
Tumor 8999 of fasted rat	26 ± 6
Tumor 8999 of refed rat	31 ± 9

[a] Methods are given in Criss (1969, 1973a).

tissue types cAMP intracellularly propagates or mimics the stimulatory signal from the protein hormones which interact primarily at the cellular surface (Robison *et al.,* 1968; Kuo and Greengard, 1969; Greengard and Costa, 1970; Tao *et al.,* 1970; Majumder and Turkington, 1971). Cyclic AMP binds to specific cytoplasmic proteins. The binding allows activation of any of several protein kinases in a variety of tissue types (Fig. 3). The protein kinases phosphorylate several different intracellular proteins. They regulate energy metabolism in liver, muscle, and adipose tissue by activating the key phosphorylases and lipases and inactivating the synthetases. They may regulate gene response by phosphorylation of nuclear histones and non-histone proteins (latter is personal communication from Dr. Gary Stein). Thus, the stimulation of a hormonally responsive tissue by its trophic hormone is transmitted through a cAMP system which includes: membrane receptors, membrane-bound adenyl cyclases, cAMP, cytoplasmic cAMP-binding proteins, protein kinases, and cAMP-phosphodiesterases. The specificity within such a system would appear to reside in the membrane receptors, membrane-bound adenyl cyclases, cAMP-binding proteins, protein kinases, possibly a protein kinase inhibitor, and the phosphodiesterases.

Several components of the cAMP system have been examined in neoplastic tissues. Certain adrenal tumors contained multiple instead of single membrane receptors (see Hinshaw and Ney, Chapter 10, this volume). Adenyl cyclase activity and cAMP levels were lower in tumors growing *in vitro* (Heidrick and Ryan, 1971; Makman, 1971). Increased levels of cAMP are associated with *in vitro* growth confluency in both normal and neoplastic cells, but neoplastic cells appear to be more growth sensitive to cAMP than normal cells (Heidrick and Ryan, 1970). Neoplastic liver tissue was found to have a decreased level of a high K_m phosphodiesterase and an increased levels of a low K_m phosphodiesterase (Rhoads *et al.*, 1972; Clark *et al.*, 1973). The overall response of the cAMP system in hepatomas to the trophic hormone glucagon was greatly decreased when compared to its corresponding response in adult differentiated liver tissue (Butcher *et al.*, 1972). The modification in the response of any of the components of the cAMP system, which regulates specificity of action, could allow unlimited growth potential. Examination of the many components of the cAMP system in neoplastic tissues is currently in progress in several laboratories.

B. Intracellular Steroid-Binding Proteins

Specific intracellular binding proteins have been observed for most steroid hormones. These protein receptors are found specifically in their target tissues (Edelman and Fimognari, 1968; Gardner and Tomkins, 1969;

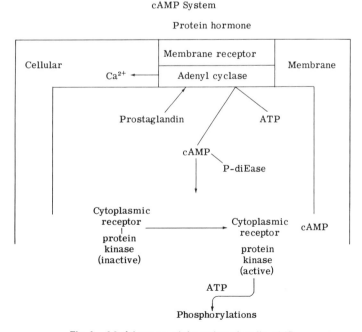

Fig. 3. Model system of the action of cyclic AMP.

Notides, 1970; Shrader *et al.*, 1972). Based on studies in the chick oviduct and immature rat uterine systems, the steroid immediately enters into the target cell, binds to a steroid receptor in the cytoplasm, enters the nucleus as a steroid-protein complex, and eventually is associated with nuclear chromatin (Jensen *et al.*, 1968; Means and O'Malley, 1972; Shrader *et al.*, 1972). This sequence of events results in derepression or decoding of specific genetic units (Fig. 4). The specificity within such a system would appear to reside in the binding proteins.

Implication of modifications in the steroid-binding system in tumors can be observed from several laboratories. Lymphoma cell lines which were resistant to cortisol killing had less cortisone-binding protein than parent lines which were sensitive to cortisol (Baxter *et al.*, 1971). Potential carcinogenic interference of the binding of cortisol to cortisol binders of liver tissue has been reported (Singer and Litwack, 1971; Litwack *et al.*,

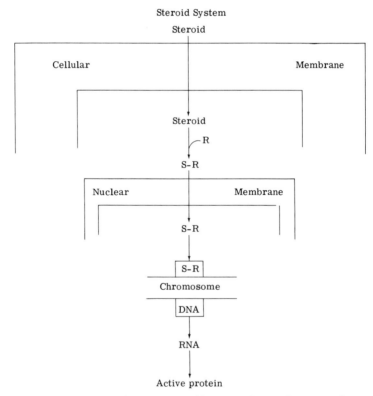

Fig. 4. Model system of the action of steroid hormones. R, protein receptor; S, steroid hormone.

1972). Hormone-dependent rat mammary carcinomas have a high affinity estradiol-binding protein that the hormone-independent carcinomas do not have (McGuire and Julian, 1971). If the steroid binders are directly involved in the genetic expression of their target tissues, modification within the chain of events leading from the initial binding of hormone to protein receptor to the newly synthesized and active gene products (e.g., active enzymes or protein derepressors) could be involved in altering the metabolic state of the tissue such that the result might lead to unchecked growth and malignancy.

C. A Common Class of Receptors?

Very recently, reports from Litwack and his colleagues, illustrate that the cAMP system and the steroid receptor systems of hormone action may not be mutually exclusive of one another. This group has isolated a class of cytoplasmic proteins from liver tissue which binds both cortisol and cAMP (Filler and Litwack, 1973). They have shown this class of proteins to inhibit protein kinase activity. Since this class of proteins also binds 3-methyl-cholanthrene and dimethaminoazobenzene (two potent carcinogens), there has now been identified a possible "common" class of molecules in which the actions of protein hormones (or catecholamines), steroid hormones (at least for cortisol), and two chemical carcinogens are centered. This is an area of neoplasia which requires intensive investigation. It may be possible in the near future to directly correlate carcinogenic action with direct modification of genetic expression at the molecular level.

Therefore, data continues to accumulate which indicates that some of the earliest events in the development of the metabolism of neoplastic tissues must involve a modification in the expression of the genotype of normal tissues. *Derepressive interception* would appear to be an expression which could describe such modified events (Fig. 5). It allows one to center his attention on any changes which might occur during the normal decoding of genes and would include the events within transcription and translation. This is particularly important since hormones may exert a controlling in-

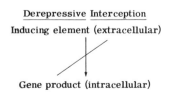

Derepressive Interception

Inducing element (extracellular)

Gene product (intracellular)

Fig. 5. Model of the concept derepressive interception.

fluence at both levels of gene expression. Since we are now able to fairly well define the sequence of events (from hormone to gene loci) which occurs during the molecular action of both protein and steroid hormones, and since some data is already available to illustrate certain modifications in those sequences have occurred in neoplastic tissues, it is encouraging to believe that we may soon begin to pinpoint some of the early molecular lesions which lead to neoplastic development.

VII. Summary

Development and establishment of the Morris "minimal deviation" rat hepatoma system has allowed extensive investigation of cancer metabolism. It has provided international investigators with transplantable lines of tumors of all grade of differentiation. Results from 13 years of studies of the Morris hepatoma system have provided the following picture of tumor metabolism: carbohydrate degradation is increased. Protein, DNA, and RNA synthesis is increased. Lipid synthesis and degradation is decreased. Protein, DNA, and RNA degradation is decreased. These trends were established by measuring the levels of key pathway enzymes and following metabolic flux through those pathway systems.

The poorly differentiated hepatoma cell is a rapidly growing and dividing cell and derives most of its energy needs from carbohydrate degradation. Increases in the activity levels of several cytoplasmic substrate-level phosphorylating enzymes and decreases in the activity levels of several mitochondrial substrate-level phosphorylating enzymes gives the hepatoma cell an advantage in phosphorylating ADP without the large need for mitochondrial oxidation. Also, a decrease in the potential of the malate–aspartate and glycerophosphate redox shuttle systems, decrease in any potential adenylate homeostasis in the outer mitochondrial compartment, and increase in the recycling of NADH within the glycolytic pathway could explain the decreased need of mitochondrial involvement in the extraction of energy for the tumor cell's functioning. That all of these enzymatic shifts are advantageous to the tumor cell which has high energy requirements can be observed from the measurable increase in adenylate energy charge in the poorly differentiated hepatoma cells.

Not only have numerous enzymatic shifts occurred within the hepatoma system, but many isozymic changes have been reported. In general, the poorly differentiated hepatomas have isozymes which are common to fetal liver and/or muscle tissues. Concomitantly with the isozyme shift, one usually finds alterations in intracellular controls such that many of the feedback and feedforward metabolite modulations which are observed in normal adult liver are not present in the poorly differentiated hepatomas.

In all of these above cited changes in hepatoma metabolism, we are, in reality, simply listing changes which occur during tumor progression, not during tumor formation. Because, if one examines the mostly highly differentiated of the Morris hepatomas he is hard pressed to find any of these changes. The enzymatic and isozymic shifts are products of tumor progression. If we examine only the highly differentiated Morris hepatomas (which we can at least define as a very, very early stage in tumor formation), we can observe modifications in the controis of genetic expression as monitored by changes in the activity levels of certain inducible enzymes.

It would appear that early stages of neoplastic development encompass modifications of hormone and/or dietary metabolite controlled expression of genes. *Derepressive interception* is a phrase which describes an interruption in the normal sequence of events which occurs between the event of a hormone acting at the cellular membrane surface (or at cytoplasmic binding level) to the event of the synthesis of a new active protein molecule.

We are now beginning to define more exactly the chain of events which occurs in a tissue that is responsive to a hormone. Many protein hormones interact at the cellular membrane and initiate a sequence of events inside the cell which results in: (1) immediate alterations in energy metabolism via activation and inactivation of key phosphorylases, synthetases, and lipases; and (2) possible production of new active proteins via activation of histone and non-histone proteins which are assoicated with chromatin. Many steroid hormones interact through intracellular binding proteins. Since the steroid–protein complex is directly associated with the chromosomes of the cell, its action is thought to involve a derepression of genetic activity. It has also recently been shown that the two hormone systems may share a common class of proteins. Therefore, since very early neoplastic changes may involve modifications in the hormonally controlled expression of genes, and since a well-defined molecular sequence of events depicting hormonal action is emerging, a new phase of cancer metabolism has begun which could lead to the identification of possible distinct molecular lesions which could result in neoplastic expression.

ACKNOWLEDGMENTS

I would like to express my deepest thanks to Dr. Sidney Weinhouse, who was paramount in initiating and perpetuating these studies, to Dr. Gerald Litwack, whose counsel has always been extremely beneficial, and to Dr. Harold Morris, without whose advice and generous supply of tumor tissue these studies could not have been accomplished. I wish to also thank the many people who also directly contributed to these works: Dr. Virginia Sapico, Mr. Ron Filler, Miss Emilia Siojo, Mr. Seth Alper, Miss Laura Fiddelke, Mrs. Dorothy Fitzgerald, Dr. Tapas Pradhan, Dr. Paul Chun, and Mrs. Caroline Easely.

REFERENCES

Aisenberg, A. C. (1961a). *Cancer Res.* **21,** 295–303.

Aisenberg, A. C. (1961b). *Cancer Res.* **21,** 304–309.

Aisenberg, A. C. (1961c). "The Glycolysis and Respiration of Tumors," Academic Press, New York.

Atkinson, D. E. (1966). *Annu. Rev. Biochem.* **35,** 85–118.

Atkinson, D. E. (1968a). *Biochemistry* **7,** 4030–4034.

Atkinson, D. E. (1968b). *In* "Metabolic Roles of Citrate" (T. W. Goodwin, ed.), pp. 23–40. Academic Press, New York.

Atkinson, D. E. (1969a). *Annu. Rev. Microbiol.* **23,** 47–68.

Atkinson, D. E. (1969b). *In* "Exploitable Molecular Mechanisms and Neoplasia" (University of Texas, M.D. Anderson Hospital and Tumor Institute), pp. 397–413. Williams & Wilkins, Baltimore, Maryland.

Baxter, J. D., Harris, A. W. Tomkins, G. M., and Cohen, M. (1971). *Science* **171,** 189–191.

Borst, P. (1962). *Biochim. Biophys. Acta* **57,** 256–269.

Boxer, G. E., and Devlin, T. M. (1961). *Science* **134,** 1495–1501.

Bruni, A. (1966). *In* "Regulation of Metabolic Processes in Mitochondria" (J. M. Tager *et al.,* eds.), Vol. 7, pp. 275–292. Amer. Elsevier, New York.

Butcher, F. R., Becker, J. E., and Potter, V. R. (1971). *Exp. Cell Res.* **66,** 321–328.

Butcher, F. R., Scott, D. F., Potter, V. R., and Morris, H. P. (1972). *Cancer Res.* **32,** 2135–2140.

Chappell, J. B., and Crofts, A. R. (1966). *In* "Regulation of Metabolic Processes in Mitochondria" (J. M. Tager *et al.,* eds.), Vol. 7, pp. 293–316. Amer. Elsevier, New York.

Clark, J. F., Morris, H. P., and Weber, C. (1973). *Cancer Res.* **33,** 356–361.

Criss, W. E. (1969). *Biochem. Biophys. Res. Commun.* **35,** 901–905.

Criss, W. E. (1970). *J. Biol. Chem.* **245,** 6352–6356.

Criss, W. E. (1971a). *Arch. Biochem. Biophys.* **144,** 138–141.

Criss, W. E. (1971b). *Cancer Res.* **31,** 1523–1542.

Criss, W. E. (1973a). *Cancer Res.* **33,** 51–56.

Criss, W. E. (1973b). *Cancer Res.* **33,** 57–64.

Criss, W. E. (1973c). *Cancer Res.* **33,** 1023–1029.

Criss, W. E. (1973d). *Amer. J. Obstet. Gynecol.* **116,** 753–761.

Criss, W. E., Litwack, G., Morris, H. P., and Weinhouse, S. (1970a). *Cancer Res.* **30,** 370–375.

Criss, W. E., Sapico, V., and Litwack, G. (1970b). *J. Biol. Chem.* **245,** 6346–6351.

Duée, E. D., and Vignais, P. V. (1969). *J. Biol. Chem.* **244,** 3920–3931.

Edelman, I., and Fimognari, G. M. (1968). *Recent Progr. Horm. Res.* **24,** 1–44.

Filler, R., and Criss, W. E. (1971). *Biochem. J.* **122,** 533–555.

Filler, R., and Litwack, G. (1973). *Fed. Proc., Fed. Amer. Soc. Exp. Biol.* **00,** (abstr.).

Gardner, R. S., and Tomkins, G. M. (1969). *J. Biol. Chem.* **244,** 4761–4767.

Goranson, E. S., and Tilser, G. J. (1955). *Cancer Res.* **15,** 626–631.

Granner, D., Chase, L. R., Aurbach, G. D., and Tomkins, G. M. (1968). *Science* **162,** 1018–1020.

Greengard, O. (1969). *Science* **163,** 891–895.

Greengard, P., and Costa, E. (1970). *In* "Role of Cyclic AMP in Cell Function," p. 67. Raven Press, New York.

Greenstein, J. P. (1956). *Cancer Res.* **16,** 641–653.

Haslam, J. M., and Krebs, H. A. (1968). *Biochem. J.* **107,** 656–667.

Heidrick, M. L., and Ryan, W. L. (1970). *Cancer Res.* **30,** 376–378.

Heidrick, M. L., and Ryan, W. L. (1971). *Cancer Res.* **31,** 1313–1315.

Henderson, P. J. F., and Lardy, H. A. (1970). *J. Biol. Chem.* **245**, 1319–1328.

Heuson, J. C., and Legros, N. (1972). *Cancer Res.* **32**, 226–232.

Heuson, J. C., Waelbroeck, C., Legros, N., Gallez, G., Robyn, C., and L'Hermite, M. (1972). *Gynecol. Invest.* **2**, 130–137.

Jensen, E. V. Suzuki, I., Kawashima, T., Stumpf, W. E., Jungblut, P. W., and DeSombre, E. R. (1968). *Proc. Nat. Acad. Sci. U.S.* **59**, 632–638.

Johnson, M. J. (1941). *Science* **94**, 200–202.

Jost, J. P., and Pitot, H. C. (1970). *Cancer Res.* **30**, 387–392.

Kaplan, N. O. (1963). *Bacteriol. Rev.* **27**, 155–169.

Kessler, I. (1970). *J. Nat. Cancer Inst.* **44**, 673–686.

Killington, R. A., Williams, A. E. Ratcliffe, N. A., Whitehead, T. P., and Smith, A. (1971). *Brit. J. Cancer* **25**, 93–105.

Knox, W. E. (1967). *Advan. Cancer Res.* **10**, 117–161.

Knox, W. E. (1972). *Amer. Sci.* **60**, 480–488.

Kodama, M., and Kodama, T. (1970). *Cancer Res.* **30**, 221–227.

Kopelovich, L., Sweetman, L., and Nisselbaum, J. S. (1970). *J. Biol. Chem.* **245**, 2011–2017.

Kuo, J. F., and Greengard, P. (1969). *Proc. Nat. Acad. Sci. U.S.* **64**, 1349–1355.

Lee, K. L., Reel, J. R., and Kenny, F. T. (1970). *J. Biol. Chem.* **245**, 5806–5812.

Liao, C. L., and Atkinson, D. E. (1971a). *J. Bacteriol.* **106**, 31–36.

Liao, C. L., and Atkinson, D. E. (1971b). *J. Bacteriol.* **106**, 37–44.

Litwack, G., Morey, K. S., and Ketterer, B. (1972). *In* "Effects of Drugs on Cellular Control Mechanisms" (B. R. Rabin and R. B. Freedman, eds.), pp. 105–130. Macmillan, New York.

Lo, C. H., Cristofalo, V. J., Morris, H. P., and Weinhouse, S. (1968). *Cancer Res.* **28**, 1–10.

Lynen, F. (1941). *Justus Liebigs Ann. Chem.* **546**, 120–141.

McGuire, W. L., and Julian, J. A. (1971). *Cancer Res.* **31**, 1440–1445.

Majumder, G. C., and Turkington, R. W. (1971). *J. Biol. Chem.* **246**, 5545–5554.

Makman, M. H. (1971). *Proc. Nat. Acad. Sci. U.S.* **68**, 2127–2130.

Means, A. R., and O'Malley, B. W. (1972). *Metab., Clin. Exp.* **21**, 357, 370.

Meisner, H., and Klingenberg, M. (1968). *J. Biol. Chem.* **243**, 3631–3639.

Meisner, H., Palmieri, F., and Quagliariello, E. (1972). *Biochemistry* **11**, 949–955.

Miller, A. L., and Atkinson, D. E. (1972). *Arch. Biochem. Biophys.* **152**, 531–538.

Morris, H. P. (1963). *Progr. Exp. Tumor Res.* **3**, 370–411.

Morris, H. P. (1965). *Advan. Cancer Res.* **9**, 277–302.

Morris, H. P., and Wagner, B. P. (1968). *Methods Cancer Res.* **4**, 125–152.

Nisselbaum, J. S., and Bodansky, O. (1969). *Cancer Res.* **29**, 360–365.

Notides, A. C. (1970). *Endocrinology* **87**, 987–992.

Olson, R. E. (1951). *Cancer Res.* **11**, 571–585.

Opie, L. H., Mansford, K. R. L., and Owens, P. (1971). *Biochem. J.* **124**, 475–490.

Otani, T., and Morris, H. P. (1968). *Cancer Res.* **28**, 2092–2097.

Palmieri, F., Quagliariello, E., and Klingenberg, M. (1970). *Eur. J. Biochem.* **17**, 230–243.

Pfaff, E., and Klingenberg, M. (1968). *Eur. J. Biochem.* **6**, 66–79.

Pitot, H. C. (1966). *Annu. Rev. Biochem.* **35**, 335–368.

Pitot, H. C. (1968). *Cancer Res.* **28**, 1880–1887.

Pitot, H. C., and Cho, Y. S. (1965). *Progr. Exp. Tumor Res.* **7**, 158–223.

Pitot, H. C., and Jost, J. P. (1967). *Nat. Cancer Inst., Monog.* **26**, 145–166.

Pitot, H. C., Peraino, C., Lamar, C., and Kennan, A. C. (1965). *Proc. Nat. Acad. Sci. U.S.* **54**, 845–851.

Potter, V. R., and Ono, T. (1961). *Cold Spring Harbor Symp. Quant. Biol.* **26**, 335.

Puckett, C. L., and Shingleton, W. W. (1972). *Cancer Res.* **32**, 789–790.

Racker, E. (1965). "Mechanisms in Bioenergetics." Academic Press, New York.

Rhoads, A. R., Morris, H. P., and West, W. L. (1972). *Cancer Res.* **32**, 2651–2655.

Robison, G. A., Butcher, R. W., and Sutherland, E. W. (1968). *Annu. Rev. Biochem.* **37**, 149–174.

Salzberg, D. A., and Griffin, A. C. (1952). *Cancer Res.* **12**, 294.

Sapico, V., Litwack, G., and Criss, W. E. (1970). *Biochim. Biophys. Acta* **258**, 436–445.

Scott, D. F., Butcher, F. R., Potter, V. R., and Morris, H. P. (1972). *Cancer Res.* **32**, 2127–2134.

Shrader, W. T., Toft, D., and O'Malley, B. W. (1972). *J. Biol. Chem.* **247**, 2401–2410.

Singer, S., and Litwack, G. (1971). *Cancer Res.* **31**, 1364–1368.

Siperstein, M. D., and Fagan, V. M. (1966). *Cancer Res.* **26**, 7.

Tao, M., Salas, M. L., and Lippmann, F. (1970). *Proc. Nat. Acad. Sci. U.S.* **67**, 408–414.

Vangerov, M. and McKee, R. W. (1955). *Fed. Proc., Fed. Amer. Soc. Exp. Biol.* **14**, 296.

Veech, R. L., Raihman, L., and Krebs, H. A. (1970). *Biochem. J.* **117**, 499–503.

Walker, P. R., and Potter, V. R. (1972). *Advan. Enzyme Regul.* **10**, 339–364.

Warburg, O. (1930). "The Metabolism of Tumors." Arnold, London.

Watanabe, M., Potter, V. R., Reynolds, R. D., Pitot, H. C., and Morris, H. P. (1969). *Cancer Res.* **29**, 1691–1698.

Waterhouse, C., and Kemperman, J. H.(1971). *Cancer Res.* **31**, 1273–1278.

Weber, G. (1963). *Advan. Enzyme Regul.* **1**, 321–340.

Weber, G., and Lea, M. A. (1966). *Advan. Enzyme Regul.* **4**, 115–145.

Weber, G., Singhal, R. L., and Srivastava, S. K. (1965). *Advan. Enzyme Regul.* **3**, 369–387.

Weinhouse, S. (1955). *Advan. Cancer Res.* **3**, 269–325.

Weinhouse, S. (1966). *Gann* **1**, 99–116.

Wenner, C. E. (1960). *Proc. Amer. Ass. Cancer Res.* **3**, 161.

Wenner, C. E. (1967). *Advan. Enzymol.* **29**, 321–390.

White, H. B., III., and Kaplan, N. O. (1969). *J. Biol. Chem.* **244**, 6031–6039.

Williamson, J. R., Browning, E. T., and Olson, M. S. (1968). *Advan. Enzyme Regul.* **6**, 67–100.

Wu, C., and Morris, H. P. (1970). *Cancer Res.* **30**, 2675, 2684.

Wu, C., Bauer, J. M., and Morris, H. P. (1971). *Cancer Res.* **31**, 12–18.

CHAPTER VII

INTERACTION OF THYROTROPIN-RELEASING HORMONE WITH PITUITARY CELLS IN CULTURE

PATRICIA M. HINKLE AND ARMEN H. TASHJIAN, JR.

I. Introduction

Regulation of the synthetic and secretory functions of the anterior pituitary gland is a complex process and is controlled at several loci. For some pituitary hormones, a product of the target endocrine gland exerts direct feedback control on the tropic hormone. For example, thyroxine acts directly on thyrotrophs to decrease the release of thyrotropin, and hydrocortisone depresses the secretion of ACTH. In addition, a major site of control occurs at the level of the hypothalamus. Neural cells in hypothalamic nuclei synthesize factors which stimulate or inhibit the release and synthesis of the various pituitary hormones. These hypothalamic-releasing and -inhibiting factors reach the adenohypophysis through a portal vascular system. The past few years have seen unparalleled progress in understanding the chemistry, action, and synthesis of these hypothalamic-releasing factors. Several of them have been isolated and chemically characterized; all of the factors identified thus far are peptides. Progress in this area has been the subject of a number of recent reviews (McCann and Porter, 1969; Burgus and Guillemin, 1970; Reichlin *et al.*, 1972; Blackwell and Guillemin, 1973; Schally *et al.*, 1973).

In vivo studies on the mechanism of action of hypothalamic-releasing and -inhibiting factors are often difficult to interpret for a number of reasons. In the intact animal, the concentration of a pituitary hormone in peripheral plasma is affected by numerous influences which are difficult to control individually. Once secreted, the circulating hormone is also subject to a variety of metabolic fates which can alter its apparent concentration in plasma. Hypothalamic peptides also tend to be unstable in blood, and it is unclear how much of a systemically injected dose reaches the pituitary gland in an intact form. Since it is now clear that several hypothalamic-releasing and -inhibiting factors affect more than one hormone in the intact animal, there must be multiple target cell types for these factors in the pituitary gland itself. Finally, the concentrations of releasing factors in portal blood are not yet known, and it has only recently been reported that it is possible to measure their concentrations in peripheral plasma and in urine.

All of these considerations emphasize the usefulness of *in vitro* systems in which the actions of hypothalamic factors can be studied under carefully controlled conditions. Clonal strains of hormone-producing pituitary cells in culture offer the advantage of being a single, responsive type of cell. Problems with the instability of hypothalamic peptides can be eliminated or at least monitored directly. Measurement of the response of pituitary cells is more precise and accurate in culture, and it is possible to distinguish between effects on hormone synthesis and release.

Nevertheless, it must be emphasized that experiments performed in culture, whether with primary explants of normal pituitary tissue or with established cell strains, serve only as a complement to studies in the animal. The environment of pituitary cells in culture is clearly unphysiological, and any results obtained in these systems must be carefully substantiated in animals. However, we believe that the use of GH$_3$ cells in culture provides an example of how a cell culture system can be of value in studies of the actions of a hypothalamic-releasing factor.

II.   Properties of GH$_3$ Cells

GH$_3$ cells are a clonal strain of functional rat pituitary cells. The cells were established from a prolactin- and growth hormone-producing rat pituitary tumor and adapted to culture by the technique of alternate passage between the animal host and culture (Tashjian *et al.,* 1968b).

The GH$_3$ strain was established in 1965 and the cells have been continuously propagated since that time. GH$_3$ cells are neoplastic and will produce tumors when injected into rats of the Wistar/Furth strain. They are aneuploid with a modal chromosome number of 69 (Sonnenschein *et al.,* 1970); the diploid number of chromosomes for the rat is 42.

GH$_3$ cells can be grown in monolayer, roller bottle, or suspension culture

(Bancroft and Tashjian, 1971). In our laboratory they are usually grown in either Ham's F 10 medium (monolayer) or Eagle's minimum essential medium (Spinner), in all cases supplemented with 15% horse serum and 2.5% fetal calf serum. Under these conditions the cells double in number every 48 to 72 hours in both monolayer and suspension cultures; the growth rate has not changed significantly in 8 years. GH_3 cells are viable after freezing in 10% glycerol in liquid nitrogen for periods of at least 5 years; the cells can be reestablished in culture with no detectable changes in properties.

GH_3 cells are functional pituitary cells in that they synthesize and secrete into the culture medium both growth hormone and prolactin. Growth hormone and prolactin are simple proteins with molecular weights of approximately 21,000 daltons. The hormones synthesized by GH_3 cells are indistinguishable from the authentic rat hormones in terms of both biological activity and immunological properties (Tashjian *et al.*, 1968a, 1970; Tashjian, 1969). The concentrations of intracellular and secreted prolactin and growth hormone are determined by microcomplement fixation immunoassays which are specific for each hormone (Tashjian *et al.*, 1968a, 1970). The amounts of hormone secreted into the medium by GH_3 cells are large (Table I), 2–30 μg/mg cell protein/24 hours. The intracellular

TABLE I

Hormone Production by Several Strains of
GH Cells[a]

| Strain | Hormone production (μg/mg cell protein/24 hr) | |
	Growth hormone	Prolactin
GH_3	20	8
GH_12C_1	2	<0.05
GH_4	<0.06	30

[a] Hormone production is defined as the amount of hormone that accumulates in the medium over a defined period of time divided by the amount of cell protein at the time of collection. Hormone production is usually measured in 24–72-hour samples. Growth hormone and prolactin are stable in the culture medium and are measured by microcomplement fixation.

concentrations of hormones are small, equivalent to the amount secreted in 15–30 minutes (growth hormone) or 1–2 hours (prolactin) (Tashjian *et al.*, 1970). The synthesis of prolactin and growth hormone represents 1–3% of the total protein synthesized by the cells under basal conditions, and under some circumstances the synthesis of a hormone may account for as much as 15% of the total protein synthesized. GH_3 cells are not known to synthesize any other hypophyseal hormones; they do not produce thyrotropin, LH, FSH, or ACTH. Growth hormone and prolactin are the only proteins known to be secreted by these cells.

In addition to the GH_3 strain, several other cell strains are available which synthesize either growth hormone or prolactin but not both (Table I). The GH_1 $2C_1$ strain was derived from the same pituitary tumor as GH_3 cells. This strain produces only growth hormone under all conditions which have been examined (Sonnenschein *et al.*, 1970; Tashjian *et al.*, 1973). The GH_4 cell strain arose spontaneously in 1970 from the GH_3 line. GH_4 cells synthesize prolactin alone under basal conditions, but the cells can be stimulated by hydrocortisone to produce growth hormone (Tashjian *et al.*, 1973). Mazurkiewicz (1973) has described another strain of cells which arose spontaneously from GH_3 cells in his laboratory. These cells, like the GH_4 line, produce prolactin but not growth hormone. The strain isolated by Mazurkiewicz, however, has been found to produce immunologically reactive ACTH in response to the addition of vasopressin to the culture medium. The vasopressin-induced synthesis of ACTH is a finding that may be expected to provide useful insights into the mechanisms underlying the ectopic production of ACTH by neoplastic cells.

The availability of these various cell strains has proved useful in designing experiments on the control of hormone production. On the other hand, it must be recognized that GH_3 cells can give rise to functionally different substrains for reasons which are not understood. This problem is minimized if the experimenter maintains cells in the frozen state which can be placed back into culture and which retain (for a time at least) the original spectrum of hormone-producing properties. The need for constant monitoring of hormone production is, however, obvious.

A large number of factors which influence the production of growth hormone and prolactin by GH_3 cells have been identified and have been the subject of several recent reviews (Tashjian and Hoyt, 1972; Dannies and Tashjian, 1973a; Tashjian *et al.*, 1973). Many of the effects observed in GH_3 cells have also been found in animals or in primary explants of normal anterior pituitary glands. Among the agents which affect hormone production by GH_3 cells are hydrocortisone, estradiol, depolarizing concentrations of potassium ion, 2-Br-α-ergocryptine methane sulfonate (CB 154), dibutyryl-cAMP*, and TRH. The remainder of this review will deal with the effects of TRH on GH₃ cells.

III.   TRH Affects Prolactin as Well as Thyrotropin

TRH, thyrotropin-releasing hormone, was the first hypothalamic factor whose structure was elucidated. It was purified as the activity which caused the release of thyrotropin from the pituitary gland. TRH is a tripeptide: pGlu–His–ProNH₂ (Burgus *et al.,* 1969; Folkers *et al.,* 1969). It is apparently synthesized enzymatically in the hypothalamus (Mitnick and Reichlin, 1971, 1972). Synthetic TRH became available shortly after its structure was determined and it was first reported by Tashjian *et al.* in 1971 that the addition of nanomolar concentrations of TRH to cultures of GH₃ cells caused an increase in the production of prolactin and a decrease in growth hormone production. This was the first report that a hypothalamic-releasing factor lacked complete target hormone specificity. The prolactin-stimulating activity of TRH has subsequently been confirmed *in vivo.* Plasma concentrations of prolactin, as well as thyrotropin, increase markedly after the injection of TRH in many species, e.g., rat, goat, cow, monkey, sheep, human. The prolactin-releasing activity of TRH has been studied most extensively in humans, where the doses of TRH required to elicit a prolactin response are as low or lower than the doses required to elevate plasma thyrotropin, and the magnitudes of the two responses are similar. The prolactin-stimulating activity of TRH has been the subject of recent reviews (Bowers *et al.,* 1973; Dannies and Tashjian, 1974). These results all suggest that TRH may be a regulator not only of thyrotropin, but also of prolactin.

It had been anticipated that each hypothalamic-releasing factor would cause the release of a single pituitary hormone. However, in addition to TRH, each of the other hypothalamic-releasing and -inhibiting factors that have now been isolated has been shown to affect the release of more than one hormone. A single decapeptide causes the release of both luteinizing hormone and follicle-stimulating hormone (see Blackwell and Guillemin, 1973; Schally *et al.,* 1973). Growth hormone release-inhibiting factor (somatostatin) (Brazeau *et al.,* 1973) inhibits the release of growth hormone and also blocks the TRH-mediated stimulation of thyrotropin, but not prolactin, release (Vale *et al.,* 1973a,b).

---

* The abbreviations used are TRH, thyrotropin-releasing hormone; cAMP, adenosine 3′, 5′ cyclic monophosphate; dibutyryl-cAMP, N^6, $O^{2'}$-dibutyryl adenosine 3′, 5′-cyclic monophosphate.

The physiological significance of the multiple sites of releasing factor action is at present unclear. It has recently become possible to measure the concentrations of two releasing factors in plasma, urine, and in hypophyseal portal blood (Arimura *et al.*, 1973; Bassiri and Utiger, 1973; Keye *et al.*, 1973; Koch *et al.*, 1973; Montoya *et al.*, 1973; Nett *et al.*, 1973; Seyler and Reichlin, 1973). As new data become available on the concentrations of releasing factors in plasma in different physiological states, it may be expected that the physiology of the hypothalamic–hypophyseal axis will be more clearly understood.

The TRH-mediated decrease in growth hormone production by GH_3 cells is a highly reproducible, dose-dependent phenomenon (Section VII). This activity of TRH has not been confirmed *in vivo*. In acute experiments in which the release of stored growth hormone has been measured, TRH has been shown to have either no effect or a stimulatory effect on growth hormone (Carlson and Mariz, 1973).

The anterior pituitary gland contains at least two types of cells which respond to TRH: thyrotrophs and lactotrophs. Growth hormone-producing cells may also respond *in vivo*. On the other hand, GH_3 cells are a clonal, TRH-responsive cell strain. TRH itself is stable in the medium of GH_3 cultures (Hinkle and Tashjian, 1973), in contrast to its instability in plasma (Nair *et al.*, 1971; Bassiri and Utiger, 1972). Thus the GH_3 system offers useful properties for examining the actions of TRH.

IV.   Effects of TRH on GH_3 Cells

A. *Prolactin and Growth Hormone Production*

The major biological effect of TRH on GH_3 cells is to increase the rate of production (see Table I) of prolactin by the cells. When GH_3 cells are treated with nanomolar concentrations of TRH for several days there is a 2- to 5-fold increase in the amount of prolactin produced, and the response exhibits a typical log dose-response relationship (Fig. 1). The concentrations of TRH required to produce this effect are comparable to the doses required to obtain a TSH response in other systems. The increase in prolactin production reaches a maximum "induced" level in 24 to 48 hours (Tashjian *et al.*, 1971; Tashjian and Hoyt, 1972). Prolactin production remains elevated as long as TRH is present in the culture medium. Furthermore, the effect of TRH is maintained for some time after its removal from the culture medium. If GH_3 cells are treated with 28 n*M* TRH for 6 hours, the amount of prolactin produced by the cells is significantly greater in treated than in control cultures for at least 4 days after the peptide has been removed from the medium (Tashjian *et al.*, 1973). The rate of

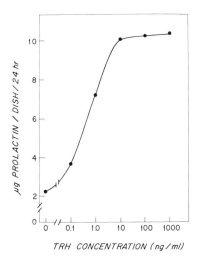

TRH CONCENTRATION (ng/ml)

Fig. 1.   Effects of various concentrations of TRH on prolactin production by GH₃ cells. Replicate dishes were incubated for 24 hours with TRH at the concentrations shown. Each point gives the mean of duplicate determinations. Reproduced from Tashjian *et al.* (1971).

prolactin production eventually returns to control levels so that it is not necessary to postulate that the peptide leads to a heritable alteration in the cells.

TRH also causes a 50–75% decrease in the rate of growth hormone production by GH_3 cells. The reduction in growth hormone production exhibits the same dependence on the concentration of TRH as the prolactin response (Section VII). The decrease in growth hormone production occurs at the same time as the increase in prolactin, and growth hormone levels remain depressed as long as TRH is present in the medium (Tashjian *et al.*, 1971).

The effects of TRH on prolactin and growth hormone in GH_3 cells are highly specific. TRH leads to no change in the rate of growth of the cells, measured by the increase in total protein, even in experiments of three weeks duration. Furthermore, its addition to cultures causes no change in the rate of protein synthesis measured by the ability of the cells to incorporate radioactively labeled amino acids into material precipitable by trichloroacetic acid. TRH does not act nonspecifically to increase the rate of production of all exportable proteins, because it has no effect on the production of albumin by an established strain of hepatoma cells (Tashjian *et al.*, 1971). Finally, TRH has no detectable effect on the GH_12C_1 strain of growth hormone-producing pituitary cells which does not synthesize prolactin either basally or under the influence of TRH.

B. Prolactin Synthesis and Degradation

The increase in the accumulation of prolactin in the medium of TRH-treated cultures, which we have called "production," is of sufficient magnitude and duration that it must be the result of an increase in the net amount of the hormone in the system. Since prolactin is stable in the culture medium, the increase caused by TRH cannot be due to enhanced stability of prolactin after secretion. The effect of TRH must, therefore, occur by either of two processes: an increase in the rate of *de novo* synthesis of prolactin; or a decrease in the rate of its intracellular degradation. In order to distinguish between these two possibilities, the rate of prolactin synthesis was measured directly (Dannies and Tashjian, 1973b). Newly synthesized proteins were radioactively labeled by the addition of [^{3}H]leucine to the culture medium. Intracellular prolactin or prolactin in the culture medium was isolated by immunoprecipitation with specific rabbit anti-prolactin serum. The precipitation was carried out in the presence of unlabeled carrier prolactin and sufficient antiserum to place the serological reaction in slight antibody excess. The immune precipitate was dissolved in buffer containing sodium dodecyl sulfate and mercaptoethanol, conditions which lead to dissociation of the antigen–antibody complex. Radioactively labeled prolactin was then separated from any labeled protein contaminants which had coprecipitated by electrophoresis on acrylamide gels in sodium dodecyl sulfate. The pattern of radioactivity in such a gel is shown in Fig. 2; the amount of newly synthesized prolactin was determined from the radioactivity in the peak which coelectrophoresed with standard rat prolactin.

The rate of prolactin synthesis was measured by this method in control cultures and in cultures which had been maximally stimulated with TRH (Fig. 3). The increase in the rate of prolactin synthesis in the TRH-treated cultures was identical to the increase in prolactin accumulation after TRH treatment (Table II). Thus increased synthesis accounts entirely for increased accumulation. TRH causes no change in the rate of degradation of prolactin. Prolactin is secreted into the culture medium about 1 hour after it is synthesized in both control and TRH-treated cultures (Dannies and Tashjian, 1973b). TRH causes an increase in the rate of synthesis of prolactin 3–4 hours after it is added to GH$_3$ cultures (Dannies and Tashjian, 1974).

The degradation of prolactin has been measured directly in two ways (Dannies and Tashjian, 1973b). Cultures were incubated with [^{3}H]leucine to label prolactin. The incorporation of radioactive label was then stopped by either of two methods: (1) Radioactive medium was removed, the cells were washed, and medium containing a large excess of unlabeled leucine was added to cultures to chase the radioactive leucine; or (2) Cyclohexi-

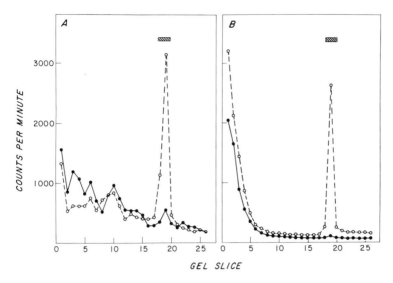

Fig. 2. Sodium dodecyl sulfate disc gel electrophoresis of immunoprecipitates. *A*. Immunoprecipitates from cell sonicates of GH₄C₃ cells that were labeled with [³H]leucine for 1 hour. *B*. Immunoprecipitates from medium of GH₄C₃ cells that were labeled with [³H]leucine for 3 hours. The bars at the top of the figures indicate the position of standard rat prolactin which was run in separate gels and identified by staining with amido black. The symbols are rat serum albumin and rabbit anti-rat serum albumin (●——●), and rat prolactin and rabbit anti-rat prolactin (○----○). Reproduced from Dannies and Tashjian (1973b).

mide was added to stop protein synthesis. The amount of radioactive prolactin was measured at intervals after these treatments. In both experiments there was no measurable decrease in intracellular, labeled prolactin for 3 hours, indicating that degradation of prolactin is negligible during this period. The feature of this system which allows effects on synthesis to be clearly differentiated from effects on degradation is the fact that prolactin is secreted from the cells rapidly and, therefore, escapes the processes of intracellular degradation. In the course of these experiments, it was found that there are two pools of leucine in GH₃ cells. Amino acids from proteins degraded intracellularly are used preferentially in new protein synthesis (Mortimore *et al.*, 1972; Dannies and Tashjian, 1973b). The existence of multiple pools for amino acids points out the importance of caution in interpreting "pulse-chase" experiments in eukaryotic cells.

C. Populations of Hormone-Producing Cells

The experiments described above demonstrate that TRH increases prolactin synthesis by GH₃ cells. However, it has been shown in two labora-

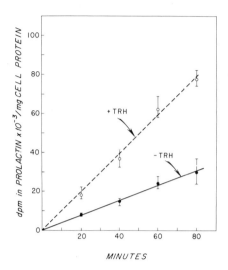

Fig. 3. Appearance of labeled prolactin in GH₃ cells with and without TRH. TRH was added to the cells 3 days before the start of the labeling experiment and [³H]leucine was added at zero time. Each point is the average of triplicates; bars indicate the range. The symbols are control cells (●——●) and cells treated with 28 n*M* TRH (○----○). Reproduced from Dannies and Tashjian (1973b).

tories that in unsynchronized cultures of GH₃ cells, only a fraction of the cells contain immunoreactive prolactin (Hoyt and Tashjian, 1973; Mazurkiewicz, 1973). In fact, Mazurkiewicz (1973) has reported that different cells in his GH₃ cultures contain growth hormone or prolactin, but that no cell contains both hormones. This is somewhat unexpected because our GH₃ cells have been cloned repeatedly from single cells. In all cases the resulting populations have been found to make both prolactin and growth hormone as soon after cloning as it is possible to measure hormone production (∼ 10⁴ cells). Thus it was possible that TRH increases synthesis merely by increasing the fraction of cells in the culture which synthesize prolactin and not by increasing the rate of prolactin synthesis. This possibility was ruled out by staining preparations of fixed GH₃ cells with antiserum to prolactin using an immunoperoxidase method (Sternberger *et al.*, 1970) to visualize cells containing prolactin. The percentages of prolactin-producing cells in control cultures and in cultures which had been treated with either hydrocortisone or TRH were essentially the same (Table III), although the intracellular concentrations of prolactin differed over an 8-fold range in these three populations of GH₃ cells (Hoyt and Tashjian, unpublished data).

D. Prolactin and Growth Hormone Release

The effects of TRH on the release of stored hormones has been measured directly by labeling intracellular proteins with ^{3}H and then following the rate at which radioactive prolactin and growth hormone are secreted when either fresh control medium or medium containing TRH is added to the cultures. Release was followed by conventional acrylamide gel electrophoresis which readily separates prolactin and growth hormone.

TRH causes an increase in the amount of prolactin secreted in 30 minutes following its addition to the medium (Table IV). The enhanced release of stored prolactin exhibits the same dependence on TRH concentration as does the increased synthesis due to TRH. TRH-mediated stimulation of prolactin release is also enhanced if theophylline is added simultaneously (Gautvik et al., 1974). TRH did not change the amount of labeled growth hormone accumulated in the medium in 30 minutes following TRH treatment (Table IV).

When TRH is added to cultures there is an immediate decrease in the intracellular concentration of prolactin due to the burst of hormone release caused by the tripeptide. However, after three days of treatment with 100 ng/ml of TRH, intracellular prolactin concentrations become elevated (290%) while those of growth hormone are unchanged (Tashjian and Hoyt, 1972).

TABLE II

Increase in Incorporation of [^{3}H]Leucine into Prolactin and Increase in Prolactin Production Caused by TRH[a]

	Ratio of prolactin (+TRH/−TRH)	
Experiment no.	[^{3}H]Leucine in intracellular prolactin[b]	Production of prolactin[c]
I	2.5 ± 0.02	2.4 ± 0.12
II	3.7 ± 0.33	3.2

[a] Reproduced from Dannies and Tashjian (1973b).

[b] Measured as [^{3}H]leucine incorporation into prolactin in TRH-treated and control cells at various times (Fig. 3). Mean values ± SE.

[c] Measured by microcomplement fixation.

TABLE III

Cytochemical Distribution of Prolactin in Monolayer Cultures
of GH$_3$ Cells[a]

Treatment	No. of cells counted	Prolactin-positive cells (% of total)	Relative intracellular [prolactin]
Control	3675	35	1.0
TRH	4866	45	4.0
Hydrocortisone	4439	33	0.5

[a] Unsynchronized monolayer cultures of GH$_3$ cells were treated for
36 hours with TRH (28 nM) or for 5 days with hydrocortisone (5 μM).
The cultures were incubated for 3 hours with 10^{-6} M colchicine prior
to fixation. Prolactin-containing cells were stained as described by
Hoyt and Tashjian (1973). Intracellular concentrations of prolactin
were measured by microcomplement fixation (R. F. Hoyt, Jr. and A.
H. Tashjian, Jr., unpublished data).

E. Cell Morphology

The morphology of GH$_3$ cells which have been treated with TRH for
6–20 hours differs markedly from control cultures. TRH causes the cells to
become flattened and more adherent to the surface of the culture vessel.
TRH-treated cells also have a smoother surface membrane. These changes

TABLE IV

Effect of TRH on Release of Prolactin and Growth Hormone[a]

Treatment	Hormone released (cpm/mg cell protein)	
	Prolactin	Growth hormone
Control	200 ± 80	430 ± 100
+ TRH (0.3 μM)	780 ± 70	455 ± 45

[a] Replicate dishes of GH$_3$ cells were incubated for 30 minutes at 37°C with [^{3}H]lysine (50 mCi/ml F 10 medium without serum). TRH was then added and the incubation continued for 30 minutes. The amount of radioactive prolactin
and growth hormone in the medium was then determined by
electrophoresis on acrylamide gels at pH 9.3. Values shown
are the means and ranges of duplicate determinations.

are clearly visible in the phase-contrast microscope, but they are more vividly apparent in scanning electron photomicrographs (Figs. 4 and 5).

V.   TRH Receptors in GH_3 Cells

TRH labeled with tritium in the prolineamide position has been used to study the mechanism of TRH action in GH_3 cells (Hinkle and Tashjian, 1973). The binding of TRH to a single target cell can be studied with GH_3 cells in contrast to studies with whole pituitary tissue which contains at least two types of responsive cells, thyrotrophs and lactotrophs. When [³H]TRH is added to monolayer cultures of GH_3 cells, radioactivity becomes tightly associated with the cells and cannot be removed by extensive

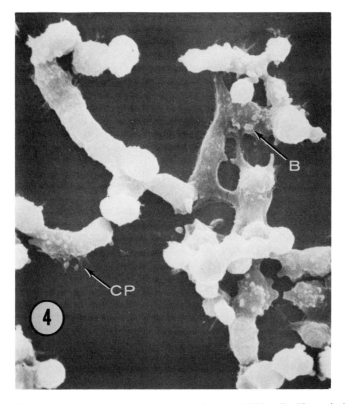

Fig. 4. Scanning electron micrograph of untreated, control GH_3 cells. The majority of the cells are drawn up, away from the substratum; the surfaces of these cells are irregularly rugated and are drawn outward into prominent "buds" or clublike appendages (B). Note the fine, cytoplasmic processes (CP) that bind occasional cells to the glass substratum. ×1000. Reproduced from Tashjian and Hoyt (1972).

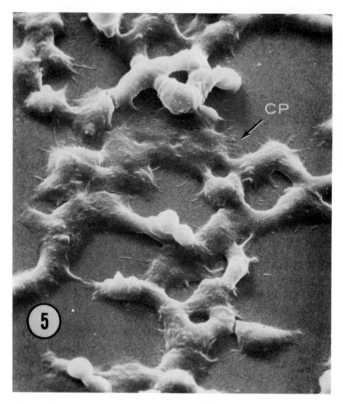

Fig. 5. A scanning electron micrograph of GH₃ cells treated with TRH, 10 ng/ml, for 20 hours. Most of the cells are flattened firmly against the substratum. These cells are not attenuated, as are the occasional firmly bound cells in control cultures; they are substantial in appearance and are bound firmly to the substratum by numerous fine, branching cytoplasmic processes (CP) that extend outward from the basal regions of each cell. The surfaces of these cells are quite smooth in contrast to those of control preparations (Fig. 4). Budlike surface projections are seen only rarely. × 1000. Reproduced from Tashjian and Hoyt (1972).

washing. The amount of TRH bound to cells reaches a maximum in less than 2 minutes at high TRH concentrations (1μM), and in approximately 30 minutes at 2.8 nM TRH. The presence of specific receptors for TRH was established by demonstrating: that the TRH-binding curve resembles the dose-response curve for the biological activity of TRH, stimulation of prolactin synthesis; and that binding of TRH is specific for the cell strain which responds biologically (Fig. 6). Half-maximum binding of TRH to GH₃ cells occured at a higher TRH concentration (11 nM) than the half-maximum biological effect (2 nM). This difference may be in part the result of experimental error, but it is similar to differences found in many receptor systems and has led to the concept of "spare receptors"; i.e., that the biological effects of the agonist are maximal before receptors are fully saturated. At saturation, there are 130,000 molecules of TRH bound per GH_3 cell. If not all cells in the population produce prolactin and growth hormone (Section IV,C), it is possible that only a fraction of the cells bind

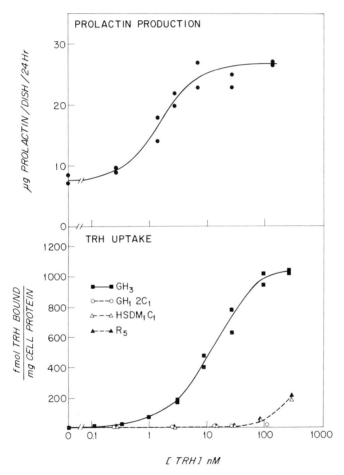

Fig. 6. Dependence of TRH binding and prolactin production on TRH concentration. Lower figure: Replicate dishes of cells were incubated with indicated amounts of TRH for 1 hour and the amount of [³H]TRH bound to the cells determined. $GH_1 2C_1$ cells are a clonal strain of rat pituitary cells that produce growth hormone but do not produce prolactin. R_5 and $HSDM_1C_1$ are clonal strains of rat and mouse fibroblasts, respectively. Upper figure: Replicate dishes of GH_3 cells were treated with the indicated concentrations of TRH for 3 days and the amount of prolactin measured in the medium by microcomplement fixation. Reproduced from Hinkle and Tashjian (1973).

TRH and that the number of receptors per responsive cell is higher than this average value.

Gourdji *et al.* (1973) have studied the binding of [^{3}H]TRH to GH$_3$ cells and obtained results similar to ours, except that they report a class of nonsaturable, low affinity binding sites which were not evident with our GH$_3$ cultures (Hinkle and Tashjian, 1973). In addition, these workers carried out an autoradiographic analysis of the binding of [^{3}H]TRH. Grains were found in each GH$_3$ cell but were present over the entire cell and not localized on the plasma membrane. After crude fractionation of GH$_3$ cells which had been treated with [^{3}H]TRH, radioactivity was found in cytoplasmic, nuclear, and membrane fractions (Brunet *et al.*, 1974). However, because of possible artifacts arising from redistribution of the small peptide during fixation for autoradiography, as well as during cell fractionation, we believe that further studies are necessary to establish the location of TRH receptors in GH$_3$ cells.

Some of the properties of the TRH receptor in GH$_3$ cells have been investigated using a Millipore filter assay to measure binding in a cell free system (Hinkle and Tashjian, 1973). The saturation kinetics of TRH binding *in vitro* are shown in Fig. 7, from which a dissociation constant of 25 nM was determined for the TRH-receptor complex at 0°C. There appears to be only one class of TRH-binding sites on this single, TRH-responsive cell strain. Receptor activity is found almost exclusively in membrane fractions of the cells and is destroyed by treatment with proteolytic enzymes, detergents, or phospholipases A and C, which are ex-

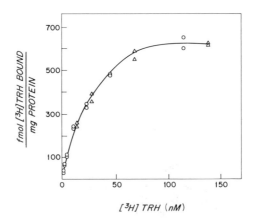

Fig. 7. Binding of TRH to GH$_3$ homogenates. GH$_3$ homogenate [(O) 106 μg or (Δ) 50 μg protein] was incubated with the indicated concentrations of [^{3}H]TRH for 2 hours at 0°C. The amount of TRH bound to receptor was measured as described by Hinkle and Tashjian (1973). Reproduced from Hinkle and Tashjian (1973).

TABLE V

Properties of the GH$_3$ Cell TRH Receptor[a]

>95% Receptor activity associated with membranes	
Inactivated by:	Pronase, trypsin, phospholipases A and C, Triton X-100, NP 40, SDS
Stable to:	RNase, DNase, phospholipase D
TRH-binding activity:	No effect of EDTA (20 mM); no effect of Mg^{2+} (0–36 mM); no effect of Ca^{2+} (0–10 mM); inhibition by Ca^{2+} (>10 mM) pH optimum = 7.5
Dissociation constant of TRH–receptor complex = 25 nM	
TRH-binding capacity = 0.74 pmole/mg cell protein	
Half-time for dissociation of TRH–receptor complex = 2–3 hours	

[a] Data were obtained using a filter assay method to measure the binding of [^{3}H]TRH to GH$_3$ homogenates (Hinkle and Tashjian, 1973).

pected to disrupt the integrity of membrane structures (Table V). TRH-binding activity is reported to be associated with the plasma membrane fraction of bovine pituitary glands (Labrie *et al.*, 1972), but is apparently not located exclusively on the plasma membranes of mouse pituitary tumor tissue (Vale *et al.*, 1973d). Binding of TRH to the GH$_3$ receptor does not require divalent cations and exhibits a pH optimum of 7.5 indicating that the uncharged species of TRH binds to the receptor (Table V).

VI. Involvement of cAMP

It has frequently been suggested that hypothalamic-releasing factors, like other peptide hormones, act at the plasma membranes of target cells to stimulate adenylate cyclase activity, and that cAMP acts as a second messenger in the cells. At this time the evidence implicating cAMP as a second messenger for TRH is indirect and tentative. Poirier *et al.* (1972) have shown that both adenylate cyclase activity and TRH-binding activity are located in the plasma membrane fraction of bovine anterior pituitary cells, but the total purification in these experiments was only 40-fold.

Initial experiments designed to test the second messenger hypothesis in GH cells have yielded the following results. Addition of TRH to cultures of GH cells led to a 2-fold increase in the intracellular concentration of cAMP (Table VI). The increase in cAMP caused by TRH in GH cells occured within 5 minutes and was therefore rapid enough to account for the earliest known effect of TRH in the cells, stimulation of prolactin release. In addition, the increase in cAMP concentration depended on the concentration of TRH in a dose-related manner which was reasonably similar to that for the binding of TRH to the cells. In recent experiments, however, it has been possible to demonstrate that TRH can stimulate prolactin release under conditions in which there is no measurable increase in the intracellular concentration of cAMP.

The question of whether cAMP can mimic TRH actions in the GH₃ cell system has also been investigated. The most rapid action of TRH is also produced by the cyclic nucleotide. Dibutyryl-cAMP stimulates prolactin release by GH cells (Fig. 8). The extent of this stimulation is the same as that caused by TRH, and release is enhanced by theophylline in both TRH- and dibutyryl-cAMP-treated cultures.

It is not possible to test the effects of theophylline in experiments of 1 to 3 days duration because it is toxic to the cells under these circumstances. The long term effects of dibutyryl-cAMP alone have been examined though. Dibutyryl cAMP stimulates prolactin synthesis to about the same extent as TRH, but it also causes a 3- to 4-fold increase in growth hormone production while TRH leads to a 50–75% decrease in growth hormone. These data are summarized in Table VII.

It is not known why dibutyryl-cAMP and TRH have opposite effects on

TABLE VI

Effect of TRH on the Concentration of cAMP
in GH₃ Cells[a]

	Intracellular cAMP (pmole/mg cell protein)	
Treatment	GH_4C_1	GH_12C_1
Control	15.2 ± 1.4	14.0 ± 5.2
+TRH (0.3 μM)	28.5 ± 1.9	15.5 ± 1.3

[a] Intracellular concentrations of cAMP were measured by the method of Steiner et al. (1969) 15 minutes after the addition of TRH. The GH_4C_1 strain is a prolactin-producing clone of GH_4 cells which responds to TRH; GH_12C_1 cells do not produce prolactin or respond to TRH (Section II) (Gautvik et al., 1974).

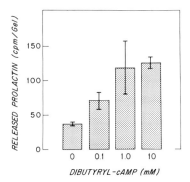

Fig. 8. Effect of dibutyryl cAMP on prolactin release. Replicate dishes of GH_3 cells were incubated with [^{3}H]leucine (50 μCi/ml complete F 10 medium) for 30 minutes at 37°C. The indicated concentrations of dibutyryl cAMP were then added and the incubations continued for 30 minutes. The amount of radioactive prolactin in the medium was then measured as described by Dannies and Tashjian (1973b). Values given are the mean and range of duplicate determinations (Gautvik *et al.*, 1974).

growth hormone production by GH cells. This fact, in addition to the observation that TRH can stimulate prolactin release in the absence of a measurable increase in cAMP concentrations, makes it clear that the second messenger hypothesis cannot account for all of the actions of TRH in GH cells.

VII. Activity of TRH Analogs

The GH_3 system has been used to study the activity of peptide analogs of TRH supplied by Abbott Laboratories. Analog studies are useful both for defining the structural requirements of the TRH receptor and also for identifying antagonists or highly active peptides of potential clinical importance. The advantage of the GH_3 cell system for such studies is that it is possible to measure conveniently both the biological activity of a peptide and also its affinity for the TRH receptor. Biological activity is measured as the ability of a peptide to stimulate prolactin or decrease growth hormone production; binding activity is measured as the ability to compete with radioactively labeled TRH for binding to the receptor. The system allows determination of the intrinsic activity of a peptide under conditions where degradation is not a problem and there are not multiple target cell types.

An example of the type of biological data obtained with TRH analogs is given in Fig. 9, which shows the effects on prolactin and growth hormone production of peptides with substitutions for the histidine of TRH. The N^{3im}-methyl derivative is more active than TRH, stimulating prolactin and decreasing growth hormone production at 7-times lower concentrations

TABLE VII

Effects of TRH and Dibutyryl cAMP on Hormone Production
by GH₃ Cells[a]

	Hormone production (% of control)	
	Prolactin	Growth hormone
TRH (0.3 μM)	370	26
Dibutyryl cAMP (1 mM)	350	360

[a] The amount of prolactin and growth hormone produced by GH₃ cells was measured in control cells and in cells treated for 3 days with doses of TRH or dibutyryl cAMP which produce maximum responses. Values shown are the mean of duplicate determinations (Tashjian and Hoyt, 1972).

than TRH. This peptide was first shown to have enhanced thyrotropin-releasing activity by Vale *et al.* (1971). Its high affinity for the TRH receptor on GH₃ cells has been confirmed by Vale *et al.* (1973c). The lysine and arginine substituted peptides are inactive. The binding activity of these analogs is shown in Fig. 10. Competition experiments were carried out using a TRH concentration which is two-thirds saturating, a condition which gives both high sensitivity and substantial binding of labeled TRH. The binding results are in agreement with the biological data. The N^{3im}-methyl histidyl derivative again competes for binding at lower concentrations than TRH, while the lysine and arginine peptides are inactive. The enhanced activity of the methylated derivative is not a pK_a effect. At the pH of these experiments, 7.6, more than 90% of both TRH (p$K_a = 6.25$) and methyl-TRH (p$K_a = 5.95$) are in free base form (Grant *et al.*, 1972a), and pH studies have indicated that it is the unprotonated species of TRH which binds to the TRH receptor in this system (Hinkle and Tashjian, 1973).

Using these methods the activity of more than 40 TRH analogs has been measured in the GH₃ system and the results are summarized in Table VIII, which shows both the concentration of peptide required to give a half-maximum biological response and the apparent dissociation constant of the analog–receptor complex. In all cases, those peptides with measurable activity caused the same maximum responses as TRH, both in biological and binding experiments. All peptides which stimulated prolactin synthesis also decreased growth hormone production, and the two effects exhibited the same concentration dependence, suggesting that these actions involve either the same or very similar receptors (e.g., see Fig. 9). Finally, although the biological activities of peptides varied over a large range, the biological potencies could, in all cases, be explained solely by the altered affinity of the peptide for the TRH receptor. No TRH antagonists were found.

From the data in Table VIII, it can be seen that the TRH receptor in GH₃ cells is highly selective. The ring structure of the N-terminal pyro-glutamyl residue is important for activity, but peptides with minor substitutions in the ring retain considerable TRH-like activity. The receptor appears to be even more selective for the C-terminal residue, and only the methyl and ethyl amides of proline retain as much as 1% of the activity of the parent molecule.

It is not known whether the TRH receptors on lactotrophs and thyro-trophs are similar. The affinity of TRH for receptors on prolactin-pro-ducing GH₃ cells is similar to the affinity of TRH for receptors from bovine anterior pituitary glands (Labrie *et al.*, 1972) and a murine thy-rotropin-secreting tumor (Grant *et al.*, 1972b). The amounts of TRH needed to elicit a thyrotropin response are similar to those required to give a prolactin response both in humans (Section III) and in primary cultures of rat pituitary cells (Vale *et al.*, 1973c). In addition, the activity of TRH

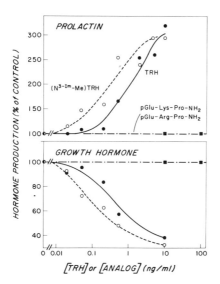

Fig. 9. Effects of TRH analogs on prolactin and growth hormone production by GH₃ cells. Replicate dishes were incubated for 7 days with TRH or TRH analogs at the concentrations shown. Each point gives the mean of duplicate determinations of the amount of growth hormone and prolactin in media collected from the last 3 days of treatment. (●———●) TRH; (O----O)N^{3im}-methyl-TRH; (■— . —■) pGlu-Lys-ProNH₂ and pGlu-Arg-ProNH₂.

TABLE VIII

Activity of TRH Analogs in the GH$_3$ System[a]

Peptide	Half-maximum prolactin-stimulation [peptide] (nM)	Apparent K_{diss} peptide-receptor (nM)
(TRH structure)	2	25
(structure)	4	120
(structure)	6	200
(structure)	250	1,000
Gln-His-ProNH$_2$	—	5,400
pGlu-N^{3-im}-methyl-His-ProNH$_2$	0.3	4.7
pGlu-Arg-ProNH$_2$	>1,000	>5,000
pGlu-Lys-ProNH$_2$	>1,000	>5,000
pGlu-His-Pro	~4,000	~13,000
pGlu-His-ProNHCH$_3$	50	1,000
pGlu-His-ProNHCH$_2$CH$_3$	40	500
pGlu-His-ProN(CH$_3$)$_2$	>1,000	>30,000
pGlu-His-NH$_2$, -MetNH$_2$, -GlyNH$_2$, -LeuNH$_2$, -ValNH$_2$, -TrpNH$_2$, PheNH$_2$	>500	>2,500

[a] The concentration of a peptide necessary to obtain a half-maximal stimulation of prolactin production was determined from data such as that shown in Fig. 9, and the apparent dissociation constant of the peptide–receptor complex from data such as that shown in Fig. 10 (Hinkle et al., 1974).

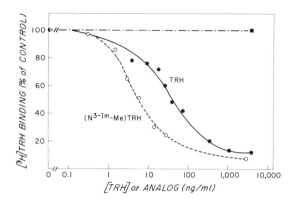

Fig. 10.   Competition of TRH analogs with [³H]-TRH for binding to GH₃ homogenates. Incubation mixtures contained: 18 ng/ml [³H]-TRH and the indicated concentrations of (●————●) unlabeled TRH; (O----O) N^{3im}-methyl-TRH; (■—·—·—·—■) pGlu-Lys-ProNH₂ and pGlu-Arg-ProNH₂. Binding assays were carried out as described by Hinkle and Tashjian (1973).

analogs in the GH₃ system parallels closely their activity in tests of thyrotropin-releasing activity (Hinkle *et al.*, 1974). These data all suggest that TRH receptors on thyrotropin-producing cells are similar, or perhaps identical, to TRH receptors on prolactin-producing cells.

VIII.   Summary

Hormone-producing pituitary cells in culture provide a system in which factors controlling hormone synthesis and release can be examined in a carefully controlled environment. GH₃, a clonal strain of rat growth hormone- and prolactin-producing cells, has been used to investigate the actions of the hypothalamic tripeptide, thyrotropin-releasing hormone (TRH). TRH stimulates prolactin production and decreases growth hormone production by GH₃ cells. The prolactin-stimulating activity of TRH has been confirmed in animals. TRH acts by increasing the rate of *de novo* prolactin synthesis. TRH also increases the rate at which stored prolactin is secreted. TRH causes a morphological change but does not significantly affect the percent of prolactin-producing cells in unsynchronized cultures. TRH binds to specific membrane receptors.

Intracellular cAMP concentrations are elevated by TRH. Like TRH, dibutyryl-cAMP causes increased prolactin synthesis and release, but the two compounds have opposite effects on growth hormone production. The system has been used to study the intrinsic activity of peptide analogs of

TRH; both the biological activities and the affinities of analogs for the TRH receptor have been measured.

ACKNOWLEDGMENT

The research described in this report was supported in part by a grant from the National Institute of Arthritis, Metabolism and Digestive Diseases (AM11011). We are grateful to Ms. Diane Jensen and Ms. Anne Downing for expert assistance, and to Dr. Eugene Woroch of Abbott Laboratories for supplying TRH analogs.

REFERENCES

Arimura, A., Sato, H., Kumasaka, T., Worobec, R. B., Debeljuk, L., Dunn, J., and Schally, A. V. (1973). *Endocrinology* **93**, 1092.

Bancroft, F. C., and Tashjian, A. H., Jr. (1971). *Exp. Cell Res.* **64**, 125.

Bassiri, R., and Utiger, R. D. (1972). *Endocrinology* **91**, 657.

Bassiri, R., and Utiger, R. D. (1973). *J. Clin. Invest.* **52**, 1616.

Blackwell, R. E., and Guillemin, R. (1973). *Annu. Rev. Physiol.* **35**, 357.

Bowers, C. Y., Friesen, H. G., and Folkers, K. (1973). *Biochem. Biophys. Res. Commun.* **51**, 512.

Brazeau, P., Vale, W., Burgus, R., Ling, N., Butcher, M., Rivier, J., and Guillemin, R. (1973). *Science* **179**, 77.

Brunet, N., Gourdji, D., Tixier-Vidal, A., Pradelles, Ph., Morgat, J. L., and Fromageot, P. (1974). *FEBS Lett.* **38**, 129.

Burgus, R., and Guillemin, R. (1970). *Annu. Rev. Biochem.* **139**, 499.

Burgus, R., Dunn, T., Desiderio, D., and Guillemin, R. (1969). *C.R. Acad. Sci.* **269**, 1870.

Carlson, H., and Mariz, I. (1973). *Program Endocrine Soc. Meet.* p. A141 (abstr. no. 186).

Dannies, P. S., and Tashjian, A. H., Jr. (1973a). *In* "Tissue Culture: Methods and Applications" (P. F. Kruse, Jr. and M. K. Patterson, Jr., eds.). p. 561. Academic Press, New York.

Dannies, P. S., and Tashjian, A. H., Jr. (1973b). *J. Biol. Chem.* **248**, 6174.

Dannies, P. S., and Tashjian, A. H., Jr. (1974). *Isr. J. Med. Sci.* (in press).

Folkers, K., Enzmann, F., Boler, J., Bowers, C. Y., and Schally, A. V. (1969). *Biochem. Biophys. Res. Commun.* **37**, 123.

Gautvik, K. M., Dannies, P. S., and Tashjian, A. H., Jr. (1974). Submitted for publication.

Gourdji, D., Tixier-Vidal, A., Morin, A., Pradelles, P., Morgat, J.-L., Fromageot, P., and Kerdelhue, B. (1973). *Exp. Cell Res.* **82**, 39.

Grant, G., Ling, N., Rivier, J., and Vale, W. (1972a). *Biochemistry* **11**, 3070.

Grant, G., Vale, W., and Guillemin, R. (1972b). *Biochem. Biophys. Res. Commun.* **46**, 28.

Hinkle, P. M., and Tashjian, A. H., Jr. (1973). *J. Biol. Chem.* **248**, 6180.

Hinkle, P. M., Woroch, E. L., and Tashjian, A. H., Jr. (1974). *J. Biol. Chem.* (in press).

Hoyt, R. F., Jr., and Tashjian, A. H., Jr. (1973). *Anat. Rec.* **175**, 374.

Keye, W. R., Jr., Kelch, R. P., and Jaffe, R. B. (1973). *Program Endocrine Soc. Meet.* p. A146 (abstr. no. 196).

Koch, Y., Wilcheck, M., Fridkin, M., Chobsieng, P., Zor, U., and Linder, H. R. (1973). *Biochem. Biophys. Res. Commun.* **55**, 616.

Labrie, F., Barden, N., Poirier, G., and DeLean, A. (1972). *Proc. Nat. Acad. Sci. U.S.* **69**, 283.

McCann, S. M., and Porter, J. C. (1969). *Physiol. Rev.* **49**, 240.

Mazurkiewicz, J. E. (1973). *Anat. Rec.* **175**, 382.

Mitnick, M. A., and Reichlin, S. (1971). *Science* **172**, 1241.

Mitnick, M., and Reichlin, S. (1972). *Endocrinology* **91**, 1145.

Montoya, E., Seibel, M. J., and Wilber, J. (1973). *Program Endocrine Soc. Meet.* p. A138 (abstr. no. 180).

Mortimore, G. E., Woodside, K. H., and Henry, J. E. (1972). *J. Biol. Chem.* **247,** 2776.

Nair, R. M. G., Redding, T. W., and Schally, A. V. (1971). *Biochemistry* **10,** 3621.

Nett, T. M., Akbar, A. M., Hopwood, M. L., and Niswender, G. D. (1973). *Program Endocrine Soc. Meet.* p. A149 (abstr. no. 201).

Poirier, G., Labrie, F., Barden, N., and Lemaire, S. (1972). *FEBS Lett.* **20,** 283.

Reichlin, S., Martin, J. B., Mitnick, M. A., Boshans, R. L., Grimm, Y., Bollinger, J., Gordon, J., and Malacara, J. (1972). *Recent Progr. Horm. Res.* **28,** 229.

Schally, A. V., Arimura, A., and Kastin, A. J. (1973). *Science* **179,** 341.

Seyler, L. E., Jr., and Reichlin, S. (1973) *J. Clin. Endocrinol. Metab.* **37,** 197.

Sonnenschein, C., Richardson, U. I., and Tashjian, A. H., Jr. (1970). *Exp. Cell Res.* **61,** 121.

Steiner, A. L., Kipnis, D. M., Utiger, R., and Parker, C. (1969). *Proc. Nat. Acad. Sci. U.S.* **64,** 367.

Sternberger, L. A., Hardy, P. H., Jr., Cuculis, J. J., and Meyer, H. G. (1970). *J. Histochem. Cytochem.* **18,** 315.

Tashjian, A. H., Jr. (1969). *Biotechnol. Bioeng.* **11,** 109.

Tashjian, A. H., Jr., and Hoyt, R. F., Jr. (1972). *In* "Molecular Genetics and Developmental Biology" (M. Sussman, ed.), p. 353. Prentice-Hall, Englewood Cliffs, New Jersey.

Tashjian, A. H., Jr., Levine, L, and Wilhelmi, A. E. (1968a). *Ann. N.Y. Acad. Sci.* **148,** 352.

Tashjian, A. H., Jr., Yasumura, Y., Levine, L., Sato, G. H., and Parker, M. L. (1968b). *Endocrinology* **82,** 342.

Tashjian, A. H., Jr., Bancroft, F. C., and Levine, L. (1970). *J. Cell Biol.* **47,** 61.

Tashjian, A. H., Jr., Barowsky, N. J., and Jensen, D. K. (1971). *Biochem. Biophys, Res. Commun.* **43,** 516.

Tashjian, A. H., Jr., Hinkle, P. M., and Dannies, P. S. (1973). *In* "Endocrinology" (R. O. Skow, ed.) p. 648. Exerpta Medica/American Elsevier, Amsterdam, ICS No. 273.

Vale, W., Rivier, J., and Burgus, R. (1971). *Endocrinology* **89,** 1485.

Vale, W., Brazeau, P., Rivier, C., Rivier, J., Grant, G., Burgus, R., and Guillemin, R. (1973a). *Fed. Proc., Fed. Amer. Soc. Exp. Biol.* **32,** 211.

Vale, W., Brazeau, P., Rivier, C., Rivier, J., Grant, G., Burgus, R., and Guillemin, R. (1973b). *Program Endocrine Soc. Meet.* p. A118 (abstr. no. 139).

Vale, W., Blackwell, R., Grant, G., and Guillemin, R. (1973c). *Endocrinology* **93,** 26.

Vale, W., Grant, G., and Guillemin, R. (1973d). *In* "Frontiers in Neuroendocrinology" (W. F. Ganong and L. Martini, eds.), p. 375. Oxford Univ. Press, London and New York.

CHAPTER VIII

RECEPTORS AND MECHANISMS OF ACTION OF ANDROGENS IN PROSTATES

SHUTSUNG LIAO AND TEHMING LIANG

I. Introduction

One of the most popular approaches employed to study the biochemical processes of steroid hormone actions has been to find the effects of these "chemical messengers," as Starling (1905) defined the term "hormones," on enzyme activities in experimental animals and in isolated enzyme systems. Such an approach led eventually to the discovery of cyclic AMP, which appears to act as a second chemical messenger in mediating the action of many peptide hormones (Robison *et al.,* 1971). For steroid hormones, however, this approach has been rather disappointing.

An alternative approach to an understanding of the molecular mechanism of steroid hormone action is to study the fate of a steroid hormone after it has been generated in or administered to animals. This approach involves the study of the transformation and inter- and intracellular transport of hormones, as well as their interaction with various cellular components. The most significant progress made in this area of research has been that by Jensen and his co-workers. About fifteen years ago, these investigators found that the uterus and vagina have a striking ability to retain 17β-estradiol *in vivo* (Jensen and Jacobson, 1962). The high affinity of these estrogen-responsive tissues for 17β-estradiol was found to be estrogen-specific, could be inhibited by several anti-estrogenic compounds, and was not observed for nontarget tissues. The pioneering work eventually (in the middle 1960's) led to the discovery of what one may call cellular estrogen receptors that apparently play central roles in the selective tissue retention and functions of estrogens (Jensen and DeSombre, 1972; Gorski *et al.*, 1969). Several years later, specific cellular receptors were found for androgens and also for other steroid hormones. This article summarizes the efforts made in recent years in the search for and understanding of the nature of androgen receptors in the target tissues. The finding of a specific androgen-binding macromolecule that appeared to be a cellular receptor came about soon after the observation that 5α-dihydrotestosterone (DHT), a metabolite of testosterone, could be selectively retained by the nuclear chromatin of rat ventral prostate (Anderson and Liao, 1968; Bruchovsky and Wilson, 1968a). Since most of our understanding of the androgen receptors have been with the DHT-binding proteins in this accessory genital organ, these investigations will be described in some detail.

II.   Androgen Retention by Prostate Cells

A. *Tissue Retention*

In the rat uterus, 17β-estradiol, the major blood estrogen, is retained without metabolic conversion (Jensen and Jacobson, 1962). Testosterone, the major blood androgen, however, goes through rapid and multiple transformations in the liver and target organs. Early investigations of androgen retention were also complicated by the need to use large amounts of androgens labeled with low specific radioactivities. Nevertheless, some of the earlier studies indicated the ability of rat ventral prostate and seminal vesicles to accumulate radioactive androgens (see a review by Liao and Fang, 1969). One of the important observations made in these studies was that whereas large amounts of conjugated metabolites are present in blood and liver, the prostate and seminal vesicles accumulate mainly unconjugated androgen metabolites (Pearlman and Pearlman, 1961; Harding and Samuels, 1962; Tveter and Aakvaag, 1969).

When testosterone with high specific radioactivity became available, the high affinity of the target tissues toward androgen could be demonstrated clearly (Tveter and Attramadal, 1968; Fang *et al.*, 1969). The retention of radioactive androgen by the ventral prostate of rats was very distinct over $\frac{1}{2}$ to 3 hours (see also Rennie and Bruchovsky, 1973) from the time of injection of [³H]testosterone (Fig. 1). About 50% of the amount retained disappeared in about 6 hours, but some trace of radioactivity could be observed over 12 to 16 hours. When radioisotopes were analyzed for testosterone, androstenedione, and 5α-dihydrotestosterone (DHT; Fig. 2), only DHT was found in the ventral prostate and seminal vesicles after 3 hours. No retention of DHT could be seen in the liver, spleen, lung thymus, and diaphragm; this observation suggests that the male accessory glands have the ability to retain DHT (Fig. 3).

B. Nuclear Retention

The prolonged retention of DHT by rat ventral prostate appears to be due to the selective retention of DHT by the prostate cell nuclei (Anderson

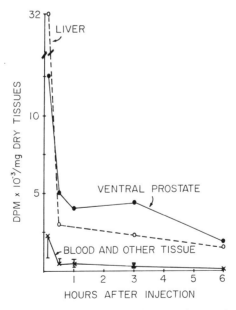

Fig. 1. Retention of radioisotopes by tissues of castrated rats injected with [³H]testosterone. Male rats (body weight 300 gm) were castrated, and 4 days later 50 μCi (1.44 μg) of [7α-³H]testosterone were injected intraperitoneally. The radioactivity per wet weight of tissue was higher in the ventral prostate than in blood, spleen, lung, thymus, and diaphragm. (From Fang *et al.*, 1969.)

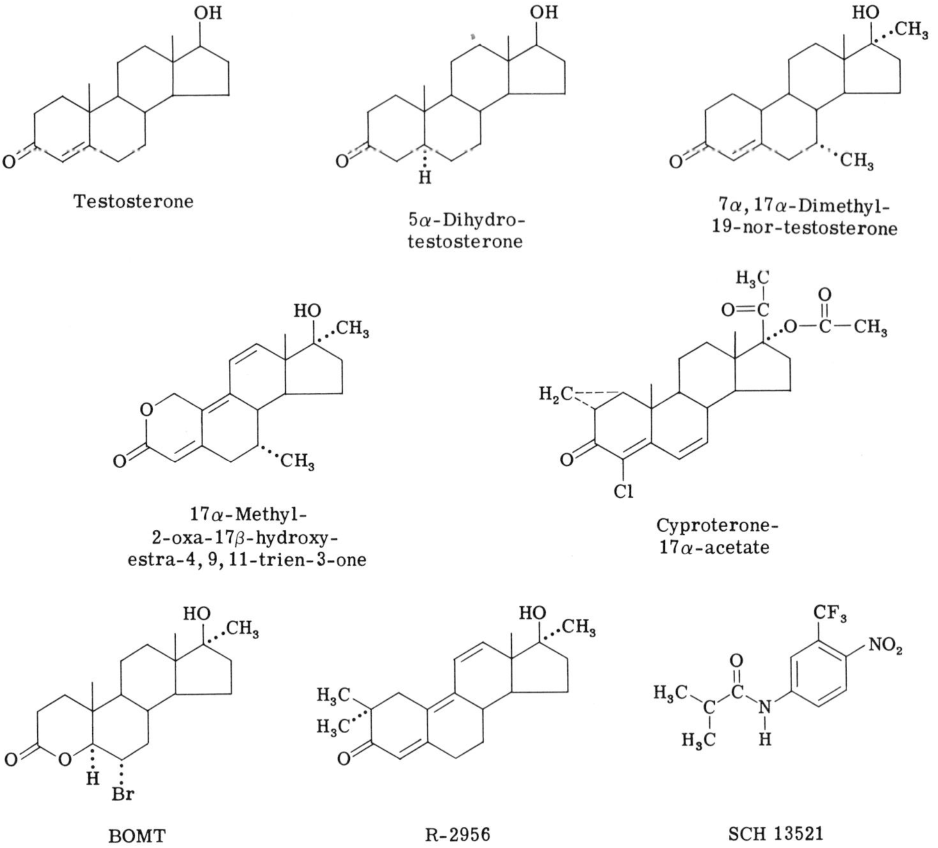

Testosterone

5α-Dihydro-
testosterone

7α,17α-Dimethyl-
19-nor-testosterone

17α-Methyl-
2-oxa-17β-hydroxy-
estra-4, 9, 11-trien-3-one

Cyproterone-
17α-acetate

BOMT

R-2956

SCH 13521

Fig. 2.   Structures of some androgens and anti-androgens.

and Liao, 1968; Bruchovsky and Wilson, 1968a), as demonstrated by biochemical or autoradiographic studies (Sar *et al.*, 1970; Tveter and Attramadal, 1969). Maximum nuclear labeling appeared at 1 hour and remained for about 3 hours. The retention of DHT by prostate cell nuclei could be reproduced *in vitro* by incubating minced prostate gland with [³H]testosterone or [³H]androstenedione (Anderson an Liao, 1968). After incubation, about 75 to 95% of the radioactivity associated with isolated nuclei was found to be due to DHT (Table I).

Some minor activity due to testosterone often appeared, but no other steroid could be found in prostate nuclei *in vivo* or during incubation of the minced tissue, even though the cytoplasm of the same tissue contained at least five other metabolites of [³H]testosterone (Anderson and Liao, 1968).

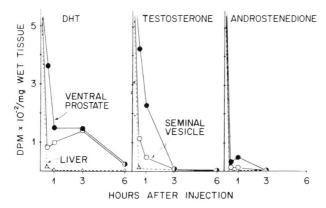

Fig. 3. Selective retention of major androgens by ventral prostate and seminal vesicles of castrated rats injected with [³H]testosterone. Note that, from 1 to 6 hours after the injection, ³H-DHT is the major androgen retained. (See Fig. 1 for experimental conditions.)

Cell nuclei of liver and other tissues less sensitive to androgens was not found to retain DHT to any significant extent, despite the fact that these tissues were able to reduce testosterone to DHT. Furthermore, non-androgens such as 17β-estradiol or cortisol were not retained by prostate nuclei.

TABLE I

Retention of Radioisotopes by Isolated Nuclei of Minced Rat Tissues Incubated with [³H]Testosterone for 30 Minutes at 37°C[a]

Tissues	Radioactivity of isolated nuclei (dpm/100 μg DNA)	Distribution of radioactivity[b]		
		Testosterone (%)	DHT (%)	Androstenedione (%)
Brain	105	96.2	2.8	0.0
Thymus	78	93.5	0.0	2.1
Diaphragm	53	78.2	2.1	17.6
Liver	60	73.4	0.0	4.5
Ventral prostate	1250	17.3	78.2	1.0

[a] From Anderson and Liao (1968).

[b] Steroids extracted from nuclei were subjected to thin-layer chromatography, and the percentage distribution of radioactivity associated with the three steroid spots was calculated. Note that only ventral prostate retained a large quantity of radioactivity that was mainly due to ³H-DHT.

C. DHT as a Functional Form of Androgen

The finding that prostate nuclei have a high affinity for DHT immediately raised the possibility that this steroid may be the active form of the cellular androgen. Some pertinent observations in support of this view are (a) DHT retention occurs in the cell nuclei, where androgens have a rapid effect on RNA synthesis (Liao *et al.*, 1965; Liao and Fang, 1969). (b) attempts to detect testosterone receptor and to show the stimulation of RNA synthesis by testosterone in isolated nuclear systems were not succesful, suggesting that testosterone may have to be metabolized to an active form. (c) DHT is more active than testosterone in a number of bioassay systems, including that measuring the growth of rat prostates (Dorfman and Shipley, 1956; Huggins and Mainzer, 1957; Saunders, 1963), suggesting that the action of testosterone may be mediated by DHT.

In rat ventral prostate, the formation of DHT from testosterone is catalyzed by a NADPH-dependent Δ^4-3-ketosteroid 5α-oxidoreductase. This enzyme is located in the microsomal fraction and is apparently tightly bound to the endoplasmic reticulum membranes (Shimazaki *et al.*, 1965; Ofner, 1968). Cell nuclei isolated and purified from rat ventral prostate also contain a large quantity of this enzyme (Anderson and Liao, 1968; Bruchovsky and Wilson, 1968a), which may be located in nuclear membrane sites (Moore and Wilson, 1972). The prostate reductase probably is responsible for the generation of the major portion of DHT in the target cells. A recent study revealed, however, that as much as 10 to 30% of the blood androgens in young male mammals is DHT (Ito and Horton, 1970; Tremblay *et al.*, 1970). Since DHT can be taken up by prostate cells as readily as testosterone, the blood supply of DHT should not be ignored.

III. Androgen Receptors for DHT in Prostate

A. Cytosol Receptors

With the new concept that DHT may be the active androgen, the search for specific proteins that bind DHT was initiated in many laboratories (Bruchovsky and Wilson, 1968b; Liao, 1968; Fang and Liao, 1969; Fang *et al.*, 1969; Mainwaring, 1969a,b; Unhjem *et al.*, 1969; Baulieu and Jung, 1970). In cytosol preparations of rat ventral prostate, there are several proteins that bind DHT preferentially over testosterone. One of these proteins (named β-protein) precipitates from the cytosol when ammonium sulfate is added 40% saturation (Fang and Liao, 1971). β-Protein exhibits an extremely high affinity and specificity toward DHT (see later sections). Another protein (named α-protein) that binds DHT firmly, but also binds progesterone, 17β-estradiol, and testosterone (but not cortisol) to some extent, can be sedimented from the solution if the ammonium sulfate concentration is raised to 70% saturation. For convenience, the complexes of DHT and α- or β-protein were designated as complex I or complex II, respectively. Both complex I and complex II have sedimentation constants of about 3 to 3.5 S if measured in a 0.4 M KCl solution (Fang et al., 1969; Fang and Liao, 1971). In the absence of KCl, complex II, but not complex I gradually aggregates to larger forms. The larger complex can be dissociated by the addition of KCl to 0.4 M, and complex II can be recovered in the vicinity of the 3 S fraction. As will be described later, complex II, but not complex I can be retained by prostate cell nuclei. The possibility that complex I is a precursor or a degradation product of complex II has not been excluded.

Analogous to the 17β-estradiol-receptor complex of the rat uterus, ^{3}H-DHT-protein complexes having sedimentation constants of 8 to 9 S have been detected in the cytosol preparation of rat ventral prostate (Mainwaring, 1969b; Unhjem et al., 1969; Baulieu and Jung, 1970; Tveter et al., 1971). In 0.4 M KCl solution, the 8 S complex also dissociates into components of about 3 to 4 S that are apparently identical with complex II described above. Baulieu et al. (1971) reported that their 8–10 S complex also binds testosterone to a significant extent, but not 17β-estradiol or 5α-androstane-3α (or 3β) 17β-diol. The aggregation of the small DHT-binding unit (3 to 4 S protein) to some of the larger complexes appears to involve other cellular components, since recentrifugation or purification of complex II tends to minimize the extent of aggregation (Liao et al., 1971c).

It was reported earlier that the measurable 8 S receptor protein disappears rapidly within a day after the rats have been castrated (Baulieu and Jung, 1970; Mainwaring, 1970). Such a rapid loss of DHT-receptor protein was not observed by Liao et al., (1971c) if the receptor protein was protected from degradation by the addition of DHT at the time of tissue homogenization. Sullivan and Strott (1973) also showed recently that the loss of receptor from prostate cells is gradual and closely follows the rate of regression of the prostate after the animals have been deprived of androgens. The immediate action of DHT after it reaches a target cell is therefore dependent on the existing cellular receptor rather than on a specific DHT-dependent induction of the receptor protein.

B. Cytoplasmic Membrane-Bound Receptors

The prostate microsomal fraction in rats injected with [3H]testosterone also retains ^{3}H-DHT to some extent. When such a microsomal fraction is extracted with a 0.4 M KCl solution, a ^{3}H-DHT-protein complex that has a sedimentation constant of about 3 S can be obtained (Liao and Fang, 1969, 1970). The microsomal ³H-DHT-binding protein is very similar to the cytosol β-protein in its steroid specificity, heat sensitivity, sedimentation properties, and ability to be retained by prostate nuclear chromatin. The amount of microsomal DHT-binding protein in prostate cells with well-developed endoplasmic reticulum membranes can be about 30 to 50% of the total β-protein found in the prostate cytosol fraction (Liao, 1973). This protein may thus be responsible at least in part for the retention of DHT by the microsomal fractions of prostates (Kowarski et al., 1969). As will be described later, some of these receptor-like proteins may be bound to certain ribonucleoprotein particles.

C. Nuclear Receptor and Its Origin

The ³H-DHT retained by prostate cell nuclei or chromatin in vivo appears to bind to a protein that can be extracted with 0.4 M to 0.6 M KCl solution (Bruchovsky and Wilson, 1968b; Liao and Fang, 1969; Mainwaring, 1969a). The sedimentation constant of the DHT-bound protein is about 3 S (Fang and Liao, 1969; Fang et al., 1969), which appears to be somewhat smaller than the 5 S 17β-estradiol-receptor complex of uterine nuclei (Jensen and DeSombre, 1972). More than 80% of the nuclear DHT retained in vivo can be recovered as the 3 S protein-bound form. The nuclear ³H-DHT protein complex shares all properties described above for the cytosol complex II and the microsomal complex, suggesting that they may be closely related, if not identical.

The salt extracts of prostate cell nuclei isolated from castrated rats contain very few proteins that bind DHT tightly. Incubation of the isolated prostate nuclei with radioactive DHT also did not result in significant formation of the DHT-protein complex. If the nuclei are incubated with ³H-DHT in the presence of a whole cytosol preparation however, one can obtain the ³H-DHT-protein complex from the reisolated nuclei. The prostate nuclear DHT-receptor protein, therefore, originates in the cytoplasm (Fang et al., 1969; Liao and Fang, 1969).

One can prepare ³H-complex II and then mix it with prostate nuclei to show that the appearance of the nuclear complex is accompanied by a stoichiometric reduction in the soluble cytosol ³H-complex II. Interestingly, the complex I (or α-protein) that cannot be retained by prostate nuclei strongly reduces the nuclear retention of complex II (Fig. 4).

D. Androgen-Mediated Translocation of a Cytoplasmic Protein to Cell Nuclei

Since the retention of 17β-estradiol or DHT by their target cell nuclei is dependent on a cytoplasmic receptor protein, the receptor protein may

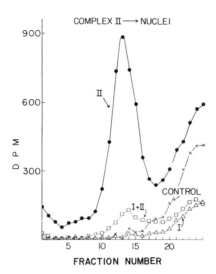

Fig. 4. Selective retention of the prostate ³H-DHT-protein complex II by isolated prostate nuclei. α-Protein (20 mg protein) and β-protein (9 mg protein) fractions, either alone or in combination (I and II), were mixed with 1.25 μCi of ³H-DHT in 1.4 ml of 0.02 *M* Tris-HCl, pH 7.5, containing 1.5m*M* EDTA and kept at −20°C for 20 hours. After thawing, they were incubated with a prostate 600 *g* nuclear pellet (0.5 mg DNA). Nuclei were reisolated, extracted, and the ³H-DHT-protein complex was analyzed by sucrose (with 0.4 *M* KC1) gradient centrifugation. The control tube contained only the nuclear sediments and the radioactive androgen during the incubation. (From Fang and Liao, 1971.)

simply function as a carrier of the hormone to regulate its concentration at various cellular sites. On the other hand, one may also visualize the binding of a steroid to a specific protein as a necessary step in the translocation of the protein to another cellular locus where the receptor protein (or the protein in a complex with the steroid), rather than the steroid alone, functions.

For uterine estrogen receptor systems, 17β-estradiol was shown to play a key role in the temperature-dependent transformation of a 4 S cytosol receptor to a 5 S entity. The latter rather than the 4 S material can be retained by the uterine nuclei (Jensen and DeSombre, 1972). This transformation of the receptor protein is believed to be related to the earlier observation, by autoradiographic techniques, that the nuclear retention but not the tissue uptake of the [³H]estrogen requires the incubation of uteri at a high temperature (37°C).

The temperature-dependent nuclear retention of ³H-DHT was first realized in the autoradiographic study (Sar *et al.*, 1970) and in the tissue incubation experiments with ³H-DHT (Fang *et al.*, 1969). Nuclear retention occurs to a limited extent at 2°C, but is greatly enhanced at 37°C (see Table II). Working with cell-free systems in showing the retention of the

TABLE II

Retention of ^{3}H-DHT-Receptor Complex by Cell Nuclei of Rat Ventral Prostate[a]

Incubation temperature (°C)	^{3}H-DHT	Radioactivity associated with receptor protein in nuclei during incubation of	
		Minced tissue (dpm/100 μg DNA)	Homogenate (dpm/100 μg DNA)
0	—[b]	55	33
0	+	528	1295
10	+	1339	1674
20	+	2142	2323
30	+	1876	1700
40	+	534	353

[a] Sprague-Dawley male rats (weighing 300 to 450 gm) were castrated 18 hours before they were killed. Minced prostates (see Fang et al., 1969) or prostate homogenates (see Fang and Liao, 1971) were incubated with ^{3}H-DHT for 20 minutes at the temperature shown. Nuclei were isolated, and the ^{3}H-DHT-receptor complex was extracted and analyzed by gradient centrifugation. The radioactivity associated with the 3 S protein fractions was measured.

[b] ^{3}H-DHT was omitted from the incubation mixture, but was added after nuclear extract had been obtained.

cytoplasmic ^{3}H-complex II (see above), Fang and Liao (1971) also observed that nuclear retention is more efficient at 37°C than at 0°C (Table II). It was also demonstrated that very little of the cytoplasmic receptor protein could be retained by the cell nuclei if DHT was omitted during incubation of the nuclei with cytoplasmic protein fractions (Fig. 5). The binding of DHT to β-protein (to form complex II), is clearly necessary for the cytoplasmic receptor protein to bind to the cell nuclear sites.

IV.   Chemical Nature of DHT-Receptor Complex

A. Receptor Proteins

Since the biological functions of the various cellular steroid-receptor proteins have not been clearly demonstrated, the identification of the receptor proteins for various steroid hormones has been based on their binding to

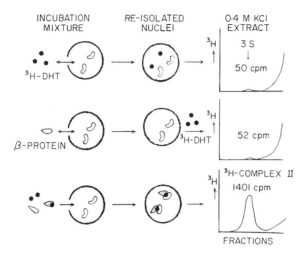

Fig. 5. DHT-dependent retention of a cytoplasmic receptor protein by prostate cell nuclei. The prostate β-protein was labeled with ³H-DHT and incubated with a prostate cell nuclear fraction. Nuclei were reisolated, and the ³H-DHT-receptor complex retained by the nuclei was extracted and analyzed by sucrose gradient (with 0.4 M KCl) solution to determine the amount of the complex sedimented at the 3 S region (lower row). For comparison, we omitted ³H-DHT from one of the incubation tubes (middle row) to see whether the unlabeled β-protein can be retained by the cell nuclei. This was done by labeling the nuclear extract directly and analyzing it by gradient centrifugation. In another control tube, prostate nuclei were incubated with ³H-DHT in the absence of β-protein (upper row), to show that very little receptor protein is present in the prostate nuclei of rats castrated 18 hours before they were killed.

specific radioactive steroids. Thus, it is difficult to determine the relationships, in the target cells, among various forms of receptor proteins for steroids. Gradient centrifugation has been the most useful and popular technique for the characterization of steroid-receptor complexes since its first application by Toft and Gorski (1966) for the 17β-estradiol receptor. However, various artefacts affect the sedimentation constants of a radiometric amount of receptor protein in a crude extract, and thus often complicate their evaluation. Like the estrogen-receptor complex (Chamnes and McGuire, 1972) various forms of the prostate ³H-DHT-receptor complex with sedimentation constants ranging from 3 to 12 S or higher can be observed if conditions such as pH, temperature, or concentration of salt, polyion (including poly A), etc., are altered. It is not certain at this time which forms of the complex are those present *in vivo*.

Other descriptions of the cytosol DHT-receptor protein have also been based on studies using crude preparations. It is generally recognized that the receptor protein is an acidic protein, that its steroid-binding ability is unstable at temperatures above 30°C (10 minutes), and that it may have a molecular weight of the order of about 30,000 (the 3 S unit). The affinity constant of the β-protein for DHT is at least of the order of 10^{10} M^{-1} (Fang et al., 1969). A recent calculation from a partially purified preparation gave 10^{12} M^{-1}. More reliable information on the chemical properties of the receptor protein can be obtained only when a more highly purified material is available for analysis. So far, attempts to purify the androgen-receptor complex have not been very successful (Mainwaring and Mangan, 1971; Rennie and Bruchovsky, 1972a).

B. Steroid Binding

DHT associates with the receptor protein through noncovalent bindings. It has been proposed that a large part of the DHT molecule is physically enveloped in the receptor protein (Fang and Liao, 1971; Liao et al., 1971c, 1972). Such a suggestion was originally based on the observation that ^{3}H-DHT, once bound to β-protein, does not exchange readily with a several-hundredfold concentration of nonradioactive DHT while maintained for many hours at 0°C. Such an exchange can be brough about, however, by freezing and thawing of the complex.

More recently, we investigated the nature of the receptor binding of an androgen by studying the structural requirements for tight binding of a steroid to the receptor proteins (Liao et al., 1973b). To explain the low affinity of testosterone for β-protein, we considered that the steroid-binding site(s) on the receptor protein may be in a narrow hole that can accommodate a flat molecule like DHT, but not testosterone. [Molecular models (Fig. 6) as well as X-ray crystallographic studies (Cooper et al., 1968) suggested that, in Δ ^{4}-androstenes, ring A of the steroid nucleus bends appreciably to the α side of the relatively flat carbon skeleton of the rest of the steroid nucleus.] The bulkiness at the ring A areas may interfere with the ability of testosterone to approach the binding site. If the angular methyl group at C-10 is removed, such a steric hindrance may be eliminated. In fact, some of the 19-nortestosterone derivatives which are very potent androgens bind firmly to β-protein (Table III). Among them are 17α-methyl-2-oxa-17β-hydroxy-estra-4,9,11-triene-3-one and related compounds (Fig. 7). By having conjugated double bonds which extend from ring A to C, these androgens are indeed very flat molecules with gross solid geometric structures more like that of the saturated androgen, DHT, than that of testosterone (Fig. 6).

The receptor-binding affinity of 19-nortestosterone appears to increase somewhat if a methyl group is present at the 17α-position; but the stimulation is most dramatic if the methyl substitution is at the 7α position.

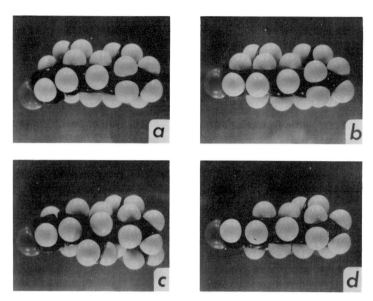

Fig. 6. CPK models of androgens. Corey-Pauling atomic models with Koltun connectors were used to construct (*a*) testosterone, (*b*), DHT, (*c*) $7\alpha,17\alpha$-dimethyl-19-nortestosterone, and (*d*) 2-oxa-17β-hydroxy-estra-4,9,11-trien-3-one. These are side views, with ring A oxygens at the far left and the α-faces of the steroid facing downward. (From Liao *et al.*, 1973b.)

Since $7\alpha,17\alpha$-dimethyl-19-nortestosterone has an apparent affinity to β-protein several times higher than that of 5α-dihydrotestosterone, it is very likely that the receptor protein contains a specific local site (M site) that interacts with the 7α-methyl group (Liao *et al.*, 1972, 1973b).

The importance of the 17β-hydroxy group for receptor binding is evident from the fact that androstanedione, 5α-androstan-3-one, and the 17α isomer of DHT do not bind tightly to the prostate receptor, nor are they retained by prostate cell nuclei (Table III). This could be the reason for the high potency of the 17β-hydroxylated androgens.

Some androgens, such as 17β-hydroxy-5α-androstane, 17α-methyl-17β-hydroxy-5α-androstane, 5α-androstane, and related compounds, do not have an oxygen atom at the C-3 and/or C-17 positions (see reviews by Liao and Fang, 1969; Vida, 1969). Since these steroids do not bind tightly to β-protein (Table III), their androgenic actions in animals may be dependent on their oxygenation. As they are not able to compete with DHT for nuclear retention during their incubation with minced prostate, such metabolic conversions might be carried out mainly outside the prostate. In the rabbit, the liver has enzyme systems to convert 17α-methyl-17β-hydroxy-5α-androstane to 17α-methyl-5α-dihydrotestosterone (Wolff and Kasuya,

TABLE III

Relative Androgenic Activities (RA) and Relative Competition Indexes (RCI)
of Various Androgens[a]

Steroid	RA	RCI[f] Nuclear retention	Receptor binding
Group A[b]			
Testosterone	0.4	0.7	0.1
$7\alpha,17\alpha$-(CH$_3$)$_2$-testosterone	0.6	0.3	0.2
$7\beta,17\alpha$-(CH$_3$)$_2$-testosterone	0.1	<0.1	<0.1
5α-Dihydrotestosterone (5α-DHT)	1.0	1.0	1.0
$7\alpha,17\alpha$-(CH$_3$)$_2$-5α-DHT	1.5	0.7	0.6
$7\beta,17\alpha$-(CH$_3$)$_2$-5α-DHT	0.0	<0.1	<0.1
19-Nortestosterone (NorT)	0.2	0.7	0.9
$7\alpha,17\alpha$-(CH$_3$)$_2$-NorT (DMNT)	5.7	3.6	3.5
19-Nor-DHT (Nor-5α-DHT)	0.1	0.6	0.5
$7\alpha,17\alpha$-(CH$_3$)$_2$-Nor-5α-DHT	0.3	0.4	1.0
Group B[c]			
2-Oxa-17β-hydroxy-estra-4,9-dien-3-one	3.2[d]	—	1.4
2-Oxa-17β-hydroxy-estra-4,9,11-trien-3-one	8–12[d]	—	3.2
2-Oxa-17α-methyl-17β-hydroxy-estra-4,9,11-trien-3-one	80–120[d]	—	3.8
17α-Methyl-17β-hydroxy-estra-4,9,11-trien-3-one	24[e]	—	2.3
$3\alpha,17\beta$-Dihydroxy-5α-androstane	0.2[e]	0.2	0.0
5α-Androstane-3,17-dione	0.2[e]	0.2	0.0
5α-Androstane	—[a]	0.0	0.0
5α-Androstane-3-one	—[a]	0.0	0.0
17β-Hydroxy-5α-androstane	—[a]	0.0	0.0
3α-Hydroxy-5α-androstan-17-one	0.2[e]	0.0	0.0

[a] See Liao *et al.* (1973b).

[b] The relative activities of androgens shown in Group A were calculated from our own results with 5α-dihydrotestosterone taken as 1.0. Test steroids were injected subcutaneously into castrated rats daily for 7 days, and the wet weights of the ventral prostates were compared. The prostate weights for the control group were 11.2 ± 0.5 mg. The daily dose of 5α-dihydrotestosterone needed to maintain the weight of the ventral prostate in the steroid-injected rats at twice that of the control castrates was 0.8 ± 0.1 µg per rat (body weight:50 gm).

[c] The relative activities of androgens shown in Group B were calculated from the results of other workers. Some of these investigators used the value for 17α-methyltestosterone as 1.0 in their reports. For convenience of comparison with other data, the figures were recalculated using DHT as 1.0. The relative activity for 17α-methyltestosterone was assumed to be 0.4 (see Liao and Fang, 1969).

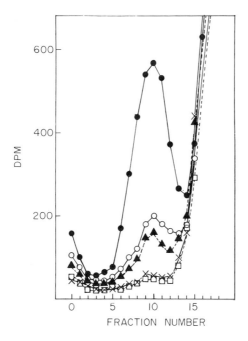

Fig. 7. Competition of the β-protein binding of ³H-DHT by dienic and trienic derivatives of 2-oxa-19-nortestosterone. A β-protein preparation (3 mg protein/ml) was incubated with ³H-DHT (0.5 nM; 48 Ci/mmole) in the presence of 1.5 nM nonradioactive DHT (○), 2-oxa-17β-hydroxy-estra-4,9,diene-3-one (▲), 2-oxa-17β-hydroxy-estra-4,9,11-triene-3-one (×), and 2-oxa-17α-methyl-17β-hydroxy-estra-4,9,11-triene-3-one (□) as competitors. The control tube (●) contained no competitor. Note that these androgens show a higher affinity toward the receptor protein even when they are highly unsaturated. These androgens are, in fact, biologically more potent than DHT (see Table III) and apparently do not require a metabolic conversion for their action.

---

[d] Calculated from Bucourt *et al.* (1971).

[e] Calculated from Feyel-Cabanes (1963).

[f] The relative competition indexes were measured by methods based on the ability of various steroids to compete with ³H-DHT for binding to β-protein in a cell-free system and for retention by prostate cell nuclei during the incubation of minced prostates. These methods are especially useful if test compounds are available only in minute quantities (<1 μg). A compound with an RCI of 1 is expected to bind to β-protein receptor with an affinity equivalent to that of DHT. A compound with an RCI higher than 1 is expected to be biologically more active than DHT. A low RCI in the β-protein binding assay for a potent androgen (like testosterone) that also shows a high RCI in the nuclear retention assay with the tissue-incubation system suggests that the biological activity of the compound is dependent on its transformation to an active form or on a process not dependent on β-protein binding.

1972). A better understanding of the importance of the ring A oxygen in androgen actions may be obtained from a study of the metabolic fate and the receptor binding of the newly discovered nonsteroidal androgen, 1,4-seco-2,3-bisnor-17β-hydroxy-5α-androstane (Zanati and Wolff, 1973).

The findings based on a study of the structural requirements for the binding of androgens to the well-defined cellular receptor (β-protein) are in accord with that based on the study of the chemical structure and end-point activity (Ringold, 1961; Wolff et al., 1964; see reviews by Liao and Fang, 1969; Vida, 1969). Both strongly suggested that there are multiple sites for the attachment of a receptor molecule to an androgen and indicated that the steric characteristics of an androgen play a more important role than the local electronic structure in the receptor binding and in the eliciting of the biological response. The enveloping of an androgen is likely to result in the reorientation of certain flexible polypeptide chains on the receptor molecule. This may result in a conformational change of the protein that is necessary for the reaction of a receptor protein with "acceptor" molecules and for triggering the hormone action.

V.   Nucleoprotein Binding of DHT-Receptor Complex

A. Deoxyribonucleoprotein Complex

Soon after the breakthrough in the understanding of the basic molecular processes involved in gene expression, androgens (Liao and Williams-Ashman, 1962) and other steroid hormones (Karlson, 1963; see review articles in Litwack, 1972) were implicated in the regulation of these processes. This prompted a study of the possible nature of the interaction of steroid hormones with nuclear components. Huggins and Yang (1962) and Dannenberg (1963) pointed out the similarity in the molecular geometry of steroids and the base pairs of the DNA helix. T'so and Lu (1964) examined the binding of steroids to purified DNA, and found that single-stranded DNA could bind steroids much more firmly than duplex DNA. More recently, Kidson et al., (1971) observed that DHT could bind to heat-denatured bovine spleen DNA more firmly than testosterone, whereas the non-androgenic 17α-hydroxy epimer of testosterone (cis-testosterone) has considerably less affinity toward denatured DNA. Various guanine-containing synthetic polyribo- (or deoxyribo-) nucleotides (poly dG, poly UG, poly G) also appear to bind various steroids more firmly than poly A, poly C, or poly U, suggesting the involvement of 2-amino groups of guanine in the binding. In a report, yet to be confirmed, Goldberg and Atchley (1966) indicated that certain steroid hormones could weaken the DNA intrastrand bonds holding the double helix.

Wilson and Loeb (1965a,b) studied the binding of radioactive androgen(s) to the cell nuclei of preen glands. The radioactivity originating from labeled testosterone injected into ducks was found to associate with euchromatin fractions that had been considered to be the major sites of RNA synthesis in karyotic cells (cf. Frenster *et al.*, 1963). Sluyser (1966a,b,c) also reported that, in rats injected with radioactive testosterone, the radioactive steroid bound preferentially to the lysine-rich histone fraction of ventral prostate rather than to the lysine-poor histone fractions. He claimed that testosterone could diminish the ability of prostatic lysine-rich histone to keep the two DNA chains from separating at raised temperatures. Mangan *et al.*, (1968) also reported that the uptake of tritiated testosterone, injected directly into the prostates of the castrated rats, by the prostate cell nuclei was mostly in the heterochromatin fractions, but that the uptake per milligram DNA in the euchromatin fractions exceeded that of the heterochromatin fractions.

Since the involvement of the receptor protein in the chromatin retention of steroid hormones became known, the binding of the steroid-receptor complexes, rather than the steroids alone, to chromatin materials have been studied intensively. The binding to DNA of various receptor complexes for 17β-estradiol (King *et al.*, 1971; Clemens and Kleinsmith, 1972), progesterone (Schrader *et al.*, 1972), and DHT (Mainwaring and Mangan, 1971; Mainwaring and Peterken, 1971; Tymoczko and Liao, 1971) has been demonstrated by techniques such as density gradient centrifugation. DNA-cellulose column chromatography, and Millipore filtration. These studies, however, have not shown that such interactions are specific for DNA or receptor. The possibility that the non-histone proteins determine the specificity by preventing such binding at various DNA sites and thus making only limited DNA regions accessible to the receptor binding has been considered (King and Gordon, 1972).

On the other hand, there are indications showing that certain non-histone proteins may be necessary for the specific DNA binding of the receptor proteins for progesterone (Spelsberg *et al.*, 1971; O'Malley *et al.*, 1972). It has been proposed that these proteins, called "acceptor" proteins, specify the DNA or chromatin sites where the steroid-receptor complexes bind specifically and where they function. In such a study, Tymoczko and Liao (1971) investigated the DNA retention of the prostate DHT-receptor complex by Millipore membrane filtration. The acceptor-like protein or proteins that enhanced retention were found in the non-histone protein fractions of rat prostate cell nuclei. By this technique, the native calf thymus DNA, but not the heat-denatured DNA appeared to be functional (Fig. 8). The acceptor protein-dependent binding of the DHT-receptor complex to poly A and poly G was also demonstrated. Poly U or poly C was found to be less effective. The extracted acceptor protein(s) was heat labile suggesting

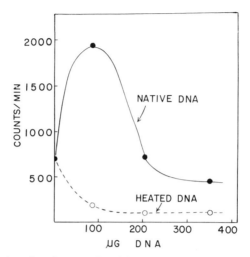

Fig. 8. DNA-dependent "acceptor" activity. A 0.4 *M* KCl extract of prostate cell nuclei (600 *μ*g protein) was incubated with a ^{3}H-DHT-receptor complex preparation (12,400 cpm/730 *μ*g protein) and an amount of calf thymus DNA as indicated. The nucleoprotein aggregates were retained by filtration through a Millipore filter and washed with 0.2 *M* KCl. The radioactivity was subsequently extracted with 0.4 *M* KCl and compared. Native DNA or DNA heated for 10 minutes at 100°C in 0.01 *M* Tris-HCl buffer, pH 7.5, containing 0.01 *M* NaCl were used. This assay method appears to measure the portion of the androgen-receptor complexes which bind to the nucleoprotein sites associated with heat-labile proteins(s). (From Tymoczko and Liao, 1971.)

that this may be the reason why prostate nuclei or nuclear chromatin lose their DHT-receptor binding ability if they are preheated at temperatures above 40°C. Liver nuclear extract appeared to contain fewer "acceptor" molecules than the corresponding prostate nuclear preparation (Tymoczko and Liao, 1971). Similar observations were made for the estrogen–uterus system (Liang and Liao, 1972).

B. Ribonucleoprotein

It was demonstrated recently that certain nuclear ribonucleoprotein (RNP) particles isolated from uteri and prostates could bind steroid-receptor complexes of their own tissues (Liao *et al.,* 1973a). In rat ventral prostate, some of these RNP particles were readily extracted from nuclei by 0.4 *M* KCl solutions, but many appeared to bind tightly to the chromatin. The chromatin-bound RNP particles could be freed by treatment of the chromatin with DNase and deoxycholate. To demonstrate the association of the nuclear particles and ^{3}H-complex II, we incubated them together and then analyzed them by gradient centrifugation (Fig. 9). The

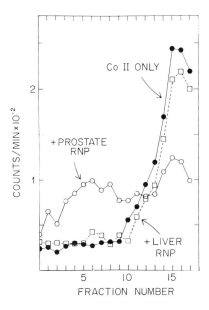

Fig. 9. Interaction of a ³H-DHT-receptor complex of ventral prostate with nuclear RNP particles of ventral prostate and liver. A ³H-complex II preparation (1800 cpm/0.17 mg protein), alone or in the presence of 0.1 unit (at 260 nm) of nuclear RNP isolated from rat ventral prostate (O) or liver (□), in 0.2 ml, was layered on the top of a centrifuge tube containing sucrose gradient (10 to 30%) solution. The gradient solution and the samples also contained 1.5 mM EDTA and 20 mM Tris-HCl buffer, pH 8.1. Gradient centrifugation was performed at 2°C and 54,000 rpm for 2.3 hours in a Spinco L2-65B ultracentrifuge with an SW 56 rotor. Fractions (0.2 ml) were collected and numbered from the bottom of the centrifuge tubes. Nuclear RNP particles were prepared as described by Hu and Wang (1971) from the chromatin sediments of nuclei which had been extracted with 1 M KCl particles of RNP were released from the sediments by treatment with RNase-free DNase I (Worthington) and 1% sodium deoxycholate. The particles were collected by centrifugation at 2°C and at 100,000 g for 2 hours.

ternary complexes appeared to have sedimentation constants of about 60 to 80 S. The ³H-DHT-receptor complex could be dissociated from the ternary comple by 0.4 M KCl or RNase treatment. Since DNase-I treatment of RNP particles did not affect the association of DHT-receptor complex with RNP particles, the interaction did not appear to involve DNA.

Preparations of RNP isolated in the same manner from rat liver were usually much less active than the prostate RNP in binding the ³H-complex II (Fig. 9). The [³H]progesterone- and [³H]17β-estradiol-binding proteins of calf uterus did not bind to RNP isolated from the chromatin of rat ventral prostate. The binding sites on the RNP particles could be saturated by the androgen-receptor complex. If one assumes that only one androgen-receptor complex can bind to an RNP particle, less than 10% of the RNP particle appears to have the binding site. A possible biological implication of this finding is discussed in the following section.

VI. Speculative Views on Receptor Cycling and Function

A. RNA Synthesis and Nuclear Retention of Receptors

One of the earliest actions of many steroid hormones on their target cells is to influence nuclear RNA synthesis (Williams-Ashman, 1965; Tata, 1966). Within one hour after testosterone has been injected into castrated rats, the nuclear RNA polymerase activity is enhanced (Liao et al., 1965). There are indications that such an effect occurs predominant at nucleolar regions of the prostate nuclear chromatin (Liao and Lin, 1967; Mainwaring et al., 1971), but whether this is preceded by a more specific RNA synthesis is not clear. The possibility that the formation of the DHT-receptor complex may be related to the stimulation of RNA synthesis was recently indicated by Anderson et al., (1972). These workers observed that cyproterone, which inhibits the formation of the androgen-receptor complex and the nuclear retention of DHT, can inhibit the synthesis of "nucleolar" RNA. This experiment strongly supports the contention that the receptor action on the nuclear activity is a dynamic phenomenon and requires a continuous supply of DHT-receptor complex to the prostate nucleus (Liao et al., 1971b).

It is widely believed that the steroid-receptor complex regulates the synthesis of specific species of RNA at nuclear chromatin sites. Whether this is achieved by the derepression of repressed genes (negative control), by providing necessary effectors (positive control), or by other means (chemical or physical alterations of the chromatin template or the products) is not clear (see Liao and Fang, 1969). Several investigators have recently reported that in the cell-free systems, 17β-estradiol together with uterine cytosol protein fractions can enhance the RNA-synthesizing ability of isolated uterine cell nuclei (Raynaud-Jammet and Baulieu,1969; Arnaud, et al., 1971; Mohla et al., 1972). A similar observation was also made recently for the DHT–prostate system (Davies et al., 1972). Earlier, it had been claimed that DHT (but not testosterone), in the absence of added cytoplasmic proteins, can stimulate the incorporation of radioactive nucleosides into RNA fractions (Bashirelahi and Villee, 1970). Since the RNA-synthesizing activity of an isolated nuclear preparation is extremely complex, a more direct demonstration of the involvement of a specific steroid-receptor complex is still needed before a final assessment of these observations can be made. Further biochemical characterization of these interesting systems may result in a better understanding of the basic mechanisms involved in the receptor actions on gene activities.

B. RNA Utilization and Receptor Cycling

Whereas considerable attention has been given to the nuclear retention of the steroid-receptor complexes in the cytoplasm of the target cells, essentially no study has been made on the release process of the steroid-receptor complexes from the cell nuclei to the cytoplasm. (One exception to this was the consideration given to the glucocorticoid receptor; see Munck et al., 1972.) In the ventral prostate, the disappearance of androgens after castration is apparently accompanied by a loss of the receptor protein from the prostate cell nuclei (Fang and Liao, 1971). Since the amounts of cytoplasmic receptor proteins for DHT decrease at a slower rate after castration, the nuclear loss of the receptor protein is probably due to the inability of the receptor protein (in the absence of DHT) to bind to the nuclear sites (Liao et al., 1971c). As noted previously, the nuclear retention of androgen-receptor complexes may be a dynamic process even in the presence of androgens, and such a process may be a part of the steroid hormone action.

Since certain nuclear RNP particles can bind a DHT-receptor complex in a specific manner, it has been suggested that some of these RNP particles may be involved in such a functional process. A hypothetical model based on this line of thinking has been presented (Liao, 1973; Liao et al., 1973a,c). In this model, a steroid hormone binds to a receptor protein in the cytoplasm and possibly induces a conformational change in the protein. The complex then enters the cell nucleus and becomes involved in the regulation of the synthesis of specific species of RNA. During such a process, the steroid receptor and possibly other regulatory or catalytic proteins involved in RNA synthesis may bind to DNA in a coordinated way at restricted portions of the nuclear chromatin. Eventually, the steroid-receptor complex may bind to the newly synthesized RNA and form a RNP particle. The steroid-receptor-bound RNP may then be processed to a mature form and enter the cytoplasm, where they may participate in protein synthesis (Fig. 10).

The role of the steroid-receptor complex in this model is seen to provide the structural specificity needed for the formation, processing, and also the function of RNP. If the steroid hormone of the cell is depleted, the receptor protein may lose its ability to bind to RNP at different stages of processing and utilization. When the steroid hormone is replenished, the receptor proteins and other protein factors may reassociate with these RNP particles at different stages of the receptor cycle. This would imply that the importance

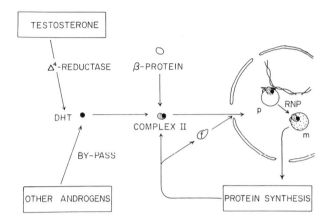

Fig. 10. A speculative model for androgen-receptor cycling. In a prostate cell, testosterone, the major blood androgen, is reduced to DHT that binds to β-protein. The DHT-receptor protein complex (complex II) then enters the cell nuclei and may participate in certain nuclear actions related to RNA production. The complex also binds to certain nuclear ribonucleoprotein (RNP) particles that may go through processes of maturation (p→m) enter cytoplasm, and possibly participate in protein synthesis. The receptor protein and DHT then may be released from the RNP particles and recycled. Some androgens may bind to the receptor protein and act without a need for a metabolic conversion (bypass) (see text for details). (From Liao *et al.*, 1973c.)

of gene transcription (RNA synthesis) in relation to gene translation (protein synthesis) for the overall function of a steroid hormone in the target cells may be dependent on the amounts of RNP particles at different stages of processing, and on their RNA and protein constituents in the target cells at the time when the hormone is supplied. If the target cells contain sufficient amounts of these RNA and protein constituents of the RNP, certain earlier actions of the hormone may simply be dependent on protein synthesis. This may explain some steroid hormone actions that have been reported to be actinomycin-D insensitive (Frieden *et al.*, 1964; Talwar *et al.*, 1965, Frieden and Fishel, 1968).

Based on the study of enzyme induction in liver by glucocorticoids, Tomkins *et al.* (1970) considered the existence of a labile "posttranscriptional repressor" that both inhibits the translation and enhances the degradation of messenger RNA. The steroid-receptor complex is thought to antagonize these functions of the repressor by interacting directly with the repressor, or by inhibiting the synthesis or speeding its inactivation. Ohno (1971) also proposed that the receptor protein for an androgen may act as a "translational block" when the androgen is not attached, by binding to certain messenger RNA's. It was suggested that androgens can interact with the RNA-binding protein and that the messenger RNA is thus released and translated. Ohno believes that the same androgen-receptor complex enters the prostate cell nuclei and activates nucleolar RNA polymerase.

VII. Androgen-Binding Proteins and Androgen Dysfunction

A. Actions of Anti-Androgens

Estrogens do not appear to bind selectively to prostate nuclei in any significant amount. Even at high concentrations, they antagonize the binding of DHT to β-protein poorly (Fang et al., 1969; Fang and Liao, 1969). In the prostate and uterus, the 17β-estradiol-binding protein is distinct from the DHT-receptor protein (Jungblut et al., 1971). At high concentrations (>10 μM), the NADPH-dependent enzymic reduction of testosterone to DHT by cell-free preparations of rat ventral prostate can be inhibited by 17β-estradiol, diethylstilbestrol, and related estrogens (Shimazaki et al., 1965).

Progesterone also binds to a cytosol protein of rat ventral prostate which can be distinguished from the DHT-receptor protein (Fang and Liao, 1971; Karsznia et al., 1969). However, progesterone can inhibit the reduction of testosterone by substrate competition during which progesterone is reduced to 5α-pregnane-3,20-dione (Voigt et al., 1970). Other steroids, including weak androgens that are substrates for the 5α-reductase system, can be expected to reduce the concentration and the nuclear retention of β-protein binding of DHT.

Many steroid anti-androgens (Fig. 2) are now known to reduce the nuclear retention of DHT in prostate cells. At 0.2 to 1 μM, cyproterone (6-chloro-17α-hydroxyl-1,2α-methylene-4, 6-pregnadiene-3,20-dione) and its 17α-acetate inhibit the binding of DHT by β-protein and prostate cell nuclei (Fang and Liao, 1969; Fang et al., 1971; see also Neumann and von Berswordt-Wallrabe, 1966; Geller et al., 1969; Stern and Eisenfeld, 1969; Whalen et al., 1969). Among other anti-androgens (Fig. 2) that appear to inhibit the receptor binding of DHT in rat prostate are S K and F 7690 (17α-methyl-β-nortestosterone; Tveter and Aakvaag, 1969), R-2956 (17β-hydroxy-2α,2β,17α-trimethyl-estra-4,9,11-triene-3-one; Baulieu and Jung, 1970), and BOMT (6α-bromo-17β-hydroxy-17α-methyl-4-oxa-5α-androstane-3-one; Mangan and Mainwaring, 1972). A new nonsteroidal anti-androgen, Sch-13521 (4′nitro-3′-trifluoro-methyl isobutranilide) made by American Schering Company (Neri et al., 1972), also strongly supresses the retention of DHT by prostate cell nuclei both *in vivo* and in tissue incubation experiments (S. Liao, et al., 1974).

B. Abnormality in Androgen-Sensitive Tissues

The levels of DHT in its normal and abnormal target cells have been studied carefully and extensively by Wilson and his co-workers. From the studies of the rate of conversion of testosterone to DHT in tissue slices of sex accessory tissues of many species and of human skin from a variety of anatomical sites (Gloyna and Wilson, 1969; Wilson and Gloyna, 1970), it has been concluded that DHT formation is not a clear obligatory feature of all androgen actions. In human subjects, Siiteri and Wilson (1970) found that the DHT content was significantly greater in hypertrophic than in normal prostates. These differences were apparently not due to the difference in the rate of DHT formation. In the periurethral area where prostatic hypertrophy usually commences, the DHT content was also two to three times greater than in the outer regions of the gland. In some cases of prostatic carcinoma, conversion of testosterone to DHT was indeed found to be very small (Giorgi et al., 1971, 1972). A similar finding was made in dogs (Gloyna et al., 1970).

The high concentration of DHT in hypertrophic areas may be due to DHT-binding proteins. Although these proteins have been found in human prostate (in normal and benign hyperplasia), a clear distinction of this protein from the steroid-binding proteins of human serum has not been made (Hansson et al., 1971; Fang, 1974). The formation of the androgen-protein complex can be inhibited by antiandrogens such as cyproterone and 17α-methyl-β-nortestosterone (S K and F 7690), but the binding of 17β-hydroxysteroid to a blood protein has also been shown to be inhibited by cyproterone (Mercier-Bodard et al., 1970; but, see also Vermeulen and Verdonck, 1970). Antiandrogen inhibition alone, therefore, may not be taken as evidence to show that the binding is due to a specific androgen receptor.

The androgen insensitivity or testicular feminization syndrome was originally suspected to be the result of a lower rate of testosterone conversion to DHT. Mauvais-Jarvis et al. (1970) showed that patients with the androgen insensitivity syndrome are about 10 times more sensitive to exogenous estrogens than normal males in regard to the increase in the level of plasma testosterone-binding proteins and the fall in urinary DHT and 5α-androstanediol. The higher plasma protein binding of testosterone may reduce the supply of testosterone to peripheral tissues. However, the androgen insensitivity in these types of patients cannot be due simply to the reduced supply of DHT to tissues that are normally androgen responsive, since DHT formation appears to be normal in many cases (Wilson and Walker, 1969; Perez-Placios et al., 1971; Rosenfield et al., 1971). In addition, in most cases the administration of DHT, like that of testosterone, does not fully restore the nitrogen retention or other typical effects of androgens (Strickland and French, 1969; Rosenfield et al., 1971). It is possible that the androgen insensitivity may be due to an alteration and dysfunction of the cellular androgen-receptor protein.

A strain of male pseudohermaphroditic rats developed by Stanley and Gumbreck was characterized by a female phenotype and a lack of androgen-dependent differentiation. In these rats, very little androgen effect can be produced in the preputial glands or other tissues by the administration of testosterone or DHT (Bardin *et al.*, 1969, 1970). The preputial tissue can convert testosterone to DHT, but does not retain DHT. In these androgen-insensitive rats, the cell nuclei of the preputial gland (Bullock and Bardin, 1970), liver, and kidney (Ritzen *et al.*, 1972b) appear to have a reduced ability to concentrate DHT. Since the *in vivo* uptake of radioactive androgens by these tissues is similar to that in normal rats, the defect in nuclear retention may be due to an abnormality in the androgen-receptor proteins or the nuclear-acceptor substances. In mice with a testicular-feminization (Tfm) mutation (Lyon and Hawkes, 1970), testosterone and DHT do not induce hypertrophy or certain enzymes of kidney as in normal animals (Dofuku *et al.*, 1971). It has been shown that the amount of DHT-binding protein in the cytoplasm and nuclei of the kidney is distinctly less in Tfm than in the normal mouse (Gehring *et al.*, 1971). The uptake of radioactive androgen by the kidney (Bullock *et al.*, 1971) and by the submandibular gland (Goldstein and Wilson, 1972) was reported to be normal in the Tfm animals, however. In fact, Wilson and Goldstein (1972) reported that supernatant of submandibular glands from Tfm animals exhibited greater capacity and higher affinity for the protein binding of androgen than did that from normal male mice.

VIII. Concluding Remarks

Many natural androgens can be metabolized to DHT in rat ventral prostate (Bruchovsky, 1971). Therefore, their androgen actions in this organ may be dependent on the same receptor mechanism that operates for DHT. We recently investigated whether the same mechanism also operates for many synthetic androgens in this tissue (Liao *et al.*, 1973b) by comparing the abilities of various synthetic androgens to compete with ^{3}H-DHT for binding to β-protein and retention by cell nuclei of rat ventral prostate. Since most of the potent androgens exhibit high binding affinities toward the receptor protein and show high retention by the nuclei (Table III), they appear to have a common receptor protein for their actions.

The findings of similar DHT-binding proteins in other androgen-sensitive tissues such as the seminal vesicles (Stern and Eisenfeld, 1969; Tveter and Unhjem, 1969; Liao *et al.*, 1971c), epididymis (Ritzen *et al.*, 1971; Blaquier, 1971; Tindall *et al.*, 1972; Danzo *et al.*, 1973), testis (Mainwaring, 1972;

Ritzen et al., 1972a; Vernon et al., 1972), kidney (Gehring et al., 1971; Ritzen et al., 1972b), androgen-sensitive tumors (Bruchovsky, 1972; Matsumoto et al., 1972; Rennie and Bruchovsky, 1972b), hair follicles (Fazekas and Sandor, 1972), sebaceous and preputial glands (Bullock and Bardin, 1970; Adachi and Kano, 1972; Eppenberger and Hsia, 1972), and uterus

TABLE IV

Androgen Actions Not Attributed to Dihydrotestosterone[a]

System	Observation[b]	Reference
Vagina, epithelial cells	3α-OH- and 3-keto-androstanes stimulate the production of mucus by the superficial cells, 3β-OH steroids affect deeper layers	Huggins et al. (1954)
Uterus	Testosterone, but not DHT, stimulates glandular secretion and increases the height of the luminal epithelium	Gonzalez-Diddi et al. (1972)
Prostate organ culture	DHT and not 3β-androstanediol increases cell proliferation, but both androgens maintain epithelial cell growth	Baulieu et al. (1968); Gittinger and Lasnitzki (1972)
Seminal vesicle	The secretory output of fructose and citric acid is stimulated more by testosterone than by DHT	Mann et al. (1971)
Muscle	No DHT-receptor protein has been detected	Aakvaag et al. (1972)
Sexual behavior	Testosterone is active, but DHT is not	McDonald et al. (1970); Whalen and Luttge (1971a)
Anovulatory sterility	Testosterone is active, but DHT is not	Whalen and Luttge (1971b)
Wolffian ducts	Differentiation is induced by testosterone when 5α-reductase activity is absent	Wilson (1973)

[a] From Liao et al. (1974).

[b] Receptor-like proteins that bind testosterone preferentially over DHT have been found in uterus (Giannopoulos, 1973), muscle (Jung and Baulieu, 1972), and brain (Perez-Palacios et al., 1970; Jouan et al., 1973). The inability of DHT in stimulating the sexual behaviour and anovulatory sterility does not appear to be due to the unavailability of DHT at the local sites. DHT as well as testosterone appear to pass the blood–brain barrier readily (Whalen and Rezek, 1972; Sar and Stumpf, 1973), and brain contains 5α-reductase to metabolize testosterone to DHT (Kniewald et al., 1971; Rommerts and Van der Molen, 1971).

(Jungblut *et al.,* 1971; cf. Giannopoulos, 1973) may also indicate the universality of the receptor mechanism.

Nevertheless, many experimental observations indicate the possibility that not all androgen actions can be attributed to the receptor mechanism involving DHT alone. Some representative cases are listed in Table IV. It is possible that there are varieties of androgen receptor molecules in various androgen-sensitive cells, or even in the same cell, functioning in a somewhat different manner.

Cyclic AMP undoubtedly is essential for the normal function and growth of steroid-sensitive cells (as is the case for other mammalian cells). The possibility that steroid hormone actions may be mediated by this or by related nucleotides has been pursued by several investigators, but undisputable experimental evidence is still lacking. In the ventral prostates of castrated rats, cyclic AMP is known to enhance certain enzyme activities *in vivo* (Singhal *et al.,* 1971), but such stimulation is not inhibited by cyproterone acetate (Mainwaring, 1974) that interferes with the receptor mechanism. Neither testosterone nor DHT stimulates the adenyl cyclase activity of rat ventral prostate *in vivo* or *in vitro* (Rosenfeld and O'Malley, 1970; Liao *et al.,* 1971a). We have found that, in the cytosol of rat ventral prostate, the cyclic AMP-binding proteins sediment as 3 S and 5 S forms. The cyclic AMP-binding proteins can be retained by prostate cell nuclei. However, DHT and cyclic AMP do not compete for the protein-binding sites. Attempts to show the effect of androgen manipulation, *in vivo* or *in vitro,* on the levels of cyclic AMP-binding proteins in nuclei and cytoplasm of the prostate have not been successful.

ACKNOWLEDGMENT

Research carried out in the author's laboratory is supported by grants AM-09461 and HD-07110 from the U.S. National Institute of Health and by a grant BC-151 from American Cancer Society, Inc.

REFERENCES

Aakvaag, A., Tveter, K. J., Unhjem, O., and Attramadal, A. (1972). *J. Steroid Biochem.* **3,** 375.

Adachi, K., and Kano, M. (1972). *Steroids* **19,** 567.

Anderson, K. M., and Liao, S. (1968). *Nature (London)* **219,** 277.

Anderson, K. M., Cohn, H., and Samuels, S. (1972). *FEBS Lett.* **27,** 149.

Arnaud, M., Beziat, Y., Guilleux, J. C., Hough, A., Hough, D., and Mousseron-Canet, M. (1971). *Biochim. Biophys. Acta* **232,** 117.

Bardin, C. W., Allison, J. E., Stanley, A. J., and Gumbreck, L. G. (1969). *Endocrinology* **84,** 435.

Bardin, C. W., Bullock, L., Schneider, G., Allison, J. E., and Stanley, A. J. (1970). *Science* **167,** 1136.

Bashirelahi, N., and Villee, C. A. (1970). *Biochim. Biophys. Acta* **202,** 192.

Baulieu, E. E., and Jung, I. (1970). *Biochem. Biophys. Res. Commun.* **38**, 599.

Baulieu, E. E., Lasnitzki, I., and Robel, P. (1968). *Nature (London)* **219**, 1155.

Baulieu, E. E., Jung, I., Blondeau, J. P., and Robel, P. (1971). *Advan. Biosci.* **7**, 179.

Blaquier, J. A. (1971). *Biochem. Biophys. Res. Commun.* **45**, 1076.

Bruchovsky, N. (1971). *Endocrinology* **89**, 1212.

Bruchovsky, N. (1972). *Biochem. J.* **127**, 561.

Bruchovsky, N., and Wilson, J. D. (1968a). *J. Biol. Chem.* **243**, 2012.

Bruchovsky, N., and Wilson, J. D. (1968b). *J. Biol. Chem.* **243**, 5953.

Bucourt, R., Nedelec, L., Torelli, V., Gase, J. C., and Vignau, M. (1971). *Horm. Steroids, Proc. Int. Congr., 3rd, 1970* Int. Congr. Ser. No. 219, p. 125.

Bullock, L., and Bardin, C. W. (1970). *J. Clin. Endocrinol. Metab.* **31**, 113.

Bullock, L. P., Bardin, C. W., and Ohno, S. (1971). *Biochem. Biophys. Res. Commun.* **44**, 1537.

Chamnes, G. C., and McGuire, W. L. (1972). *Biochemistry* **11**, 2466.

Clemens, L. E., and Kleinsmith, L. J. (1972). *Nature (London), New Biol.* **237**, 204.

Cooper, A., Lu, C. T., and Norten, D. A. (1968). *J. Chem. Soc., B,* p. 1228.

Dannenberg, V: H. (1963). *Deut. Med. Wochenschr.* **88**, 605.

Danzo, B. J., Orgebin-Crist, M.-C., and Toft, D. O. (1973). *Endocrinology* **92**, 310.

Davies, P., Fahmy, A. R., Pierrepoint, C. G., and Griffiths, K. (1972). *Biochem. J.* **129**, 1167.

Dofuku, R., Tettenborn, U., and Ohno, S. (1971). *Nature (London), New Biol.* **232**, 5.

Dorfman, R. I., and Shipley, R. A. (1956). "Androgens." Wiley, New York.

Eppenberger, U., and Hsia, S. L. (1972). *J. Biol. Chem.* **247**, 5463.

Fang, S. (1974). *In* "Normal and Abnormal Growth of the Prostates" (L. R. Axelrod, ed.). Thomas, Springfield, Illinois (in press).

Fang, S., and Liao, S. (1969). *Mol. Pharmacol.* **5**, 428.

Fang, S., and Liao, S. (1971). *J. Biol. Chem.* **246**, 16.

Fang, S., Anderson, K. M., and Liao, S. (1969). *J. Biol. Chem.* **244**, 6584.

Fazekas, A. G., and Sandor, T. (1972). *Proc. Int. Congr. Endocrinol.,* 4th, Abstract, p. 80.

Feyel-Cabanes, T. (1963). *C. R. Soc. Biol.* **157**, 1428.

Frenster, J. H., Allfrey, V. G., and Mirsky, A. (1963). *Proc. Nat. Acad. Sci. U.S.* **50**, 1026.

Frieden, E. H., and Fishel, S. S. (1968). *Biochem. Biophys. Res. Commun.* **31**, 515.

Frieden, E. H., Harper, A. A., Chin, F., and Fishman, W. H. (1964). *Steroids* **4**, 777.

Gehring, U., Tomkins, G. M., and Ohno, S. (1971). *Nature (London), New Biol.* **232**, 106.

Geller, J., Damme, O. V., Garabieta, G., Loh, A., Rettura, J., and Seifter, E. (1969). *Endocrinology* **84**, 1330.

Giannopoulos, G. (1973). *J. Biol. Chem.* **248**, 1004.

Giorgi, E. P., Stewart, J. C., Grant, J. K., and Scott, R. (1971). *Biochem. J.* **123**, 41.

Giorgi, E. P., Stewart, J. C., Grant, J. K., and Shirley, I. M. (1972). *Biochem. J.* **126**, 107.

Gittinger, J. W., and Lasnitzki, I. (1972). *J. Endocrinol.* **52**, 459.

Gloyna, R. E., and Wilson, J. D. (1969). *J. Clin. Endocrinol. Metal.* **29**, 970.

Gloyna, R. E., Siiteri, P. K., and Wilson, J. D. (1970). *J. Clin. Invest.* **49**, 1746.

Goldberg, M. L., and Atchley, W. A. (1966). *Proc. Nat. Acad. Sci. U.S.* **55**, 989.

Goldstein, J. L., and Wilson, J. D. (1972). *J. Clin. Invest.* **51**, 1647.

Gonzalez-Diddi, M., Komisaruk, B., and Beyer, C. (1972). *Endocrinology* **91**, 1130.

Gorski, J., Toft, D., Shyamala, G., Smith, D., and Notides, A. (1968). *Recent Progr. Horm. Res.* **24**, 45.

Hansson, V., Tveter, K. J., Attramadal, A., and Torgersen, O. (1971). *Acta Endocrinol. (Copenhagen)* **68**, 79.

Harding, B. W., and Samuels, L. T. (1962). *Endocrinology* **70**, 109.

Hu, A. L., and Wang, T. Y. (1971). *Arch. Biochem. Biophys.* **144**, 549.

Huggins, C., and Mainzer, K. (1957). *J. Exp. Med.* **105**, 485.

Huggins, C., and Yang, N. C. (1962). *Science* **137**, 257.

Huggins, C., Jensen, E. V., and Cleveland, A. S. (1954). *J. Exp. Med.* **100**, 225.

Ito, T., and Horton, R. (1970). *J. Clin. Endocrinol. Metab.* **31**, 362.

Jensen, E. V., and DeSombre, E. R. (1972). *Annu. Rev. Biochem.* **41**, 203.

Jensen, E. V., and Jacobson, H. I. (1962). *Recent Progr. Horm. Res.* **18**, 387.

Jouan, P., Samperez, S., and Theiulant, M. L. (1973). *J. Steroid Biochem.* **4**, 65.

Jung, I., and Baulieu, E. E. (1972). *Nature (London), New Biol.* **237**, 24.

Jungblut, P. W., Hughes, S. F., Gorlich, L., Gowers, U., and Wagner, R. K. (1971). *Hoppe-Seyler's Z. Physiol. Chem.* **352**, 1603.

Karlson, P. (1963). *Perspect. Biol. Med.* **6**, 203.

Karsznia, R., Wyss, R. H., Heinrichs, W. M. L., and Herrmann, W. L. (1969). *Endocrinology* **84**, 1238.

Kidson, C., Cohen, P., and Chin, R. C. (1971). *In* "The Sex Steroids" (K. W. McKerns, ed.), p. 421. Appleton, New York.

King, R. J. B., and Gordon, J. (1972). *Nature (London), New Biol.* **240**, 185.

King, R. J. B., Beard, V., Gordon, J., Pooley, A. S., Smith, J. A., Steggles, A. W., and Vertes, M. (1971). *Advan. Biosci.* **7**, 21.

Kniewald, Z., Massa, R., and Martini, L. (1971). *Horm. Steroids, Proc. Int. Congr., 3rd, 1970* Int. Congr. Ser. No. 219, p. 784.

Kowarski, A., Shalf, J., and Migeon, C. J. (1969). *J. Biol. Chem.* **244**, 5269.

Liang, T., and Liao, S. (1972). *Biochim. Biophys. Acta* **277**, 590.

Liao, S. (1968). *Amer. Zoologist* **8**, 233.

Liao, S. (1973). *In* "Biochemistry of Hormones" (H. V. Rickenberg, ed.). Medical and Technical Publ. Co., Oxford (in press).

Liao, S, and Lin, A. H. (1967). *Proc. Nat. Acad. Sci. U.S.* **57**, 379.

Liao, S., and Fang, S. (1969). *Vitam. Horm. (New York)* **27**, 17.

Liao, S., and Fang, S. (1970). *In* "Some Aspects of Aetiology and Biochemistry of Prostate Cancer" (K. Griffiths and C. G. Pierrepoint, eds.), pp. 105–108. Alpha Omega Alpha Publishing, Cardiff.

Liao, S., and Williams-Ashman, H. G. (1962). *Proc. Nat. Acad. Sci. U.S.* **48**, 1956.

Liao, S., Leininger, K. R., Sagher, D., and Barton, R. W. (1965). *Endocrinology* **77**, 763.

Liao, S., Lin, A. H., and Tymoczko, J. L. (1971a). *Biochim. Biophys. Acta* **230**, 535.

Liao, S., Tymoczko, J. L., and Fang, S. (1971b). *Horm. Steroids, Proc. Int. Congr., 3rd, 1970* Int. Congr. Ser. No. 219, p. 434.

Liao, S., Tymoczko, J. L., Liang, T., Anderson, K. M., and Fang, S. (1971c). *Advan. Biosci.* **7**, 155.

Liao, S., Liang, T., and Tymoczko, J. L. (1972). *J. Steroid Biochem.* **3**, 401.

Liao, S., Liang, T., and Tymoczko, J. L. (1973a). *Nature (London), New Biol.* **241**, 211.

Liao, S., Liang, T., Fang, S., Castaneda, E., and Shao, T.-C. (1973b). *J. Biol. Chem.* **486**, 6154.

Liao, S., Liang, T., Shao, T.-C., and Tymoczko, J. L. (1973c). *Adv. Exp. Med. Biol.* **36**, 232.

Liao, S., Tymoczko, J. L., Castaneda, E., and Shao, T.-C. (1974). *In* "Normal and Abnormal Growth of the Prostates" (L. R. Axelrod, ed.). Thomas, Springfield, Illinois (in press).

Liao, S., Howell, D. K., and Chang, T. M. (1974). *Endocrinology* (in press).

Litwack, G. (1972). "Biochemical Actions of Hormones," Vol. 2. Academic Press, New York.

Lyon, M. F., and Hawkes, S. G. (1970). *Nature (London)* **277**, 1217.

Mainwaring, W. I. P. (1969a). *J. Endocrinol.* **44**, 323.

Mainwaring, W. I. P. (1969b). *J. Endocrinol.* **45**, 531.

Mainwaring, W. I. P. (1970). *Biochem. Biophys. Res. Commun.* **40**, 192.

Mainwaring, W. I. P. (1972). *Proc. Int. Congr. Endocrinol., 4th, 1972*abstract, p. 80.

Mainwaring, W. I. P. (1974). *In* "Normal and Abnormal Growth of Prostates" (L. R. Axelrod, ed.). Thomas, Springfield, Illinois (in press).

Mainwaring, W. I. P., and Mangan, F. R. (1971). *Advan. Biosci.* **7,** 165.

Mainwaring, W. I. P., and Peterken, B. M. (1971). *Biochem. J.* **125,** 285.

Mainwaring, W. I. P., and Mangan, F. R., and Peterken, B. M. (1971). *Biochem. J.* **123,** 619.

Mangan, F. R., and Mainwaring, W. I. P. (1972). *Steroids* **20,** 331.

Mangan, F. R., Neal, G. E., and Williams, D. C. (1968). *Arch. Biochem. Biophys.* **124,** 27.

Mann, T., Rowson, L. E. A., Baronos, S., and Karagiannidis, A. (1971). *J. Endocrinol.* **51,** 707.

Matsumoto, K., Kotch, K., Kasai, H., Minesita, T., and Yamaguchi, K. (1972). *Steroids* **20,** 311.

Mauvais-Jarvis, P., Bercovici, J. P., Crepy, O., and Gauthier, F. (1970). *J. Clin. Invest.* **49,** 31.

McDonald, P., Tan, H. S., Beyer, C., Sampson, C., Newton, F., Kitching, P., Brien, B., Greenhill, R., Baker, R., and Pritchard, D. (1970). *Nature (London)* **227,** 964.

Mercier-Bodard, C., Alfsen, A., and Baulieu, E. E. (1970). *In* "Karolinska Symposia on Research Methods in Reproductive Endocrinology," 2nd Symp., p. 204.

Mohla, S., DeSombre, E. R., and Jensen, E. V. (1972). *Biochem. Biophys. Res. Commun.* **46,** 661.

Moore, R. J., and Wilson, J. D. (1972). *J. Biol. Chem.* **247,** 958.

Munck, A., Wira, C., Young, D. A., Mosher, K. M., Hallahan, C., and Bell, P. A. (1972). *J. Steroid Biochem.* **3,** 567.

Neri, R., Florance, K., Koziol, P., and Van Cleave, S. (1972). *Endocrinology* **91,** 427.

Neumann, F., and von Berswordt-Wallrabe, R. (1966). *J. Endocrinol.* **35,** 363.

Ofner, P. (1968). *Vitam Horm. (New York)* **26,** 271.

Ohno, S. (1971). *Nature (London)* **234,** 134.

O'Malley, B. W., Spelsberg, T. C., Schrader, W. T., Chytil, F., and Steggles, A. W. (1972). *Nature (London)* **235,** 141.

Pearlman, W. H., and Pearlman, M. R. J. (1961). *J. Biol. Chem.* **236,** 1321.

Perez-Palacios, G., Castaneda, E., Gomez-Perez, F., Perez, A., and Gual, C. (1970). *Biol. Reprod.* **3,** 205.

Perez-Palacios, G., Morato, T., Perez, A. E., Castaneda, E., and Gual, C. (1971). *Steroids* **17,** 471.

Raynaud-Jammet, C., and Baulieu, E. E. (1969). *Comp. Rend.* **D268,** 3211.

Rennie, P., and Bruchovsky, N. (1972a). *J. Biol. Chem.* **247,** 1546.

Rennie, P., and Bruchovksy, N. (1972b). *Proc. Int. Congr. Endocrinol; 4th, 1972,* Abstract, p. 79.

Rennie, P., and Bruchovsky, N. (1973). *J. Biol. Chem.* **218,** 3288.

Ringold, H. J. (1961). *In* "Mechanism of Action of Steroid Hormones" (C. A. Villee and L. L. Engel, eds.), p. 200. Pergamon, Oxford.

Ritzen, E. M., Nayfeh, S. N., French, F. S., and Dobbins, M. C. (1971). *Endocrinology* **89,** 143.

Ritzen, E. M., Dobbins, M. C., French, F. S., and Nayfeh, S. N. (1972a). *Proc. Int. Congr. Endocrinol., 4th, 1972* p. 79.

Ritzen, E. M., Nayfeh, S. N., French, F. S., and Aronin, P. A. (1972b). *Endocrinology* **91,** 116.

Robison, G. A., Butcher, R. W., and Sutherland, E. W. (1971). "Cyclic AMP." Academic Press, New York.

Rommerts, F. F. G., and Van der Molen, H. J. (1971). *Biochim. Biophys. Acta* **248,** 489.

Rosenfeld, M. G., and O'Malley, B. W. (1970). *Science* **168,** 253.

Rosenfield, R. L., Lawrence, A. M., Liao, S., and Landau, R. L. (1971). *J. Clin. Endocrinol. Metab.* **32,** 625.

Sar, M., and Stumpf, W. E. (1973). *Endocrinology* **92,** 251.

Sar, M., Liao, S., and Stumpf, W. E. (1970). *Endocrinology* **86,** 1008.

Saunders, F. J. (1963). *Nat. Cancer Inst., Monogr.* **12,** 139.

Schrader, W. T., Toft, D. O., and O'Malley, B. W. (1972). *J. Biol. Chem.* **247,** 2401.

Shimazaki, J., Kurihara, H., Ito, Y., and Shida, K. (1965). *Gunma J. Med. Sci.* **14,** 313 and 326.

Siiteri, P. K., and Wilson, J. D. (1970). *J. Clin. Invest.* **49,** 1737.

Singhal, R. L., Parulekar, M. R., and Vijayvargia, R. (1971). *Biochem. J.* **125,** 329.

Sluyser, M. (1966a). *J. Mol. Biol.* **19,** 591.

Sluyser, M. (1966b). *J. Mol. Biol.* **22,** 41.

Sluyser, M. (1966c). *Biochem. Biophys. Res. Commun.* **22,** 236.

Spelsberg, T. C., Steggles, A. W., and O'Malley, B. W. (1971). *J. Biol. Chem.* **246,** 4188.

Starling, E. H. (1905). *Lancet* **2,** 339.

Stern, J. M., and Eisenfeld, A. J. (1969). *Science* **166,** 233.

Strickland, A. L., and French, F. S. (1969). *J. Clin.Endocrinol. Metab.* **29,** 1284.

Sullivan, J. N., and Strott, C. A. (1973). *J. Biol. Chem.* **218,** 3202.

Talwar, G. P., Modi, S., and Rao, K. N. (1965). *Science* **150,** 1315.

Tata, J. R. (1966). *Progr. Nucleic Acid Res. Mol. Biol.* **5,** 191.

Tindall, D. J., French, F. S., and Nayfeh, S. N. (1972). *Biochem. Biophys. Res. Commun.* **49,** 1391.

Toft, D., and Gorksi, J. (1966). *Proc. Nat. Acad. Sci. U.S.* **55,** 1574.

Tomkins, G. M., Martin, D. W., Jr., Stellwagen, R. H., Baxter, J. D., Mamont, P., and Levinson, B. B. (1970). *Cold Spring Harbor Symp. Quant. Biol.* **35,** 635.

Tremblay, R. R., Beitins, I. Z., Kowarski, A., and Migeon, C. J. (1970). *Steroids* **16,** 29.

Ts'o, P. O. P., and Lu, P. (1964). *Proc. Nat. Acad. Sci. U.S.* **51,** 17.

Tveter, K. J., and Aakvaag, A. (1969). *Endocrinology* **85,** 683.

Tveter, K. J., and Attramadal, A. (1968). *Acta Endocrinol. (Copenhagen)* **59,** 218.

Tveter, K. J., and Attramadal, A. (1969). *Endocrinology* **85,** 350.

Tveter, K. J., and Unhjem, O. (1969). *Endocrinology* **84,** 963.

Tveter, K. J., Unhjem, O., Attramadal, A., Aakvaag, A., and Hansson, V. (1971). *Advan. Biosci.* **7,** 193.

Tymoczko, J. L., and Liao, S. (1971). *Biochim. Biophys. Acta* **252,** 607.

Unhjem, O., Tveter, K. J., and Aakvaag, A. (1969). *Acta Endocrinol. (Copenhagen)* **62,** 153.

Vermeulen, A., and Verdonck, L. (1970). *In* "Karolinska Symposia on Research Methods in Reproductive Endocrinology," 2nd Symp., p. 239.

Vernon, R. G., Dorrington, J. H., and Fritz, I. B. (1972). *Proc. Int. Congr. Endocrinol., 4th 1972* abstract, p. 79.

Vida, J. A. (1969). "Androgens and Anabolic Agents." Academic Press, New York.

Voigt, W., Fernandez, E. P., and Hsia, S. L. (1970). *J. Biol. Chem.* **245,** 5594.

Whalen, R. E., and Luttge, W. G. (1971a). *Horm. Behav.* **2,** 117.

Whalen, R. E., and Luttge, W. G. (1971b). *Endocrinology* **89,** 1320.

Whalen, R. E., and Rezek, D. L. (1972). *Steroids* **20,** 717.

Whalen, R. E., Luttge, W. G., and Green, R. (1969). *Endocrinology* **84,** 217.

Williams-Ashman, H. G. (1965). *Cancer Res.* **25,** 1096.

Wilson, J. D. (1973). *Endocrinology* **92,** 1192.

Wilson, J. D., and Gloyna, R. E. (1970). *Recent Progr. Horm. Res.* **26,** 309.

Wilson, J. D., and Goldstein, J. L. (1972). *J. Biol. Chem.* **247,** 7342.

Wilson, J. D., and Loeb, P. M. (1965a). *In* "Developmental and Metabolic Control Mechanisms and Neoplasia," p. 375. Williams & Wilkins, Baltimore, Maryland.

Wilson, J. D., and Loeb, P. M. (1965b). *J. Clin. Invest.* **44,** 1111.

Wilson, J. D., and Walker, J. D. (1969). *J. Clin. Invest.* **48,** 371.

Wolff, M. E., and Kasuya, Y. (1972). *J. Med. Chem.* **15,** 87.

Wolff, M. E., Ho, W., and Kwok, R. (1964). *J. Med. Chem.* **7,** 577.

Zanati, G., and Wolff, M. E. (1973). *J. Med. Chem.* **16,** 90.

Chapter IX

STRUCTURE, SYNTHESIS, AND TRANSCRIPTION OF MITOCHONDRIAL DNA IN NORMAL, MALIGNANT, AND DRUG-TREATED CELLS

MARGIT M. K. NASS

I.   Introduction: Why Do We Study Mitochondrial DNA?

One of the major advances in molecular biology within the past decade has been the finding that cytoplasmic organelles, in particular the mitochondria and chloroplasts, are not merely the sites of respiration and energy transduction but contain the components of a unique genetic apparatus which may function, at least in part, separately from the nuclear genetic system. As a consequence of this work it is now known that mitochondria contain specific DNA molecules capable of replication and have their own equipment to transcribe this DNA into RNA and translate RNA into proteins in association with mitochondria-specific ribosomes and transfer RNA. This mitochondrial genetic apparatus has many similarities with microbial genetic systems. The biogenesis and function of the mitochondria depend on the joint operation of the nuclear–cytoplasmic and the mitochondrial genetic system.

One of the prime factors that stimulated interest in this field was the discovery between 1962 and 1965 that mitochondria contain DNA. By applying combined electron microscopical and cytochemical methods, Nass and Nass (1962; M. M. K. Nass and S. Nass, 1963; Nass et al., 1965; S. Nass and M. M. K. Nass, 1963) have demonstrated the presence of DNA fibrils within the matrix of mitochondria of all major animal phyla and a plant species. Mitochondrial DNA of animal cells has since been shown to consist of circular, double-stranded molecules, with a molecular weight of 9 to 10 million daltons (Nass, 1966; Sinclair and Stevens, 1966; Van Bruggen et al., 1966). This molecule is theoretically capable to code for not more than 32 polypeptides of molecular weight 20,000. The structure, physico-chemical properties, replication, and informational content of this DNA have been extensively studied. A burgeoning body of literature on this subject has accumulated in the past few years (for reviews, see Borst and Kroon, 1969; Nass, 1969a; Ashwell and Work, 1970; Paoletti and Riou, 1970; Wunderlich, 1971; Borst, 1972).

The identification of mitochondrial DNA has provided a molecular basis for the earlier important, but little understood genetic work of Ephrussi (1953) who discovered the yeast "petite" mutants that carry a cyto-plasmically inherited respiratory deficiency. A large body of literature now describes the molecular basis of the cytoplasmic mutation, especially the presence and consequence of abnormal types of mitochondrial DNA, which range from altered base composition to deletions and apparent absence of this DNA (see Section IX).

The recent advances in the field of mitochondrial informational systems, which add a new dimension to the function and significance of these organelles, have prompted many virologists, geneticists, pathologists, pharmacologists, and some radiologists to participate in investigations of mitochondria in mammalian cells. Mitochondrial membrane structure, respiratory function, and the components of the mitochondrial genetic apparatus, all of which appear to be closely associated, are markedly affected in many pathological conditions, including malignancy, and in many cases of drug and radiation therapy (see Section II). Disorders of mitochondria in cancer cells, for example, frequently result in marked changes of aerobic respiration and energy production which may unfavorably influence the synthetic, replicative, and repair mechanism of the cell.

There are many indications (at least in yeast and *Neurospora*) that mitochondrial DNA can mutate. It is conceivable that in some pathological conditions a defect may occur in a component(s) of the mitochondrial genetic system. The effects of viruses are pertinent in this respect (see Sections V and X). Because of the many functional links between mitochondria and other major cell organelles a defect in mitochondria may have important consequences. Conversely, because of feedback mechanisms, a defect in other parts of the cell can adversely affect the mitochondria.

The most pertinent questions and avidly pursued subjects in this particular field are at present: (1) what exactly does the organelle DNA code for? (2) What is the interaction and individual contribution of nuclear and organelle genetic systems? (3) What is the role or behavior of this second genetic system in cell differentiation, in oncogenesis, and in other pathological conditions? (4) How do hormones affect macromolecular synthesis in mitochondria? (5) Can oncogenic viruses functionally influence or develop in mitochondria? (6) How have organelle genetic systems evolved? Our studies have dealt with certain aspects of all these problems. In this paper I wish to summarize both some of our earlier and most recent work, as well as include relevant background information on mitochondrial macromolecular systems in tumor cells, a subject that in this context has not been comprehensively represented elsewhere.

II.   Mitochondrial Abnormalities in Disease and Therapy

Before proceeding with the more specific problems involving mitochondrial DNA, a brief elaboration on just what type of mitochondrial abnormalities have been observed may be informative. Although some of these changes may be related to defects in either one or both of the cellular genetic systems, many are undoubtedly due to perturbance of the supply of essential nutrients and to degenerative processes. It is hoped that the reader will be stimulated to reexamine some of these or other cases in the light of current information.

The most common manifestation of mitochondrial damage is an abnormal ultrastructure and respiratory capacity. Mitochondrial alterations are found most frequently in various types of myopathies (Luft *et al.*, 1962; Shy *et al.*, 1966; Hulsmann *et al.*, 1967; Shafiq *et al.*, 1967; Afifi *et al.*, 1972; Meijers, 1972). Mitochondrial structural injury has also been reported in hepatocytes of cases with Reyc's syndrome (Partin *et al.*, 1971), Hurler syndrome, and Sanfilippo disease (Haust, 1968). The changes were reversible during recovery from Rye's syndrome.

A diverse (and sometimes controversial) literature indicates that in many (but not all) types of malignant cells the mitochondria show structural abnormalities (Bernhard, 1958; Nass and Nass, 1964; Bernhard and Tournier, 1966; Paoletti and Riou, 1970). These usually consist of a scarcity of mitochondrial membranes (cristae) and/or a spectrum of different inclusion bodies. Many abnormalities of the internal structure of mitochondria are unstable, i.e., they are reversible if cells are cultured *in vitro*, and may be secondary phenomena. An exception was found in a hamster cell line transformed by the oncogenic adenovirus 12 (Bernhard and Tournier, 1966). The abnormal internal structure of mitochondria has now been maintained in *in vitro* culture for several years.

A plethora of papers has dealt with the respiration, oxidative phosphorylation, and glycolysis of various types of tumor cells and the mitochondria isolated from them. Since the original controversial view of Warburg implicating defective mitochondrial respiration as a causative factor in tumorigenesis (cf. Weinhouse, 1955, 1972) relatively few advances have been made except to show that both the number of mitochondria (content of mitochondrial protein) and respiratory rates are lowered in many (but not all) tumors. A study of mitochondrial content and activity of the mitochondrial enzyme β-hydroxybutyrate dehydrogenase (Ohe *et al.*, 1967) has shown that, as compared with the content of mitochondrial protein (M-protein) of liver (49 mg/gm tissue), the M-protein content for slow-growing, high-respiring, well-differentiated tumors was reduced (18–33 mg), and for rapidly growing, low-respiring, poorly differentiated tumors was lowest (9–14 mg/gm). The specific activity of the enzyme was similarly decreased. The studies also suggested that high respiration is characteristic of the well-differentiated tumor, and lowered respiration, coupled with loss of mitochondria, accompanies loss of differentiation (Ohe *et al.*, 1967; Lo *et al.*, 1968). The high aerobic glycolysis, characteristic of many highly differentiated tumors, could be decreased and respiratory ATP production increased by replacing the mitochondria of the incubation mixture with others from tissues that have a normal Pasteur effect (Lo *et al.*, 1968). In another study mitochondrial structural alterations have been compared in several types of Morris hepatomas, and it is believed that the alterations in this case are not specific for neoplasia but may be related to nutritional deficiencies and degenerative processes (Hruban *et al.*, 1972).

Mitochondrial lesions have also been shown in drug and radiation therapy. In chloramphenicol therapy, the drug induced a reversible ultrastructural modification involving an increased density of the matrix of bone marrow mitochondria (Martelo *et al.*, 1969; Smith *et al.*, 1970). Chloramphenicol is known to inhibit protein synthesis on mitochondrial and bacterial ribosomes, but not on extramitochondrial cellular ribosomes. The ready and early vulnerability of mitochondria to X-irradiation has also been stressed (Manteifel and Meisel, 1965). Following X-irradiation the mitochondria of lymphocytes reacted earlier than the other cell components and it is believed that the ultrastructural abnormalities and associated decrease of oxidative phosphorylation unfavorably influences the synthesizing and repair processes of the cell, ultimately (but not exclusively) determining the fate of the cell.

Of special interest are recent reports of the presence of virus-like particles and virus-associated macromolecular synthesis within mitochondria. This will be discussed in Sections V and X.

III.   Structure of Mitochondrial DNA

A. Membrane Association, Circular Forms, and Genetic Complexity

We have shown by electron cytochemical methods and by osmotic release of DNA molecules from isolated L-cell and ascites tumor mitochondria that a high proportion of DNA molecules is associated with inner mitochondrial membranes in several regions of a given mitochondrion (Nass and S. Nass, 1963; S. Nass and Nass, 1964; Nass, 1966, 1969b). Brief treatment with proteolytic enzymes dissociates the molecules. In confirmation, the isolation of a membrane-DNA–RNA complex of rat liver mitochondria was recently reported (Van Tuyle and Kalf, 1972).

It is now well established that mitochondrial DNA of animal cells, e.g., mouse L-cells (Nass, 1966), HeLa cells (Radloff *et al.*, 1967), amphibian oocytes (Dawid and Wolstenholme, 1967), and sea urchin (Pikó *et al.*, 1968) occur as covalently closed circular double-stranded molecules with a contour length of 4.5 to 5.5 μm corresponding to a molecular weight of $9\text{--}10 \times 10^6$ daltons. Mixing experiments with isolated M-DNA from different species demonstrated the existence of true but small size differences. The significance of such minior differences in terms of informational content is not known (Nass, 1969c). In many lower organisms and in plants, M-DNA is of higher molecular weight than in animal cells. In the case of yeast (Hollenberg *et al.*, 1970) and *Neurospora* (Clayton and Brambl, 1972) mitochondria, M-DNA appears to be a circular molecule of about five and four times, respectively, the length of the 5 μm animal M-DNA. Renaturation experiments have shown that the "genetic content" or nonrepeated base sequence of the 5 μm and 25 μm type DNA is roughly equivalent to molecular size (Hollenberg *et al.*, 1970). It is therefore possible that either the 25 μm DNA has a greater informational content than the M-DNA of animals at a higher evolutionary level or that the excess base sequences above a 5 μm unit include noncoding "spacers." This problem is at present little understood.

The 5 μm circle can theoretically code for a very limited number of proteins, approximately 32 polypeptide chains of molecular weight 20,000, which is far from sufficient for the biogenesis of an entire, complex mitochondrion. Many mitochondrial proteins are now known to be synthesized, at least in part, under nuclear control on extramitochondrial ribosomes and then transported into the organelle by an as yet unknown mechanism (see Section VIII).

In addition to the conventional monomeric DNA, dimeric and oligomeric mitochondrial DNA has been demonstrated in our and other laboratories (see Section IV). Electron micrographs of typical forms of mitochondrial DNA are shown in Fig. 1. Reannealing experiments and electron microscopy of monomeric and dimeric M-DNA from leukemic leukocytes have revealed that these dimers consist of two monomer genomes which appeared to be connected in a head-to-tail rather than a head-to-head structure (Clayton *et al.*, 1970).

B. Number and Type of DNA Molecules per Mitochondrion

Individual L-cell mitochondria contain a mixture of circular monomeric and dimeric DNA molecules, located in several discrete regions (nucleoids) within the matrix of the mitochondrion (Nass, 1969a,b). The DNA regions are diagrammatically shown in Fig. 2. L-cell mitochondria contribute only

Fig. 1. Electron micrographs of monomeric and dimeric forms of mitochondrial DNA. DNA preparations were purified by equilibrium centrifugation in cesium chloride–ethidium bromide gradients and spread by the DNA monolayer technique in the presence of 50% formamide and 0.01% cytochrome c, upon a hypophase of distilled water (Nass and Ben-Shaul, 1972). (a) Monomeric M-DNA from cultured mouse adrenal tumor cells (Y1); (b) unicircular dimeric M-DNA from L-cells; (c) catenated dimeric DNA (2 monomers interlocked at arrow) from chick embryo fibroblasts transformed by T5, a thermosensitive mutant of Rous sarcoma virus, and grown at the permissive temperature of 36°C. Bar = 0.5 μm.

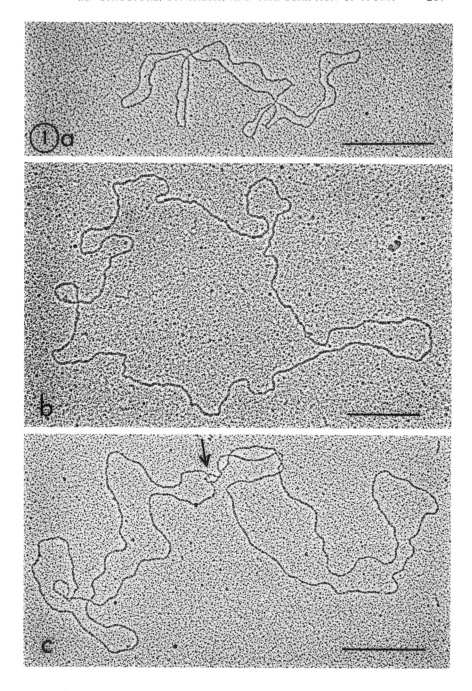

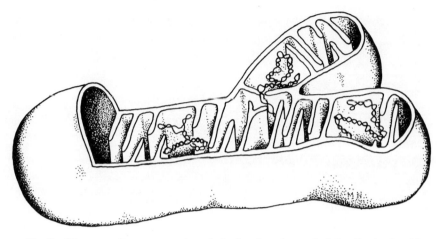

Fig. 2. Diagrammatic representation of the interior of a typical L-cell mitochondrion showing the possible arrangement of DNA molecules in various regions or "nucleoids" of the organelle. (From Nass, 1969a.)

about 0.1% of total cellular DNA. The quantity of M-DNA per mitochondrion may vary, averaging 7×10^{-17} gm DNA or 2 to 8 DNA molecules per organelle. There appears to be a direct proportionality between DNA content and size of mitochondrion. The long filamentous and branching types of organelles tend to have a larger number of DNA-containing regions than the short forms. This relationship has been formulated quantitatively by Bahr (1971).

M-DNA of embryonic cells and cultured mammalian cells contain at least twice as much DNA per milligram of mitochondrial protein (≥ 1 μg DNA/mg protein) than M-DNA of more differential tissues, such as rat liver. A range of 0.9 to 1.8 μg/mg has been reported for M-DNA of embryonic and placental tissues of various rodents (Nass *et al.,* 1965; cf. Nass, 1969a).

C. Mitochondrial DNA Content of Malignant Cells

Both electron microscopic and biochemical analyses have shown that the concentration of mitochondrial DNA in most tumor cells is several times higher than that of normal cells and similar or slightly higher than that of embryonic cells (cf. Nass, 1969a). An ultrastructural study of ascites tumor cells (Nass and Nass, 1964) has shown that M-DNA was more conspicuous than in other cell types and was visible in an abnormal form which often surrounded a globular body in structurally damaged mitochondria. There appeared to be a step-wise destruction of mitochondria leading to the formation of vesicular structures in the cytoplasm which frequently contained the globular bodies characteristic of degenerating mitochondria and also contained clusters of virus-like particles. Leduc et al. (1966) found similar condensed masses of M-DNA fibers in a hamster cell line transformed by adenovirus 12. The masses of M-DNA fibers appeared periodically each time the cells were subcultured.

Similar observations of a greater M-DNA concentration in many tumor cells have been made by biochemical analyses. For example, my studies with ascites tumor cells have shown that the DNA content based on mitochondrial protein is greater (2.5 μg/mg) than that of cultured L-cells (1.1 μg/mg) and rat liver (0.6 μg/mg). Values of the order of 5 μg DNA/mg M-protein have been reported for hepatoma, Walker and Jensen sarcoma of rat, drug-induced (diethylnitroseamine) sarcoma of mouse, and polyoma virus-induced sarcoma of hamster (Wunderlich et al., 1966). The significance and possible pitfalls in expressing DNA values for tumor mitochondria relative to mitochondrial protein, as done by most investigators, have been discussed (Nass, 1969a).

D. Physiochemical Properties and Base Composition

The sedimentation, denaturation, and renaturation of covalently closed and nicked mitochondrial DNA are comparable to the properties of circular DNA's of some viruses. Covalently closed M-DNA of L-cells contains 33 $\pm$ 2 supercoils or 3.7 helical turns per 10^6 molecular weight as determined by electron microscopy (Nass, 1969c). Refined analytical methods have revealed small differences in the degree of supercoiling (superhelix density) of M-DNA obtained from different cell types and after treatment in vivo with intercalating drugs (Smith et al., 1971). Covalently closed circular M-DNA is usually isolated free from nicked circular and linear DNA by equilibrium centrifugation in cesium chloride–ethidium bromide gradients, in which these molecules due to their different dye-binding properties band at different densities (Radloff et al., 1967). (See also Figs. 6 and 7.)

Rat liver M-DNA (Nass and Buck, 1970) and some other M-DNA's, e.g., HeLa M-DNA (Aloni and Attardi, 1971a,b), can be separated into complementary single-stranded heavy and light strands (on the basis of different base composition) by equilibrium centrifugation in alkaline cesium chloride. We have identified in the respective peak fractions intact heavy and light single-stranded DNA molecules in the electron microscope. The separated strands have been used for genetic mapping experiments (see Section VII, B).

Studies in many laboratories have shown that the guanine and cytosine content of M-DNA may be lower, similar, or higher than that of nuclear

DNA in different organisms. In mammalian cells this difference is very small (Nass, 1969c), so that mitochondrial and nuclear DNA cannot be well resolved in preparatory cesium chloride gradients. M-DNA of higher animal cells is therefore usually isolated as the covalently closed circular fraction in cesium chloride–ethidium bromide gradients.

A number of studies are underway in different laboratories on heteroduplex formation of co-annealed mitochondrial DNA's from different organisms. These studies and our own preliminary observations indicate that the base sequence homology of different M-DNA's may vary considerably and that highest homologies are generally found in closely related organisms, although exceptions have been reported in closely related species of amphibians (Dawid, 1972a).

E. Undermethylation of Mitochondrial DNA

Information has been lacking as to whether mitochondrial DNA of animal cells is methylated. We have therefore undertaken a study (Nass, 1973a) to compare the methylation patterns of mitochondrial and nuclear DNA's of several mammalian cell lines by four methods: (1) *In vivo* incorporation of [methyl-^{3}H]methionine; (2) *in vivo* incorporation of [^{32}P]orthophosphate and a combination of (1) and (2); (3) *in vivo* incorporation of [^{3}H]deoxycytidine; and (4) *in vitro* methylation of DNA's with [^{3}H]S-adenosyl-methionine as methyl donor and DNA methylase preparations from L-cell nuclei. The cell lines were L-cells, BHK_{21}/C_{13}, C_{13}/B_4 (BHK cells transformed by the Bryan strain of Rous sarcoma virus), and PyY (BHK cells transformed by polyoma virus). DNA bases were separated chromatographically.

Mitochondrial DNA was found to be undermethylated in all cell types studied and by all methods used. With 5-methylcytosine (5-MC) and 6-methylaminopurine as markers, the only methylated base detected was 5-methylcytosine. A representative experiment using method (2) is shown in Fig. 3. The level of 5-MC in M-DNA as compared with that in N-DNA was estimated as one-fourth to one-fourteenth in various cell lines. The estimated 5-MC content per circular M-DNA molecules (MW 10×10^6) was equal or less than 12 5-MC residues for L-cells and 24, 30, and 36 5-MC residues for BHK, B4, and PyY cells, respectively. Relative to cytosine residues, the estimate was 1 5-MC per 500 C residues of M-DNA and 1 5-MC per 36 C residues of N-DNA from L-cells. The values for 5 MC of M-DNA are presumed to be maximal. Polyoma virus-transformed cells as compared with other cells had the highest 5-MC content of both M- and N-DNA as estimated by method (3). No methylation of N-DNA was observed in confluent cells.

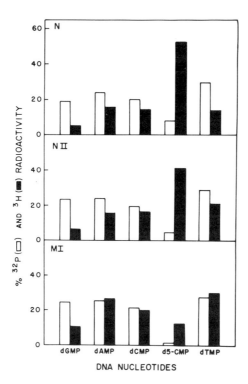

Fig. 3. Methylation patterns of nuclear and mitochondrial DNA. L-cells were labeled for 47 hours with methyl-[³H]methionine and [³²P]orthophosphate in the presence of 1 mg sodium formate/ml (to reduce introduction of [³H]methyl through the one-carbon pool). Mitochondria, nuclei, and their respective DNA fractions were isolated and, after enzymatic hydrolysis of the DNA, the nucleotides were analyzed by paper chromatography.

The only methylated base observed was 5-methylcytosine, in this case analyzed as 5-methyldeoxycytidine monophosphate (d5-CMP). N, nuclear DNA isolated by the phenol method; NII, DNA that is at least 95% nuclear DNA, isolated from crude mitochondrial fractions that had a portion of N-DNA entrapped; (NII was separated as the upper band of cesium chloride–ethidium bromide gradients); MI, purified covalently closed mitochondrial DNA, isolated as the lower band of cesium chloride–ethidium bromide gradients and then centrifuged in a second cesium chloride–ethidium bromide gradient. (From Nass, 1973a.)

Evidence for the presence of DNA methylase activity associated with mitochondrial fractions was also obtained. This activity could be distinguished from nuclear DNA methylase activity by differential sensitivity to mercaptoethanol. Radioactivity from [³H]S-adenosylmethionine was found only in 5-MC of DNA.

Further studies of the presence of DNA methylases in subcellular fractions under various experimental conditions may give clues as to the biological significance of DNA methylation. No common denominator has thus far emerged from a diversity of studies on methylation. If methylation is indeed an essential function in mitochondria, likely possibilities are (1) modification, similar to that found in microbial DNA (Arber and Linn, 1969; Meselson *et al.,* 1972); such modification may protect M-DNA from degradation by specific endonucleases, if present; (2) involvement in the initiation of DNA replication and/or transcription, e.g., by control of endonuclease action or by other mechanism (e.g., Sneider and Potter, 1969).

IV. The Problem of Multiple-Length Mitochondrial DNA in Malignancy

A. *Occurrence of Dimeric and Oligomeric Forms of Mitochondrial DNA*

General interest in mitochondrial DNA from a molecular point of view was kindled when Clayton and Vinograd (1967) reported a unique unicircular DNA dimer molecule peculiar to human leukemic leukocytes and I reported the same type of molecule (see Fig. 1) in mouse L-cells (Nass, 1968, 1969d). (The other type of dimer, consisting of two interlocked monomers, is the most common form of dimer and has been identified as a minor component of M-DNA in all cell types examined.) The frequency of unicircular dimers correlated with the severity of the leukemia (chronic granulocytic leukemia), and remission resulted in a marked drop in dimer content (Clayton and Vinograd, 1969). Similarly, a reversal of the accumulation of multiple-length M-DNA was demonstrable under a variety of experimental conditions (Nass, 1969d; also see next section).

The presence of the unicircular dimer and its high frequency are, however, not necessarily characteristics of malignant cells. Studies of M-DNA from Burkitt lymphoma cells revealed no unicircular dimers and a normal frequency (about 7%) of interlocked or catenated dimers (Nass, 1970a). Similar observations have been reported for two human nephroblastomas and two neuroblastomas (although some chemical and irradiation treatment was given prior to sample removal; Paoletti and Riou, 1970). It is of interest that in HeLa cells similarly only catenated dimers (10%) were observed. The latter cells also contain a spectrum of smaller circles of nuclear origin. Furthermore, the unicircular dimer is not only undetectable in some malignant cells but has also been found in mitochondrial DNA of nonmalignant human and beef thyroid glands (Paoletti *et al.,* 1972).

Most other studies have been carried out with non-human tumor cells, primarily malignant cells of rodents grown in culture; some of these cells were transformed with DNA-containing viruses. The unicircular dimer was again prevalent in some but not all cases. Besides our studies with L-cells (about 10% unicircular and interlocked dimers) and ascites tumor cells (9% catenated forms), Paoletti and Riou (1970) reported comparisons of unicircular and catenated dimer content in five systems: embryonic hamster cells transformed with the highly oncogenic adenovirus 12 (a DNA-containing virus), the same cells transformed with lightly oncogenic adenovirus 7, cells transformed with the DNA virus SV40, cells transformed spontaneously during passage, and hamster embryo cells in the first generation. It was found that the relative frequencies of catenated dimers were similar in all systems (9–13%). The frequency of unicircular dimers was equal and greatest in both of the adenovirus transformed cell lines (5%), i.e., the frequencies were unrelated to the degree of oncogenicity of the virus. Low frequencies (0.2–0.5%) were observed in the other three systems. My studies with polyoma virus-transformed BHK (hamster) cells showed a high concentration (34%) of catenated dimers and oligomers in these cells grown to confluency; control BHK cells in log phase and confluency had only 10 and 17%, respectively (see Table I).

Several examples have also been reported with cells transformed by RNA viruses. M-DNA from myeloblasts transformed by avian myeloblastosis virus (Riou and Lacour, 1971) contained 27% catenated dimers and oligomers as compared with M-DNA from control cells (4–5%). My studies with Rous virus-transformed BHK cells (Table I), showed a small increase (15–17%) of complex forms over control values (10%). Further work with Rous transformed cells is summarized in Section IV, C.

In brief, these studies have shown that (1) the unicircular dimer is not detectable in all types of malignant cells; (2) unicircular dimers, although common in malignant cells, are not unique to them since occasional unicircular dimers have been observed in nonmalignant cells; and (3) catenated dimers and unicircular dimers may exist in high frequencies in many malignant cells; however the increase is not observed in all tumors, and moreover, environmental factors (e.g., culture conditions) may cause increases in dimer and oligomer frequencies regardless of whether the cell line is derived from normal or malignant cells, as discussed in the following section.

B. Effects of Growth Conditions and Inhibitors on Dimer and Oligomer Formation

A survey of many cell types and growth conditions has been conducted (Nass, 1969d, 1970a) to obtain a more fundamental understanding of the mechanism of DNA oligomer formation. Some of these findings are summarized in Tables I and II. There was a significant increase in the content of circular dimers and oligomers of mitochondria if L-cells were allowed to

TABLE I

Proportions of Multiple-Length Forms of Mitochondrial DNA in Growing, Density-Inhibited, Virus-Infected, and Virus-Transformed Cells[a]

Cell type and experimental condition	Hours	Cell divisions no.	Total dimers (%)	Total dimers and oligomers (%)	Ratio[b]
Mouse fibroblasts (L-cells)					
Log, suspension	48	1.4	13	14	
Stationary, suspension	48	0.3	79	89	6.3
Reverted log, suspension	48	1.4	35	39	2.8
Mengovirus-infected L-cells					
Control, suspension	17	0.8		12	
Mengo-infected, suspension	17	0		24	2.0
Hamster kidney cells (BHK$_{21}$/C$_{13}$)					
Log, monolayer				11	
Confluent, monolayer				17	1.5
Polyoma virus-transformed BHK cells (PyY)					
Control (log)				10	
Control (confluent)				17	1.7
Transformed (confluent)				34	1.9 and 3.4
Rous virus-transformed cells (C$_{13}$/B$_4$)					
Control (log)				10	
Control (confluent)				17	1.7
Transformed (confluent)				15	0.9 and 1.5
Chick embryo fibroblasts					
Log				11	
Confluent				17	1.5

[a] Data summarized from Nass (1969d, 1970a).

[b] Ratio of percent dimers and oligomers in experimentals/controls.

grow from log into stationary phase and if protein synthesis was inhibited by amino acid starvation or treatment with cycloheximide and puromycin (4- to 8-fold accumulation of dimers and oligomers). Return to normal conditions of growth restored the formation of DNA monomers. Accumulations, although less pronounced than in L-cells, were also observed by us after treatment of chick fibroblasts and mouse ascites and adrenal tumor cells with cycloheximide. Relatively little or no effects on dimer or oligomer content were found in L-cells treated with vinblastine, Colcemid,

TABLE II

Proportions of Multiple-Length Forms of Mitochondrial DNA under Conditions That Inhibit Protein Synthesis[a]

Cell type and experimental condition	Hours	Cell divisions no.	Total dimers and oligomers (%)	Ratio[b]
Mouse fibroblasts (L-cells)				
Control	48	2.4	9	
Methionine starvation	48	0.5	47	5.2
Methionine resupplied	120	4.2	9	1.0
Phenylalanine starvation	48	0.2	52	5.8
Phenylalanine resupplied	48	1.7	33	3.7
Control	18	0.8	10	
Cycloheximide (25 μg/ml)	18	0.02	68	6.8
Cycloheximide (25 μg/ml)	41	0.2	30	3.0
Cycloheximide removed	144	4.6	10	1.0
Chloramphenicol (25 μg/ml)	48	1.6	18	
Chloramphenicol (150 μg/ml)	24	0.04	26	1.4
Chloramphenicol (150 μg/ml)	40	0.3	13	0.7
Control	17	0.8	20	
Puromycin (15 μg/ml)	17	0.3	57	2.8
Chick embryo fibroblasts				
Control	21		11	
Cycloheximide (25 μg/ml)	21		32	2.9
9β-D-Arabinofuranosyl adenine (5 $\times$ 10^{-4} M)[c]	24		9	1.5
Ehrlich ascites tumor (*in vivo*)				
Control			9	
Cycloheximide (3 times 1 mg injected within 40 hours)			19	2.1
Mouse adrenal tumor cells (Y1)				
Control + ACTH (0.05 U/ml)	24		12	
Cycloheximide (25 μg/ml) + ACTH	24		20	1.7

[a] Data summarized from M. M. K. Nass (1969d, 1970a, and unpublished).

[b] Ratio of percent dimers + oligomers in experimentals/controls.

[c] Inhibits N-DNA synthesis by 90%, but does not inhibit M-DNA synthesis. Similar ratio of 1.5 was obtained using the DNA inhibitor hydroxyurea (76 μg/ml) with L-cells (Nass, 1970a).

rifampicin, chloramphenicol, or mengovirus, or in cuprizone-induced giant mitochondria of rat liver (Nass, 1970a). We observed marked variations in the extent to which oligomer accumulation could be induced, depending on cell types. Our line of L-cells was thus far most responsive. L-cells were also the only cell line containing both unicircular and catenated dimers. In all other cell types examined by us only the catenated form was detected.

The data show that a few selected conditions, especially the inhibition of cytoplasmic protein synthesis, stimulate the accumulation of multiple-length DNA. An interpretation of these findings will be discussed in Section IV, D.

C. Temperature-Dependent Formation of Multiple-Length Mitochondrial DNA in Cells Transformed by a Thermosensitive Mutant of Rous Sarcoma Virus

The studies to date on the relative occurrence of multiple-length forms of mitochondrial DNA in malignant versus nonmalignant cells have suffered primarily from lack of a well-controlled cell system. For this reason I selected such ideally controlled experimental system as chick embryo fibroblast cells made malignant by temperature-sensitive mutants of oncogenic viruses (Martin, 1970; Martin *et al.*, 1971). In this system the same batch of cells can be induced to express malignant properties, then reversed to normal and back to maligant again simply by temperature switches.

Primary chick cells are infected by the temperature-sensitive mutant, T5, of the Schmidt-Ruppin strain of Rous sarcoma virus. Upon infection with mutant virus, the cells become transformed at the permissive temperature (36°C) and behave as malignant cells. They have the phenotypic appearance of malignant cells, form transformed clones in soft agar, transport 2-deoxyglucose at an elevated rate (Martin *et al.*, 1971) and have an elevated sialyl transferase activity characteristic of malignant cells (Warren *et al.*, 1973). At the nonpermissive temperature (41°C) these cells have the phenotypic appearance, rate of sugar transport, and sialyl transferase activity of normal, nontransformed cells.

The experiments summarized in Table III show a clear-cut correlation of an elevated level of catenated dimeric and oligomeric forms of mitochondrial DNA with the manifestation of transformation. The level of multiple-length DNA forms was 2 to 3 times higher in fibroblasts transformed by the wild-type strain of Rous sarcoma virus at both temperatures. In cells transformed by the T5 mutant, however, the level of multiple-length DNA was temperature dependent. At the permissive temperature (36°C) the high oligomer level characteristic of transformed cells was observed, whereas at the nonpermissive temperature (41°C) the oligomer level was charac-

TABLE III

Multiple-Length Mitochondrial DNA in Chick Embryo Fibroblasts Transformed by
Wild-Type and a Temperature-Sensitive Mutant of Rous Sarcoma Virus

Cell type	Temperature of culture (°C)	Uptake of 2-deoxyglucose cpm/mg cell protein	Total DNA molecules scored, Nr.	Total dimers + oligomers (%)[a]
CEF	36	8000	1075	6.5
CEF	41	7000	1013	6.4
CEF-SR	36	57000	439	13.2
CEF-SR	41	51000	371	12.1
CEF-T5	36	72000	1477	11.5
CEF-T5	41	12000	1364	6.4

[a] Oligomers comprised 5% or less of the total dimer population. All multiple-length DNA molecules that could be resolved were catenated forms.

Chick embryo fibroblasts were infected with virus 1 to 2 days after primary cultures were started. After growth at 36°C for 5 to 7 days transformation became manifested. Cells were then grown at two temperatures for at least 2 days in the presence of [^{3}H]-thymidine (Nass, 1973b). The uptake of [^{3}H]-2-deoxyglucose by whole cells was performed as described by Martin *et al.* (1971). For isolation of mitochondria cells were grown in roller bottles, and 2- to 5 × 10^8 cells were usually harvested by brief trypsination. Mitochondrial DNA was purified from isolated mitochondria by equilibrium centrifugation in cesium chloride–ethidium bromide gradients. DNA molecules were spread by the formamide method of the DNA monolayer technique (Nass and Ben-Shaul, 1972) and scored in the electron microscope. To avoid bias a code system was used so that the identity of samples was not known until after they were scored.

teristic of that in uninfected cells. Temperature shifts from 41° to 36°C and *vice versa* resulted in reversals of the respective levels of multiple-length DNA (Nass, 1973b). Transformation was verified by the appearance of morphological changes and a 3- to 5-fold increase in the uptake of 2-deoxyglucose. The fraction of cells synthesizing DNA as determined by autoradiography was found to be about the same in all cell types at both temperatures, suggesting that the observed changes in the levels of multiple-length DNA forms were not a consequence of changes in growth rates (Nass, 1973b).

We also observed a 2–3% increase in contour length of monomeric mitochondrial DNA from the transformed cells as compared with uninfected control cells (Nass, 1973b; M. M. K. Nass, manuscript in preparation). Experiments are in progress to determine whether this increase reflects a significant alteration of the mitochondrial genome, such as an integration of viral genetic material into mitochondrial DNA.

D. *Possible Mechanism of Origin of Multiple-Length Mitochondrial DNA*

Accumulations of dimeric and oligomeric DNA are common in microbial systems, such as bacteriophages, bacterial plasmids (extrachromosomal elements), and animal viruses (Helinski and Clewell, 1971). It is of special interest that oligomeric viral molecules accumulated after temperature shifts of mammalian cells that had been transformed by temperature-sensitive mutants of polyoma virus (Cuzin *et al.,* 1970). However, no simple correlations or answers have been found concerning the biological significance and mechanism of oligomer accumulation. The various forms may be normal intermediates in replication that accumulate due to an imbalance in normal environmental conditions or they are abnormal forms resulting strictly from errors in replication or as products of recombination. In studies with circular DNA of bacterial plasmids and bacteriophages, it appears that the interlocked and catenated dimer may arise primarily by recombination, whereas the unicircular dimers are generated mostly through atypical replication when replication does not terminate after one round (Benbow *et al.,* 1972). Genetic data that reconciliate several views have been recently presented (Doniger *et al.,* 1973). Nevertheless there is no clear-cut answer, and an extrapolation to mitochondrial DNA is at this stage largely hypothetical.

Two main conclusions concerning the formation of oligomeric mitochondrial DNA can be drawn from our experiments outlined in the previous sections. First, conditions that interfere with protein synthesis, such as amino acid deprivation and addition of puromycin or cycloheximide, lead to oligomer accumulation. Amino acid depletion and puromycin affect both the mitochondrial and cytoplasmic protein synthetic system. However, cycloheximide is more specific, i.e., it is known to inhibit cytoplasmic but not mitochondrial (or bacterial) protein synthesis in eukaryotes. The reverse is found with chloramphenicol. The responsible factor in oligomer accumulation may thus involve the extramitochondrial protein synthetic system. Second, the data with fibroblasts transformed by temperature-sensitive oncogenic viruses and, to some extent, the data with polyoma virus-transformed cells, indicate that the manifestation of transformation parallels an increase in multiple-length mitochondrial DNA.

Most of the mitochondrial enzymes, including DNA polymerase, are probably specified by nuclear genes, synthesized completely or in part on cytoplasmic ribosomes and are then transported into the mitochondrion (see Section VIII). It is proposed that an enzymes(s) involved in the replication of mitochondrial DNA or a protein involved in the control of DNA replication is manufactured in the cytoplasm and then transferred into the organelles (Nass, 1970a). Inhibition of cytoplasmic protein synthesis may lead to a deficiency of such enzyme(s), either by interference with its synthesis or by perturbation of its transfer into or integration with the mitochondrial structure. Possible candidates are specialized endonucleases or "nicking" enzymes which may cleave newly replicated DNA structures into monomeric molecules. Such endonucleases have been postulated in various models for ϕX phage DNA replication (Kiger and Sinsheimer, 1969; Dressler, 1970).

How does cell transformation fit into this scheme? It is well established that there are many clear-cut differences in the structure and function of cellular membranes in normal and malignant cells (e.g., see Burger, 1973; Warren et al., 1973). Such changes include sugar transport, as well as glycolipid and glycoprotein content and metabolism. Changes are not only confined to surface membranes but also include mitochondrial and other intracellular membranes (Soslau et al., 1974). Since the evidence suggests the existence of a mitochondrial DNA-inner membrane complex (see Section III, A), a conformational and/or functional alteration of the membrane may affect the attachment site of the DNA. Consequently, the activity or content of enzymes that are involved in DNA replication, such as the above-mentioned "nickases," may be reduced. Alternatively, the postulated distortion of the DNA-membrane complex may render the replicating DNA less accessible to, or susceptible to, the action of such enzymes. It is also possible that changes in the membrane systems affect intramitochondrial transport of specific "nickases" or of proteins involved in the control of M-DNA replication.

Future experimentation may allow testing of these possibilities. Future studies may also throw some light on the possible contribution of recombination to the formation of multiple-length forms of mitochondrial DNA.

V. Synthesis and Replication of Mitochondrial DNA in Normal, Malignant, Hormone-Treated, and Virus-Infected Cells

A mitochondria-specific DNA polymerase has been isolated from rat liver (e.g., Meyer and Simpson, 1970), wild-type and mutant yeast (Wintersberger and Wintersberger, 1970), and a rat hepatoma (Tschiersch and Graffi, 1970). The properties of mitochondrial DNA polymerases generally differ for enzymes of mitochondrial and nuclear origins. The M-DNA polymerase is more sensitive to the mutagenic dye ethidium bromide than the nuclear DNA polymerase (Meyer and Simpson, 1969). The incorporation of DNA precursors into M-DNA appears to be synthesis and not a repair process (Karol and Simpson, 1968).

Tschiersch and Graffi (1970) solubilized the respective DNA polymerases of mitochondrial and nuclear fractions from rat liver and hepatoma. The DNA polymerase extracted from rat hepatoma mitochondria was at least twice as active as the mitochondrial enzyme from rat liver and embryo. Kalf *et al.* (1971) reported that the incorporation of radioactively labeled deoxyribonucleoside triphosphates into DNA by isolated rat liver mitochondria is stimulated by soluble factors present in the postmicrosomal fraction of solid and mouse tumors and in regenerating and fetal rat liver, but not in normal liver. The identity and possible role of such factors in M-DNA replication are not known.

There is some evidence that M-DNA synthesis *in vivo* is greater in certain hepatomas than in liver. The rates of incorporation *in vivo* of [³H]thymidine into M-DNA and N-DNA of host livers from rat and hepatomas of different genetic, biochemical, and growth characteristics were compared (Chang *et al.*, 1968a). A correlation seems to exist between specific activity ratios of tumor to host liver M-DNA and growth rates. The most rapidly growing, undifferentiated tumors had 8–12 times greater ratios of M-DNA specific activities (M-hepatoma/M-host liver) than those of the relatively slower-growing, well-differentiated tumors. Actually, the latter values were low because host liver specific activities were much greater in intermediate growth than in rapid growth livers, thus lowering the tumor/host ratios for intermediate growth tumors. The specific activities of tumor mitochondria alone tended to be higher for tumors with intermediate growth rate. No correlations with growth rates were found for nuclear DNA specific activities. Comparisons of M-DNA with N-DNA specific activities (M/N ratios) were also made. M/N ratios < 1 (low mitochondrial incorporation) were found for some fast-growing hepatomas, host liver, and regenerating liver, > 1 for tumors with intermediate growth rates and respective host livers.

All these data have not been clear-cut enough, however, to allow generalizations. A survey of the literature indicates that the incorporation of [³H]thymidine into M-DNA may be greater or less than that into N-DNA, depending on a variety of factors, e.g., tissue of origin, growth rates, various qualitative differences in numbers of mitochondria of normal and some tumor cells, permeability of membranes, precursor pool sizes, and type of isotope used. In the latter case it is of interest that great differences between the incorporation of [³H]thymidine and the incorporation of [³H]cytidine into M-DNA were observed (Chang *et al.*, 1968b). The ratio of M-DNA to N-DNA specific activities in two transplantable rat hepatomas and host livers was 10–100 times greater following [³H]cytidine administration than the ratio following [³H]thymidine administration. Pool size and permeability differences may be responsible. In other cases, differences in specific activity values between tissue types were observed. These are illustrated in comparisons of the incorporation of 5-iodo-[¹³¹I]deoxyuridine into M-DNA and N-DNA of mouse liver and hepatoma, as opposed to lactating and neoplastic mammary gland (Georgatsos *et al.,* 1970).

Relatively little is known about the effects of hormones on mitochondrial DNA synthesis. Following testosterone administration, both nuclear and mitochondrial DNA synthesis of seminal vesicle and prostate in castrated rats were stimulated at about the same time 24 hours later. Consequently, neither type of synthesis was required for the early action of androgen (Doeg *et al.,* 1972). Kimberg and Loeb (1972) investigated the basis for reciprocal changes in mitochondrial size and number in livers of cortisone-treated rats. Cortisone treatment had little effect on yield of mitochondrial protein, M-DNA content, and specific activity of prelabeled M-DNA, and they suggest a process of mitochondrial fusion to account for the observed changes in mitochondrial size and number.

There have been reports that specifically mitochondrial DNA synthesis is stimulated by infection of monkey cells with SV40 virus (Levine, 1971), 3T3 cells with polyoma virus (Vesco and Basilico, 1971), and HeLa cells with herpes simplex virus (Radsak and Freise, 1972).

Inhibitors that are a great value in distinguishing mitochondrial and nuclear DNA synthesis, such as ethidium bromide and arabinosyl adenine, will be discussed in Section IX.

The temporal relations of M-DNA and N-DNA synthesis during the mitotic cycle indicate that the two DNA synthetic systems are not in phase. In many mammalian cells various workers have reported a periodicity of M- and N-DNA synthesis using electron microscope autoradiographic methods (Nass, 1967) or biochemical techniques (Koch and Stockstad, 1967; Bosmann, 1971; Pica-Mattoccia and Attardi, 1972). In L51784 cells M-DNA synthesis occured in S and G_2 phase (Bosmann, 1971). In some lower cell forms, e.g., *Tetrahymena* and slime mold, M-DNA synthesis appears continuous during the cell cycle (cf. Nass, 1969a).

Replication of mitochondrial DNA in rat liver appears to be by a semiconservative mechanism (Gross and Rabinowitz, 1969), as has been shown with various nuclear and microbial DNA's.

A variety of presumable replicative intermediates of mitochondrial DNA have been reported (Kasamatsu *et al.,* 1971; Ter Schegget *et al.,* 1971; Robberson *et al.,* 1972; Wolstenholme *et al.,* 1973). Some of these structures consist of double-stranded covalently closed DNA molecules with a single heavy-strand segment hydrogen-bonded to the circular light strand.

VI.   Mitochondrial RNA in Normal, Tumor, and Hormone-Treated Cells

Relatively few studies have been performed comparing mitochondrial RNA structure and metabolism in normal and tumor cells. There is some indication that the incorporation of ^{3}H-UTP *in vivo* into mitochondrial RNA is lowered in several rat hepatomas as compared with rat liver (Neubert and Morris, 1966).

There are few reports on effects of virus infection on M-RNA synthesis. In Chinese hamster ovary cells, nuclear synthesis of RNA was shown to be inhibited in the initial stages of infection with mengovirus, an RNA virus, but mitochondrial RNA synthesis was not (Vesco and Penman, 1969).

In studies of hormone effects, the consequences of steroid hormone action on target tissue have generally indicated that nuclear and mitochondrial RNA synthesis respond in unison. Nussdorfer and Mazzochi (1971a,b) report a corticosterone-induced inhibition of both nuclear and mitochondrial-dependent RNA and protein synthesis, as well as an ACTH-induced stimulation of nuclear and mitochondrial RNA synthesis. Differential effects following hormone treatment were found in liver. After cortisone injection into adrenalectomized rats, liver mitochondrial RNA synthesis increased at a faster rate than nuclear RNA synthesis (Mansour and Nass, 1970; Yu and Feigelson, 1970). In studies of other hormones, chronic treatment of thyroidectomized rats with physiological doses of triiodothyronine resulted in a significant increase of ^{3}H-UTP incorporation into RNA of isolated rat liver mitochondria. The newly synthesized RNA hybridized with mitochondrial DNA more efficiently than RNA labeled *in vitro* in mitochondria from thyroidectomized animals (Gadaleta *et al.*, 1972). It is suggested in the latter study that a change in the transcription of mitochondrial DNA under the influence of the hormone occurs *in vitro* and also *in vivo*.

It is apparent from this short sketch of data that proposed mechanisms or hormonal regulation of macromolecular syntheses have to account for an additional factor of complexity—the mitochondrial system.

Most studies that have been concerned with the identification of RNA species in mitochondria have employed a variety of nonmalignant cell types and HeLa cells. Ribosomes isolated from mitochondria of *Neurospora* (Küntzel and Noll, 1967) and various other higher organisms (O'Brian, 1971) as well as the RNA extracted from these ribosomes were shown to have smaller sedimentation coefficients than their cytoplasmic counterparts. No 5 S RNA component could be identified in mitochondrial ribosomes of *Neurospora crassa* (Lizardi and Luck, 1971) and in 4 S RNA fractions of hamster cells (Dubin and Montenecourt, 1970). Evidence for the presence of messenger RNA in HeLa mitochondria was recently presented (Perlman *et al.*, 1973). Mitochondria of *Neurospora* (Barnett *et al.*, 1967; Brown and Novelli, 1968), rat liver (Buck and Nass, 1968, 1969), and yeast (Accoceberry and Stahl, 1971) also contain distinct species of transfer RNA and aminoacyl-tRNA synthetases. *N*-Formylmethionyl-tRNA, known to function in the initiation of protein synthesis in bacteria, was also identified in mitochondria (e.g., Smith and Marcker, 1968). Mitochondrial RNA polymerase of *Neurospora* has recently been purified (Küntzel and Shäfer, 1971). In cytoplasmic mutants of *Neurospora crassa,* defective mitochondrial ribosome production (Rifkin and Luck, 1971) and altered species of mitochondrial transfer RNA (Brambl and Woodward, 1972) have been reported. Whether such alterations can occur in mitochondria of higher organisms is not known. This could be of considerable potential importance in certain pathological cases.

To characterize the unique mitochondrial tRNA species of rat liver, we have compared the mitochondrial and cytoplasmic aminoacyl tRNA's by chromatography on methylated albumin kieselguhr (Buck and Nass, 1968, 1969). This comparison revealed species of leucyl-, tyrosyl-, aspartyl-, valyl-, and seryl-tRNA which were found exclusively in mitochondria. It was also shown that mitochondrial and cytoplasmic aminoacyl-tRNA synthetases had different specificities; cytoplasmic synthetases were unable to acylate species of tRNA which were exclusively mitochondrial, whereas mitochondrial synthetases could acylate all cytoplasmic tRNA species examined. The studies added further support to the notion that the protein-synthesizing apparatus of the mitochondria is distinct from that operating in other areas of the cytoplasm.

VII. Transcription of Mitochondrial DNA

A. Hybridization with Species of Mitochondrial RNA

Does mitochondrial DNA transcribe organelle-specific RNA? Hybridization experiments have shown that M-DNA has indeed complementary base sequences to species of ribosomal RNA (Aloni and Attardi, 1971a; Chi and Suyama, 1970; Dawid, 1972; Wu *et al.,* 1972) and transfer RNA (Nass and Buck, 1969, 1970; Cohen and Rabinowitz, 1970). Also *N*-formylmethionyl-tRNA—typical of bacterial protein synthesis mechanisms—hybridizes with M-DNA (Halbreich and Rabinowitz, 1971). It was also suggested by pulse-labeling experiments with HeLa cells that the entire DNA molecule is transcribed and the transcript cut into smaller RNA molecules (Aloni and Attardi, 1971a).

Our studies have shown that mitochondrial tRNA species of rat liver hybridize exclusively with purified circular mitochondrial DNA (Nass and Buck, 1969, 1970). RNA–DNA hybridization was performed at low temperatures in the presence of 50% formamide. With this technique specific aminoacyl-tRNA–DNA hybridization can be followed in the presence of other species of RNA if the tRNA is acylated with radioactive amino acids. Competition experiments showed that mitochondrial aminoacyl-tRNA competed far more efficiently with mitochondrial tyrosyl-, phenylalanyl-, seryl-, or leucyl-tRNA for hybridization sites on mitochondrial DNA than did cytoplasmic aminoacyl-tRNA. No hybridization of mitochondrial aminoacyl-tRNA was observed with nuclear DNA or *Escherichia coli* DNA. The results showed that (1) mitochondrial leucyl-tRNA differs from cytoplasmic leucyl-tRNA in its primary base sequence, and (2) that M-DNA may be the template *in vivo* from which M-tRNA is transcribed.

The method of hybridization with aminoacyl-tRNA has also been of value in the identification of a yeast cytoplasmic mutant that appears to have a deletion for valyl-tRNA, i.e., lacks on its mitochondrial DNA hybridization sites for valyl-tRNA (Cohen and Rabinowitz, 1970). No alterations of mitochondrial DNA in tumor cells as compared with normal counterparts have thus far been reported. It is obvious that viable mutants may occur much less frequently in mammalian cells, which are obligate aerobes, than in yeast cells which can survive anaerobically.

B. Symmetrical Transcription of tRNA

To answer the question whether tRNA is potentially transcribed from one strand or from both strands of the circular duplex DNA molecule, we have isolated the complementary heavy (H) and light (L) strands of highly purified mitochondrial DNA by equilibrium centrifugation in alkaline cesium chloride (Fig. 4). To our surprise the hybridization studies showed that mitochondrial leucyl- and phenylalanyl-tRNA hybridized exclusively with the H strand, whereas tyrosyl- and seryl-tRNA hybridized exclusively with the L strand of M-DNA (Nass and Buck, 1970). These results are summarized in Fig. 5. The studies demonstrate "symmetrical transcription" in the case of tRNA, i.e., some species of mitochondrial tRNA may be transcribed *in vivo* from one strand and others from the complementary strand of M-DNA.

This type of transcription has recently been confirmed by others using entirely different methods and different cells (Aloni and Attardi, 1971b). The L strand as well as the H strand appear to be transcribed, but the L strand transcripts may be more unstable than those of the H strand, which explains why these workers failed to detect L strand transcription in earlier work. Wu *et al.*, (1972) attempted to visualize the relative positions of 4 S RNA genes and ribosomal RNA genes in mitochondrial DNA in the electron microscope. Mixtures of HeLa mitochondrial ribosomal RNA species and 4 S RNA–ferritin conjugates were hybridized with H and L strands of M-DNA. They found 12 S and 16 S rRNA–DNA duplex

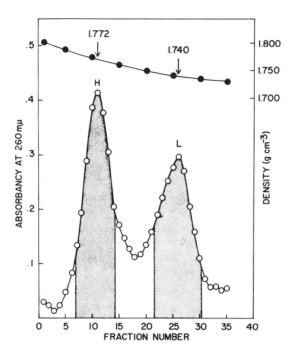

Fig. 4. Separation of heavy (H) and light (L) complementary strands of rat liver mitochondrial DNA by equilibrium centrifugation of purified MI-DNA (covalently closed M-DNA) in alkaline cesium chloride (pH 12.3). The stippled portions represent the fractions collected in the heavy and light regions of the gradient and subsequently used for hybridization studies with mitochondrial transfer RNA. (From Nass and Buck, 1970.)

regions on the H strand. By localizing electron-opaque ferritin granules, nine binding sites for 4 S RNA were detected on the H strand and three on the L strand. The sites appear to be distributed over the entire DNA molecule with relatively little clustering. It is at this time not known whether HeLa mitochondria do indeed have only 12 endogenous tRNA species. In amphibians 15 hybridizing sites for 4 S RNA have been estimated (Dawid, 1972b). If this is correct, mitochondria may either import the missing tRNA species from the cytoplasm or make proteins that lack certain amino acids. Studies of amino acid incorporation and peptide maps of mitochondrial proteins, if properly controlled for precursor pool sizes, permeability, and other factors, may give further clues. Another possibility is that certain tRNA species are present in mitochondria in very small quantities so that hybridization with crude 4 S RNA does not reveal them. The method we have used, which employs tRNA species specifically labeled in the amino acid moiety, may be of great use in further studies.

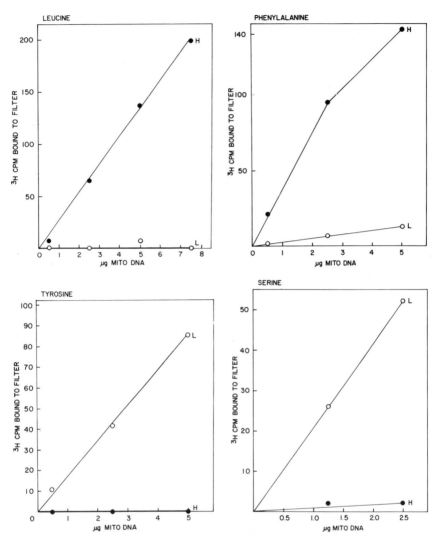

Fig. 5. Illustration of "symmetrical" transcription of mitochondrial tRNA. The hybridization of complementary heavy (H) and light (L) strands of rat liver mitochondrial DNA with mitochondrial ^{3}H-labeled phenylalanyl-tRNA, leucyl-tRNA, tyrosyl-tRNA, and seryl-tRNA was conducted as a function of increasing DNA concentration. The radioactive label was in the amino acid moiety acylated to the tRNA molecule by mitochondrial aminoacyl-tRNA synthetases so that only the hybridization of specific tRNA species is recorded and other species of RNA in the preparation remain undetected. This specificity distinguishes this method from most other studies, which use 4 S RNA containing unknown proportions of radioactively labeled transfer RNA and labeled degraded ribosomal and possibly messenger RNA.

Each hybridization vial contained one filter with heavy or light strands of DNA attached and

As a general estimate, not more than 20–30% of the mitochondrial genome is used to transcribe stable RNA species of the mitochondrial protein synthesizing apparatus. The remaining sequences may partially code for specific protein subunits (see next section) and other yet unidentified transcription products, as well as may include some spacer regions.

VIII. Mitochondrial Proteins, Protein Synthesis, and Biogenesis in Normal and Tumor Cells

The main effort has been directed toward the identification of organelle-specified or nucleus-specified protein components of the total mitochondrion or of separated inner and outer membranes. Such compounds include unspecified polypeptide fractions, subunits of specific cytochromes and enzymes, and glycoproteins. There are as yet few studies on possible alterations of mitochondrial proteins in tumor cells. A comparison of mitochondrial membrane proteins in rat liver and hepatomas by polyacrylamide gel electrophoresis was recently reported (Chang *et al.,* 1971). The profiles of these membrane proteins of hepatoma mitochondria differed from those of normal or host liver. One major protein component seemed to be missing in the tumor mitochondria, and the latter in some cases contained an additional protein component that was absent or greatly reduced in mitochondrial membranes from normal liver.

Several studies have indicated that mitochondrial protein synthesis, as measured by the incorporation of labeled amino acids into protein, is depressed in a number of tumors (Neubert and Morris, 1966) or is abnormal (Graffi *et al.,* 1965). Whether the changes observed in mitochondrial protein components and protein synthesis of hepatomas are due to alterations in mitochondrial DNA or are due to effects of the nuclear genetic system is not known.

Most studies have been concerned with the complex problem of the relative contribution of mitochondrial and nuclear–cytoplasmic protein synthesis systems to the biogenesis of mitochondrial protein components and their integration into the mitochondrial structure. The main approach has been to pulse label with radioactive amino acids in the presence or absence of specific inhibitors that preferentially inhibit mitochondrial and cytoplasmic protein synthesis (chloramphenicol and cycloheximide, respectively). Another approach has been to utilize cytoplasmic mutants of yeast that lack M-DNA and identify mitochondrial proteins that are not coded

---

0.8 ml of a solution consisting of the respective ³H-labeled aminoacyl-tRNA in 0.3 M NaCl, 0.03 M sodium citrate, pH 4.2, and 50% formamide. Incubation was for 15 hours at 33°C. (From Nass and Buck, 1970.)

for by mitochondrial DNA. It appears that less than 10% of mitochondrial proteins are synthesized on mitochondrial ribosomes and that these proteins are part of the inner membrane (Beattie, 1972). Furthermore the inner membrane enzyme complexes of the respiratory chain, such as cytochrome oxidase and ATPase and cytochrome b, are synthesized by the combined action of mitochondrial and nuclear–cytoplasmic protein synthetic mechanism. In the case of cytochrome oxidase, only a few of the electrophoretically separated polypeptides from highly purified yeast cytochrome oxidase appear to be synthesized on mitochondrial ribosomes (Schatz *et al.,* 1972). The rutamycin-sensitive ATPase of the yeast mitochondrion appears to contain at least four subunit proteins which are synthesized by the mitochondrion (Tzagoloff and Meagher, 1972). Weiss (1972) reported that two smaller subunits of cytochrome b in *Neurospora* are synthesized on cytoplasmic ribosomes and two smaller subunits with which the heme b group is associated are synthesized on mitochondrial ribosomes. The isolation of a hydrophobic peptide synthesized in rat liver mitochondria containing most of the major amino acids has also been reported (Kadenbach, 1971). It has been postulated that the limited number of proteins synthesized by the mitochondrion are of hydrophobic type (Tzagoloff, and Akai, 1972). The mitochondrial protein products were found to be easily extracted from the membrane with acidic chloroform-methanol. The organelle-made proteins presumably serve to anchor to the mitochondrial structure certain water-soluble peptides synthesized in the cytoplasm.

The majority of mitochondrial proteins are undoubtedly specified and synthesized by the nuclear-cell sap genetic system. Evidence for specific cases includes cytochrome c or at least a form of cytochrome c (Kadenbach, 1970; Davidian and Pennial, 1971), DNA polymerase (Ch´ih and Kalf, 1969), leucyl-tRNA synthetase (Gross *et al.,* 1968), and most if not all 53 structural proteins of mitochondrial ribosomal subunits of *Neurospora* (Lizardi and Luck, 1972). These and other enzymes (e.g., those involved in the citric acid cycle, glycolytic pathway, and fatty acid metabolism) must be transported into the mitochondrion by an as yet unknown mechanism. Most of the latter enzymes are associated with the outer mitochondrial membrane, the intramembrane space, or the inner matrix.

Limited information is available about the time of synthesis of mitochondrial proteins during the cell cycle. In L5178Y cells this time appears to be primarily G_1 and G_2 phases (Bosmann, 1971). In the same study evidence was also presented that glycoprotein synthesis of mitochondria occurred in G_1, S, and G_2 phases.

IX.   Ethidium Bromide as a Tool to Study the Mitochondrial Genetic System

A. Abnormal Mitochondrial DNA

The phenanthridine dye ethidium bromide (EB) is of particular interest because the mitochondria are a prime target for this drug. EB, like acriflavin or ultraviolet irradiation, induces respiratory deficient cytoplasmic mutants ("petites") in yeast (Slonimski *et al.,* 1968; Mahler *et al.,* 1971). These mutants are deficient in cytochromes a + a$_3$ and b. EB may also cause the loss of the mitochondrion-associated kinetoplast of trypanosomes (Riou, 1967). In yeast, the mutation is genetically stable or may be reversible under certain conditions (Perlman and Mahler, 1971; Mahler and Perlman, 1972). EB intercalates between the bases of double-stranded DNA (Waring, 1968) and exhibits differential binding affinities for covalently closed circular and nicked circular or linear duplex DNA (Crawford and Waring, 1967; Radloff *et al.,* 1967). This property has been applied widely to isolate and purify species of mitochondrial DNA (see also Figs. 6 and 7).

EB may also cause the actual loss of the circular kinetoplast DNA (Riou, 1968; Renger and Wolstenholme, 1970). Various EB-induced mutants of yeast have been reported, which range from mutants with an abnormal base composition that may be almost entirely "non-sense" or adenine + thymine (Bernardi *et al.,* 1968) to mutants containing mitochondrial DNA of reduced size (Goldring *et al.* 1971) or seemingly lacking M-DNA (Goldring *et al.,* 1970). Transient treatment of yeast with EB and subsequent growth without EB leads to the appearance of a mitochondrial DNA species with a lower than normal buoyant density (Perlman and Mahler, 1971).

In mammalian cells the effects of EB are not as drastic as in yeast and *Trypanosomas.* It is obviously more difficult to obtain mitochondrial mutations in mammalian cells since they require aerobic respiration for survival. Nevertheless distinct effects have been observed. The synthesis of circular mitochondrial DNA of mammalian cells is differentially inhibited over that of nuclear DNA both *in vivo* (Nass, 1970a, 1972) and *in vitro* with partially purified mitochondrial and nuclear DNA polymerases (Meyer and Simpson, 1969). Studies in this laboratory have shown that the synthesis of M-DNA of several control and virus-transformed mammalian cell lines was inhibited by EB, whereas the synthesis of nuclear DNA was actually stimulated (Nass, 1970a, 1972). This effect is of obvious potential value in studies of the function and interaction of mitochondrial and nuclear genetic systems.

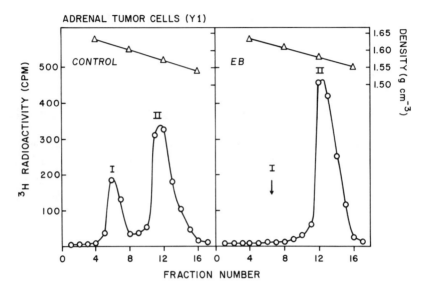

Fig. 6. Effect of the DNA intercalating dye ethidium bromide (EB) on the structure of covalently closed mitochondrial DNA (I) in cultured mouse adrenal tumor cells (Y1). Y1 cells
were set up in roller bottles (growth area 690 cm²; 2 × 10⁷ cells per bottle) and grown in the
presence of ACTH (0.05 units/ml) for 3 days. The medium was replaced and the cells prelabeled for 6 hours with [³H]thymidine (2 μCi/ml). To half of the cultures ethidium bromide (1
μg/ml) was then added and ³H-labeling continued for 48 hours (equivalent to 2 cell generations of control cells). Mitochondrial DNA was centrifuged to equilibrium in cesium chloride
gradients containing 300 μg EB/ml. DNA component II represents primarily nuclear DNA.
Component I of control mitochondria consists of mitochondrial covalently closed circular
DNA. After EB treatment this component is partially degraded and displaced (see text). Pre-
labeling of cells prior to EB treatment indicates that preexisting M-DNA, besides newly
synthesized DNA, is affected. Nuclear DNA synthesis is not inhibited by EB.

The physical structure of covalently closed M-DNA is drastically altered
upon EB treatment; there is strand breakage and some rejoining of strands,
manifested in both a greater proportion of nicked circles and linear DNA
and some closed circular DNA having a different superhelix density as compared with control cases (Nass, 1970a; Smith *et al.,* 1971). Figure 6
reveals this EB-induced partial disappearance and shift of covalently closed
mitochondrial DNA from mouse adrenal tumor cells. After 4 days of exposure to EB mitochondrial DNA of mammalian cells does not disappear
completely as in some yeast mutants but is nevertheless reduced in quantity
by about one half (Nass, 1972). Studies are in progress to determine in
greater detail the consequence of EB-induced alterations of M-DNA of
animal mitochondria.

An interesting tool in combination with the use of EB is the potential use of 9β-D-arabinofuransyl adenine (ara-a) which has been shown to have the phenotypically opposite effect of EB, namely to selectively inhibit nuclear DNA synthesis but not circular, presumably mitochondrial, DNA synthesis (Shipman *et al.,* 1972). We have confirmed this observation and determined that the DNA that is primarily labeled in the presence of ara-a can be isolated from a purified mitochondrial fraction of mouse adrenal tumor cells and chick embryo fibroblasts and is thus indeed mitochondrial DNA (Nass, 1973b). Figure 7 demonstrates this effect. With slightly higher concentrations of ara-a nuclear DNA synthesis can be completely blocked.

It is known that direct interaction with DNA is not the only site of action of EB. For example, a special affinity of EB for binding to the mitochondrial membrane may occur which causes an energy-linked transition in the membrane (Azzi and Santato, 1971). Mahler and Pearlman (1972) advanced a model for EB mutagenesis in yeast that postulates a complex between mitochondrial DNA and the inner mitochondrial membrane. An EB-generated distortion of such a complex at the at-

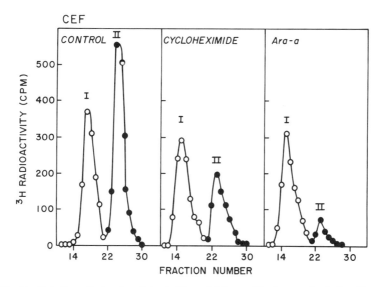

Fig. 7. Selective effects of cycloheximide and 9β-D-arabinofuranosyl adenine (Ara-a) on DNA synthesis of mitochondrial (I) and nuclear (II) DNA, as reflected by incorporation of [³H]thymidine. Growing chick embryo fibroblasts were exposed to cycloheximide (25 μg/ml) and Ara-a (5 × 10⁻⁴ M) for 24 hours in the presence of [³H]thymidine (1 μCi/ml). Mitochondria were isolated and M-DNA subjected to centrifugation in cesium chloride–ethidium bromide gradients. Data are plotted relative to equal amounts of mitochondrial protein. (From Nass, 1973b.)

tachment site of DNA may hinder DNA replication and facilitate attack by nucleases, possible repair enzymes, and/or other modifying agents. From our studies with mammalian cells we have come to similar conclusions that the DNA alterations are related to changes in the mitochondrial membrane. However, whether or not the proposed alterations in the mitochondrial membrane are organelle specific or are largely induced as a consequence of EB action on extramitochondrial metabolic processes remains to be determined.

B. Inhibitory Effects of EB on Mitochondrial Morphology and Cytochromes

A consequence of EB action has been interference with the transcription of the mitochondrial genome (Zylber et al., 1969; Fukuhara and Kujawa, 1970). Studies in this laboratory have shown that treatment of mouse L-cells with 1 μg/ml EB leads to a decrease, first of cytochromes a + a$_3$, then of b, accompanied by severe structural alterations of the mitochondria (Soslau and Nass, 1971). Figure 8 exemplifies some EB-induced morphological changes. The concentrations of cytochromes c + c$_1$, on the other hand, remained the same or actually increased in the presence of EB. The increase in these cytochromes may be an expression of the interaction of the nucleus and the mitochondrion. If only a portion of the mitochondrial complement of the cell is converted by EB into respiratory-deficient mitochondria, the nucleus may interpret this situation as a loss of mitochondria and therefore direct the synthesis of mitochondrial proteins that fall under its control. This possibility is supported by the actual increase of nuclear DNA synthesis and total mitochondrial protein per cell as a consequence of EB treatment (Nass, 1970a, 1972).

These changes have many similarities with those obtained in some of the petite mutants of yeast (Mahler et al., 1971). In mammalian cells, however, as discussed above, no viable respiratory-deficient mutant that can be propagated as a stable cell line has been found. Besides the obvious inability of mammalian cells to replicate under respiratory-deficient or anaerobic conditions it is also possible that in mammalian cells resistance to EB is more easily developed. Recently, we have isolated and characterized a mammalian virus-transformed cell line that is resistant to

---

Fig. 8. Effect of ethidium bromide on the ultrastructure of mitochondria in cultured mouse L-cells. (a) Control cells; (b) cells grown in the presence of EB (1 μg/ml) for 3 days; (c) cells grown in the presence of EB (2 μg/ml) for 3 days. Mitochondrial profiles are greatly enlarged; cristae membranes are reduced in size and number and frequently are tubular and appear to form separate circular subunits. (From Soslau and Nass, 1971.) Bar = 1.0 μm.

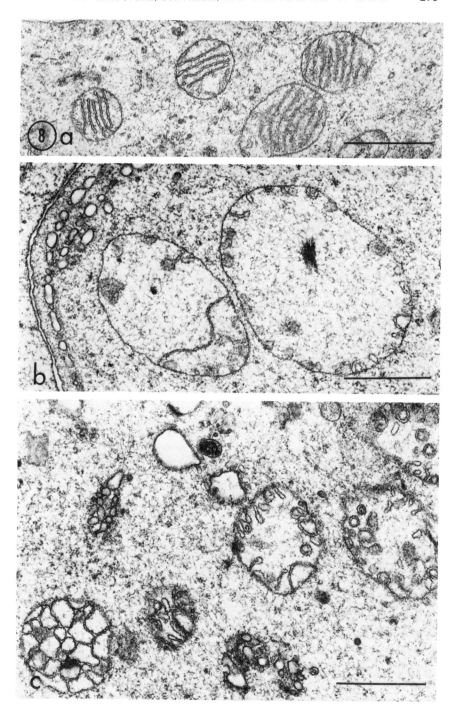

high concentrations of EB (Klietmann *et al.*, 1973). The mitochondrial DNA has normal or almost normal properties but the mitochondrial ultrastructure is altered. The EB resistance has been hereditarily transmitted for hundreds of cell generations and characterization of this apparent mutation is in progress.

C. *Inhibitory Effects on ACTH-Induced Mitochondrial Transformation and Steroid 11β-Hydroxylating Activity*

We have extended studies of EB action on the function of enzyme and membrane components to a relatively specialized enzymatic apparatus—the steroid 11β-hydroxylating enzymes associated with the inner mitochondrial membranes of adrenal cortical cells. Previous reports indicate that chloramphenicol which inhibits mitochondrial protein synthesis specifically inhibits mitochondrial morphological differentiation in ACTH-treated adrenal cortical cells without affecting the proliferation of smooth-surfaced endoplasmic reticulum (Kahri, 1970). Furthermore, the rise of mitochondrial steroid 11β-hydroxylating activity normally associated with mitochondrial transformation is also blocked by chloramphenicol (Milner, 1971). Similarly, treatment of explanted fetal adrenals with ethidium bromide (1 μg/ml for 4 days) inhibited the morphological transformation of the mitochondria normally induced by ACTH, and the steroid 11β-hydroxylating activity was either partially or completely blocked (Milner, 1972).

We have confirmed these observations using an established mouse adrenal tumor cell line, Y1 (originally cloned by Yasumura *et al.*, 1966). In these cells, however, mitochondrial ACTH induced morphological differentiation is not as pronounced as in freshly explanted adrenal cortical cells. Figures 9a and b show the reorganization of internal mitochondrial membranes under the influence of ACTH, and Figs. 9c and d reveal the inhibitory effect of EB on this transformation. Mitochondria of EB-treated cells typically do not have the condensed conformation of cristae, have relatively sparse inner membranes, and have an electron-lucent matrix. Some heterogeneity of cell response to ACTH and to EB exists in the Y1 line since a small fraction of control cells was observed that has partially transformed mitochondria (the cells do produce steroids at a low level in the absence of ACTH), and upon EB treatment some cells showed evidence of resistance to EB.

Figure 10 summarizes effects of ACTH stimulation and EB action on 11β-hydroxylating activity, as indicated by the relative conversion of [³H]deoxycorticosterone (DOC) to [³H]corticosterone (C). Since the ³H counts in progesterone were minor they are not represented here. It is apparent that this ACTH-stimulated reaction is significantly inhibited by EB.

The lesser response to EB after 5 days of treatment as compared with 3 days may indicate that partial resistance to EB may have developed or the response is within the limits of experimental variation. Further studies are required to determine whether the observed effects of EB result from inhibition of mitochondrial nucleic acid and protein synthesis or from other effects on the mitochondrial membrane.

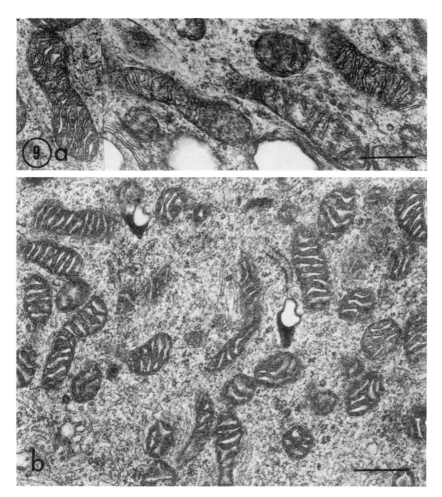

Fig. 9. Electron micrographs showing appearance of mitochondria of cultured mouse adrenal tumor cells (Y1) in the presence of adrenocorticotropin (ACTH) and ACTH plus ethidium bromide. (a) Cells grown without ACTH; (b) Cells grown in the presence of 0.01 units of ACTH/ml for 5 days; (c) and (d) cells treated with ACTH plus ethidium bromide (1 μg/ml) for 5 days. The inner mitochondrial membranes upon EB treatment are in most cells poorly developed and sometimes concentrically arranged (arrows). Bar = 0.5 μm.

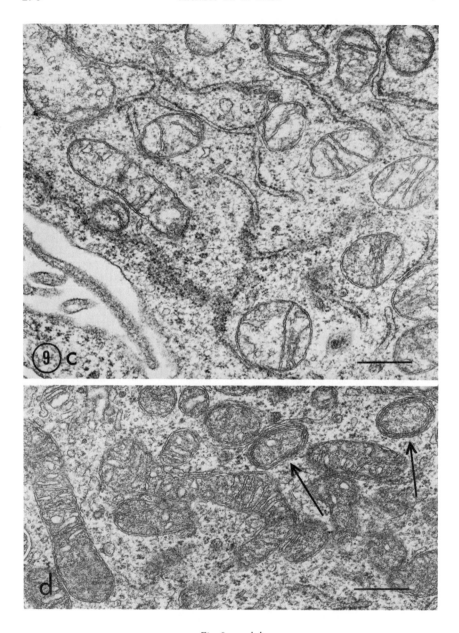

Fig. 9 c and d.

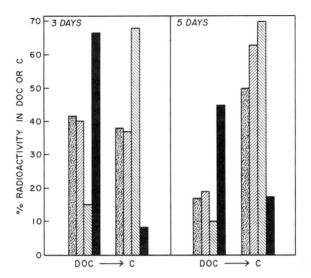

Fig. 10. Inhibitory effect of ethidium bromide on corticosterone synthesis, as reflected by the degree of conversion of [³H]deoxycorticosterone (DOC) to [³H]corticosterone (C).

The procedure is based on that of Schimmer (1969) and Roberts et al. (1964). Y1 cells were grown in small Falcon flasks in the absence of ACTH and in the presence of 0.01 and 0.05 units of ACTH per ml for 24 hours. Then 1 μg EB/ml was added to half of the dishes with ACTH. Six hours later, 1 μCi [³H]deoxycorticosterone per ml was added to all dishes and the cells incubated for 7 days with a daily replacement of the respective media. Purification of steroidal products from the collected media and thin-layer chromatography was performed essentially as described by Roberts et al. (1964). Aluminum-backed sheets coated with silica gel F254 were used and the chromatogram developed in chloroform-ethanol (95:5). The radioactivity in spots corresponding to deoxycorticosterone, progesterone, corticosterone, and 11 β-hydroxy-progesterone were cut out and counted in toluene-Liquifluor in a liquid scintillation counter. Radioactivity is presented as percent of total counts in the respective corticosteroids. Only counts in DOC and C were significant. The average of 3 determinations is recorded in each histogram. Stippled bars: no ACTH. Hatched bars: 0.01 and 0.05 units ACTH/ml. Solid bars: 1 μg EB/ml plus 0.01 units ACTH/ml. Cultures without EB show the accumulation of corticosterone, whereas EB-treated cells show little conversion of DOC to C. Cell division was reduced by about 30%. There is some variability among cells in the extent of 11 β-hydroxylation activity.

X.   Can Viruses Replicate in Mitochondria?

The existence of a DNA, RNA, protein synthesis mechanism in mitochondria has stimulated some work on the relation of viruses to mitochondria. Selected cases that indicate stimulation of mitochondrial DNA synthesis have already been discussed in Section V. In no case is it known whether mitochondrial DNA synthesis is an essential factor in the replication of a particular virus or the response of the host cell.

Hybridization experiments thus far provided no evidence that SV40 or polyoma virus DNA is integrated into mitochondrial DNA of cells transformed by these viruses (Benjamin, 1968; Sambrook et al., 1968; Kit and Minekawa, 1972).

There are scattered reports on the association of viruses with mitochondria. None have revealed whether this apparent association is a normal and essential phase in the development of a particular virus. Electron microscopy of hamster cells transformed by Rous sarcoma viruses (RSV) showed mitochondria which contained structures that were interpreted to represent viral nucleocapsids (Gazzalo et al., 1969). In a study in collaboration with Dr. C. Buck I have found numerous virus-like structures in mitochondria of RSV-infected hamster cells, as shown in Fig. 11. Intramitochondrial virus particles were also reported in a reptilian cell line, derived from a spleen tumor (Lunger and Clark, 1973). Kára et al., (1971, 1972) presented biochemical data suggesting that Rous sarcoma virus replicates inside the mitochondria and that reverse transcriptase-containing subviral particles can be isolated from mitochondria of Rous sarcoma cells (Kára et al., 1972). However, further studies with rigorously purified mitochondria are needed. More indirect studies such as effects of inhibitors of mitochondrial function on Rous sarcoma virus replication and malignant transformation have also been reported (Richert and Hare, 1972). There is suggestive evidence that some plant RNA viruses are associated with mitochondria (e.g., Hatta et al., 1971). Autoradiographic studies have shown that vaccinia viruses could replicate in enucleated L-cells (Prescott et al., 1971). Whether mitochondria were affected or involved in any way was not reported.

Bader (1972) concluded from experiments with ethidium bromide-treated virus-infected murine and avian cells that RNA-containing tumor viruses (Rauscher leukemia and Rous sarcoma) were detectable in the cytoplasm and mitochondria of both untreated and EB-treated cells, and that therefore the integrity of mitochondria is not essential for the production of these viruses. The definition of integrity, however, has been arbitrary and the use of EB as a tool in this study has been inconclusive since under the conditions used by these investigators (1 μg EB/ml) mitochondria in other cell types still contain at least half of their DNA, are partially functional, and an EB-resistant mitochondrial population may appear (Soslau and Nass, 1971; Nass, 1972). The subject of virus-related mitochondrial functions certainly requires and deserves further investigation. The question remains to be answered whether a mitochondrion-associated phase of viral development is indispensible or is merely auxiliary and can easily be carried on extramitochondrially when organelle function is impaired.

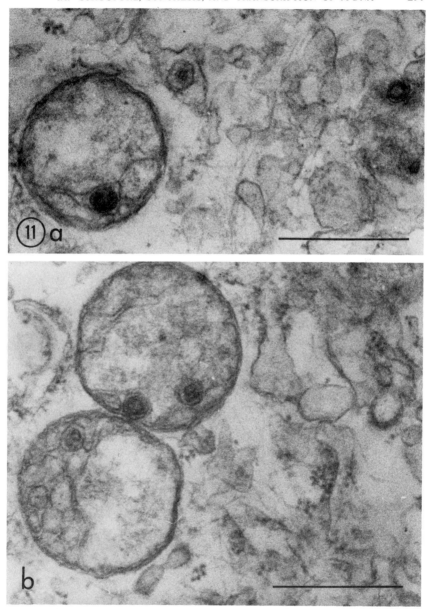

Fig. 11. Virus-like particles in mitochondria of fused hamster tumor-chick embryo cells. HAM-SR cells (Flow Laboratories), derived from a hamster tumor induced with the Schmidt-Ruppin strain of Rous sarcoma virus, were fused with chick embryo fibroblasts at a ratio of 2:1, using Sendai virus (performed by Dr. Clayton Buck). The virus-like particles are seen within the mitochondrial cristae membranes. The cristae may form a honeycomb pattern that surrounds individual particles. Similar particles are found in smooth vesicles of the cytoplasm.

XI.   Cell-Mitochondria Hybrids

Our interest in gene activity and expression of the mitochondrial genetic system has led to experiments in which mouse L-cells were allowed to phagocytically ingest isolated foreign cell organelles (Nass, 1969e, 1970b). It was found that both isolated mitochondria (e.g., from chicken) and chloroplasts of plants are taken up by the mouse cells and retained for many cell generations. In case of chloroplasts, the organelles retained membrane structure, photosynthetic activity, and intact DNA for several days within the host cells which kept on dividing. Also ethidium bromide-treated cells retained the ability to ingest cell organelles (Nass, 1970b). Although the incorporation of cell organelles into various host cells can be visualized to mimic the often postulated symbiotic origin of mitochondria from free-living organisms, such resemblance is obviously an oversimplification. [Voluminous arguments both for and against a symbiotic origin of cell organelles have been advanced (see e.g., Raff and Mahler, 1972).] The endocytic uptake of mitochondria is potentially a useful tool in attempts to "seed" normal cells with damaged or foreign mutant mitochondria and mitochondria-damaged cells with normal organelles; however, the limitations of this technique are apparent. Since the biogenesis of a mitochondrion is largely under nuclear control, the expression of nuclear genetic information of host cells must be compatible with the specific requirements of the foreign mitochondria. This limitation was revealed in recent studies. Clayton *et al.*, (1971), applying our technique of heterologous organelle uptake, found that after incorporation of human mitochondria into mouse L-cells, human mitochondrial DNA did not coexist with mouse mitochondrial DNA in the mouse host cells for longer than several days. Perhaps more promising results will be obtained if the host cells mitochondria stem from more closely related species. The lack of retention of human M-DNA was also observed by somatic cell hybridization of mouse and human cells (Clayton *et al.*, 1971; Attardi and Attardi, 1972). It is likely in this case that one or more human chromosomes that are necessary for the propagation of human mitochondria and M-DNA are lost or suppressed in the hybrids and other combinations of somatic hybridization will have to be tried.

XII.   Conclusions and Future Aims

Mitochondria are indispensible in the total function and activity of the cell. Superimposed on their previously well-known function as the site of respiration and energy transduction is the possession of a semi-autonomous, organelle-specific genetic apparatus. The DNA of the mitochondria can be distinguished from nuclear DNA by its structure, physicochemical properties, and replicative and transcriptional properties. It may be assumed from DNA renaturation studies that the entire population of mitochondrial DNA molecules has the same base sequences and, therefore, that the information content is confined to the monomer length of the DNA. There is obviously a great redundancy of this DNA per cell, which in one L-cell amounts to 500 to 2000 DNA molecules (2–8 molecules per mitochondrion; approximately 250 mitochondria per cell; see Nass, 1969a). The repetition of M-DNA may be even greater in M-DNA of many embryonic and tumor cells. Such redundancy must be of evolutionary selective advantage to allow better survival of the cell when part of the mitochondrial population is damaged by disease or other environmental limitations. It is of interest that irradiation of individual mitochondria by laser beam has shown cell survival with a small proportion of the mitochondria remaining (Berns, *et al.,* 1970, 1972).

Work to date from many laboratories indicates, but is far from complete, that mitochondrial DNA may transcribe mitochondrial ribosomal RNA and tRNA species, the latter "symmetrically," i.e., from both complementary DNA strands, and may code for the more insoluble types of protein of the inner membrane. The bulk of the enzymes are coded by nuclear genes, synthesized in the cytoplasm and transported at variable stages of completion into the mitochondrion. In at least three cases, the oligomycin-sensitive ATPase and cytochrome oxidase complex and cytochrome b, products of both genetic systems seem to be required to have functional, membrane-integrated enzymes. Future studies may indicate whether nuclear messenger RNA for mitochondrial function can not only be translated on cytoplasmic but also on mitochondrial ribosomes. The potential vulnerability of such a complex system in the incidence of disease is evident.

Are the differences observed in mitochondria of normal and tumor cells significant? Such differences have consisted mainly in differential activities of enzymes related to respiratory metabolism, differential rates of synthesis and concentrations of DNA, RNA and protein components, and both quantitative and qualitative differences, such as the preferential formation of multiple-length DNA and altered membrane protein patterns. The latter two are undoubtedly also a consequence of altered metabolic activities. Future studies must be concerned with understanding the interaction of nucleus-controlled and mitochondria-controlled processes in normal and pathological cells. Concentration merely on mitochondrial functions would be a gross oversimplification of the problem.

Such research should determine and consider critically whether any changes occur in mitochondria that are directly and significantly related to malignancy or whether mitochondrial effects are among the numerous secondary changes which fill the literature on cancer research. The studies which attempt to dissect, understand, and ultimately influence the function and possible role of mitochondria in malignancy should also aid our understanding of the function of these organelles in other pathological conditions and in normal cell function, growth and differentiation. Conversely, a better insight into normal differentiation should aid in our understanding of dysfunctions of differentiation.

The essential prerequisite for studies of pathological cells is a completely controllable experimental system. The lack of proper controls (e.g., normal cells from which certain tumors are derived) has been responsible for most of the previous, often irrelevant and contradictory, scatter of information on mitochondria of tumor and other abnormal cells. We have presented our studies with fibroblasts transformed by temperature-sensitive mutants of oncogenic viruses as an example of a well-controlled system (Section IV, C) since these cells can be induced to express malignant properties and then reversed to normal, simply by temperature switches. The nontransformed parent cells and cells transformed with wild-type virus are available for additional comparisons. Other equally favorable or better systems may become available.

Special emphasis may be placed on the following topics and experimental approaches: (1) selective use of pharmacological agents that differentiate between mitochondrial and nuclear–cytoplasmic function (e.g., EB, ara-a, hydroxyurea, cycloheximide, chloramphenicol, erythromycin, lincomycin, and others) as well as studies with thymidine kinase-deficient cells, recently shown to be positive for mitochondrial thymidine kinase (Clayton and Teplitz, 1972; Kit and Minekawa, 1972); (2) the fact that mitochondria are highly sensitive to certain drugs and to irradiation may be important in better understanding and regulating many effects (and side effects) of therapy, e.g., chloramphenicol and irradiation therapy involving bone marrow depression; (3) the molecular basis and consequences of changes in the mitochondrial and other cellular membranes (induced by viruses, hormones, drugs, etc.), with special focus on membrane–M-DNA–enzyme relations; (4) heteroduplex studies of base sequence homologies and of possible small deletions in mitochondrial DNA's of various tumors and other pathological cells; M-DNA due to its small size renders itself to easier analysis than the exceedingly large and heterogeneous nuclear DNA molecules; (5) virus-related functions in mitochondria, especially the possibility of transcription and intramitochondrial integration of genetic material from oncogenic RNA viruses; our finding of a length increase of mitochondrial DNA from Rous virus-transformed cells (see Section IV, D) may be an example of such a possibility; (6) the technique of seeding normal and diseased cells with heterologous types of mitochondria promises new approaches and answers if the factors that control organelle retention become better known. There are now many avenues open to a deeper understanding of mitochondrial function and dysfunction.

ACKNOWLEDGMENTS

This work has been supported by Grants P01-AI07005, R01-CA 13814 and Career Development Award K03-AI-08830 from the National Institutes of Health and Grant NP-93 from the American Cancer Society.

REFERENCES

Accoceberry, B., and Stahl, A. (1971). *Biochem. Biophys. Res. Commun.* **42**, 1235–1243.

Afifi, A. K., Ibrahim, M. Z. M., Bergman, R. A., Haydar, N. A., Mire, J., Bahuth, N., and Kaylani, F. (1972). *J. Neurol. Sci.* **15**, 271–290.

Aloni, Y., and Attardi, G. (1971a). *J. Mol. Biol.* **55**, 251–270.

Aloni, Y., and Attardi, G. (1971b). *Proc. Nat. Acad. Sci. U.S.* **68**, 1757–1761.

Arber, W., and Linn, S. (1969). *Annu. Rev. Biochem.* **38**, 467–500.

Ashwell, M., and Work, T. S. (1970). *Annu. Rev. Biochem.* **39**, 251–290.

Attardi, B., and Attardi, G. (1972). *Proc. Nat. Acad. Sci. U.S.* **69**, 129–133.

Azzi, A., and Santato, M. (1971). *Biochem. Biophys. Res. Commun.* **44**, 211–217.

Bader, A. V. (1972). *J. Cell Biol.* **55**, 11a.

Bahr, G. F. (1971). *Advan. Cell Mol. Biol.* **1**, 267–292.

Barnett, W. E., Brown, D. H., and Epler, J. L. (1967). *Proc. Nat. Acad. Sci. U.S.* **57**, 1775–1781.

Beattie, D. S. (1972) *Sub-Cell. Biochem.* **1**, 1–23.

Benbow, R. M., Eisenberg, M., and Sinsheimer, R. L. (1972). *Nature (London), New Biol.* **237**, 141–144.

Benjamin, T. L. (1968). *Virology* **36**, 685–687.

Bernardi, G., Carnevali, F., Nicolaieff, A., Piperno, G., and Tecce, G. (1968). *J. Mol. Biol.* **37**, 493–505.

Bernhard, W. (1968). *Cancer Res.* **18**, 491–499.

Bernhard, W., and Tournier, P. (1966). *Int. J. Cancer* **1**, 61–80.

Berns, M. W., Gamaleja, N., Olson, R., Duffy, C., and Rounds, D. E. (1970). *J. Cell. Physiol.* **76**, 207–214.

Berns, M. W., Gross, D. C. L., Cheng, W. K., and Woodring, D. (1972). *J. Mol. Cell. Cardiol.* **4**, 71–83.

Borst, P. (1972). *Annu. Rev. Biochem.* **41**, 333–376.

Borst, P., and Kroon, A. M. (1969). *Int. Rev. Cytol.* **26**, 107–190.

Bosmann, H. B. (1971). *J. Biol. Chem.* **246**, 3817–3823.

Brambl, R. M., and Woodward, D. O. (1972). *Nature (London), New Biol.* **238**, 198–200.

Brown, D. H., and Novelli, G. D.(1968). *Biochem. Biophys. Res. Commun.* **31**, 262–266.

Buck, C. A., and Nass, M. M. K. (1968). *Proc. Nat. Acad. Sci. U.S.* **60**, 1045–1052.

Buck, C. A., and Nass, M. M. K. (1969). *J. Mol. Biol.* **41**, 67–82.

Burger, M. M. (1973). *Fed. Proc., Fed. Amer. Soc. Exp. Biol.* **32**, 91–101.

Chang, L. O., Morris, H. P., and Looney, W. B. (1968a). *Brit. J. Cancer* **22**, 860–866.

Chang, L. O., Morris, H. P., and Looney, W. B. (1968b). *Cancer Res.* **28**, 2164–2167.

Chang, L. O., Schnaitman, C. A., and Morris, H. P. (1971). *Cancer Res.* **31**, 108–113.

Chi, J. C. H., and Suyama, Y. (1970). *J. Mol. Biol.* **53**, 531–556.

Ch'ih, J. J., and Kalf, G. F. (1969). *Arch. Biochem. Biophys.* **133**, 38–45.

Clayton, D. A., and Brambl, R. M. (1972). *Biochem. Biophys. Res. Commun.* **46**, 1477–1482.

Clayton, D. A., and Teplitz, R. L. (1972). *J. Cell Sci.* **10**, 293–487.

Clayton, D. A., and Vinograd, J. (1967). *Nature (London)* **216**, 652–657.

Clayton, D. A., and Vinograd, J. (1969). *Proc. Nat. Acad. Sci. U.S.* **62**, 1077–1092.

Clayton, D. A., Davis, R. W., and Vinograd, J. (1970). *J. Mol. Biol.* **47**, 137–153.

Clayton, D. A., Teplitz, R. L., Nabholz, M., Dovey, H., and Bodmer, W. (1971). *Nature (London)* **234**, 560–562.

Cohen, M., and Rabinowitz, M. (1970). *J. Cell Biol.* **47**, Part 2, 37a.

Crawford, L. V., and Waring, M. T. (1967). *J. Mol. Biol.* **25**, 23–28.

Cuzin, F., Vogt, M., Dieckmann, M., and Berg, P. (1970). *J. Mol. Biol.* **47**, 317–333.

Davidian, N., McC., and Penniall, R. (1971). *Biochem. Biophys. Res. Commun.* **44**, 15–21.

Dawid, I. B. (1972a). *Develop. Biol.* **29**, 139–151.

Dawid, I. B. (1972b). *J. Mol. Biol.* **63**, 201–216.

Dawid, I. B., and Wolstenholme, D. R. (1967). *J. Mol. Biol.* **28**, 233–245.

Doeg, K. A., Polomski, L. L., and Doeg, L. H. (1972). *Endocrinology* **90**, 1633–1638.

Doniger, J., Warner, R. C., and Tessma, I. (1973). *Nature (London), New Biol.* **242**, 9–12.

Dressler, D. (1970). *Proc. Nat. Acad. Sci. U.S.* **67**, 1934–1942.

Dubin, D. T., and Montenecourt, B. S. (1970). *J. Mol. Biol.* **48**, 279–295.

Ephrussi, B. (1953). "Nucleo-Cytoplasmic Relations in Microorganisms: Oxford Univ. Press, London and New York.

Fukuhara, H., and Kujawa, C. (1970). *Biochem. Biophys. Res. Commun.* **41**, 1002–1008.

Gadaleta, M. N., Barletta, A., Caldarazzo, M., deLeo, T., and Saccone, C. (1972). *Eur. J. Biochem.* **30**, 376–381.

Gazzalo, L., de-Thé, G., Vigier, P., and Sarma, P. S. (1969). *C. R. Acad. Sci.* **268**, 1668–1670.

Georgatsos, J. C., Antonoglou, O., and Gabrielides, C. (1970). *Arch. Biochem. Biophys.* **136**, 219–222.

Goldring, E. S., Grossman, L. I., Krupnick, D., Coyer, D. R., and Marmur, J. (1970). *J. Mol. Biol.* **52**, 323–335.

Goldring, E. S., Grossman, L. I., and Marmur, J. (1971). *J. Bacteriol.* **107**, 377–381.

Graffi, A., Butschak, G., and Schnieder, E. J. (1965). *Biochem. Biophys. Res. Commun.* **21**, 418–423.

Gross, N. J., and Rabinowitz, M. (1969). *J. Biol. Chem.* **244**, 1563–1566.

Gross, S. R., McCoy, M. T., and Gilmore, E. (1968). *Proc. Nat. Aca. Sci. U.S.* **61**, 253–260.

Halbreich, A., and Rabinowitz, M. (1971). *Proc. Nat. Acad. Sci. U.S.* **68**, 294–298.

Hatta, T., Nakamoto, T., Takagi, Y., and Ushiyama, R. (1971). *Virology* **45**, 292–299.

Haust, M. D. (1968). *Exp. Mol. Pathol.* **9**, 242–257.

Helinski, D. R., and Clewell, D. B. (1971). *Annu. Rev. Biochem.* **40**, 899–942.

Hollenberg, C. P., Borst, P., and Van Bruggen, E. F. J. (1970). *Biochim. Biophys. Acta* **209**, 1–15.

Hruban, Z., Mochizuki, Y., Sleser, A., and Morris, H. P. (1972). *Cancer Res.* **32**, 853–867.

Hulsmann, W. C., Bethlem, J., Meijer, A. E. F. H., Fleury, P., and Schellens, J. P. M. (1967). *J. Neurol., Neurosurg. Psychiat.* [N.S.] **30**, 519–525.

Kadenbach, B. (1970). *Eur. J. Biochem.* **12**, 392–396.

Kadenbach, B. (1971). *Biochem. Biophys. Res. Commun.* **44**, 724–730.

Kahri, A. I. (1970). *Amer. J. Anat.* **127**, 103–129.

Kalf, G. F., D'Agostino, M. A., and Hunter, G. R. (1971). *Cancer Res.* **31**, 2054–2058.

Kára, J., Mach, O., and Černá, (1971). *Biochem. Biophys. Commun.* **44**, 162–170.

Kára, J., Dvořák, M., and Černá, H. (1972). *FEBS Lett.* **25**, 33–37.

Karol, M. H., and Simpson, M. V. (1968). *Science* **162**, 470–473.

Kasamatsu, H., Robberson, D. L., and Vinograd, J. (1971). *Proc. Nat. Acad. Sci. U.S.* **68**, 2252–2257.

Kiger, J. A., Jr., and Sinsheimer, R. L. (1969). *J. Mol. Biol.* **40**, 467–490.

Kimberg, D. V., and Loeb, J. N. (1972). *J. Cell Biol.* **55**, 635–643.

Kit, S., and Minekawa, Y. (1972). *Cancer Res.* **32**, 2277–2288.

Klietmann, W., Sato, N., and Nass, M. M. K. (1973). *J. Cell Biol.* **58**, 11–26.

Koch, J., and Stokstad, E. L. R. (1967). *Eur. J. Biochem.* **3**, 1–6.

Küntzel, H., and Noll, H. (1967). *Nature (London)* **215**, 1340–1345.

Küntzel, H., and Schäfer, K. P. (1971). *Nature (London), New Biol.* **231**, 265–269.

Leduc, E., Bernhard, W., and Tourier, P. (1966). *Exp. Cell Res.* **42**, 597–616.

Levine, A. J. (1971). *Proc. Nat. Acad. Sci. U.S.* **68**, 717–720.

Lizardi, P. M., and Luck, D. J. L. (1971). *Nature (London), New Biol.* **229**, 140–142.

Lizardi, P. M., and Luck, D. J. L. (1972). *J. Cell Biol.* **54**, 56–74.

Lo, C., Cristofalo, V. J., Morris, H. P., and Weinhouse, S. (1968). *Cancer Res.* **28**, 1–10.

Luft, R., Ikkos, D., Palmieri, G., Ernster, L., and Afzelius, B. (1962). *J. Clin. Invest.* **41**, 1776–1804.

Lunger, P. D., and Clark, H. F. (1973). *J. Nat. Cancer Inst.* **50**, 111–117.

Mahler, H. R., and Perlman, P. S. (1972). *J. Supramol. Str.* **1**, 105–124.

Mahler, H. R., Mehrotra, B. D., and Perlman, P. S. (1971). *Prog. Mol. Subcell. Biol.* **2**, 274–296.

Mansour, A. M., and Nass, S. (1970). *Nature (London)* **228**, 665–667.

Manteifel, V. M., and Meisel, M. N. (1965). *Izv. Akad. Nauk SSSR, Ser. Biol.* **30**, T981–T988.

Martelo, O. J., Manyan, D. R., Smith, U., and Yunis, A. A. (1969). *J. Lab. Clin. Med.* **74**, 927–940.

Martin, G. S. (1970). *Nature (London)* **227**, 1021–1023.

Martin, G. S., Venuta, S., Weber, M., and Rubin, H. (1971). *Proc. Nat. Acad. Sci. U.S.* **68**, 2739–2741.

Meijers, A. E. F. H. (1972). *Acta Histochem. Suppl.* **12**, 33–334.

Meselson, M., Yuan, R., and Heywood, J. (1972). *Annu. Rev. Biochem.* **41**, 447–466.

Meyer, R. R., and Simpson, M. V. (1969). *Biochem. Biophys. Res. Commun.* **34**, 238–244.

Meyer, R. R., and Simpson, M. V. (1970). *J. Biol. Chem.* **245**, 3426–3435.

Milner, A. J. (1971). *Endocrinology* **88**, 64–69.

Milner, A. J. (1972). *J. Endocrinol.* **52**, 541–548.

Nass, M. M. K. (1966). *Proc. Nat. Acad. Sci. U.S.* **56**, 1215–1223.

Nass, M. M. K. (1967). *In* "Organizational Biosynthesis" (H. J. Vogel, J. O. Lampen, and V. Bryson, eds.), pp. 503–522. Academic Press, New York.

Nass, M. M. K. (1968). *In* "Biochemical Aspects of the Biogenesis of Mitochondria" (E. C. Slater *et al.,* eds.), pp. 27–50. Adriatrica Editrice, Bari.

Nass, M. M. K. (1969a). *Science* **165**, 25–35.

Nass, M. M. K. (1969b). *J. Mol. Biol.* **42**, 521–528.

Nass, M. M. K. (1969c). *J. Mol. Biol.* **42**, 529–545.

Nass, M. M. K. (1969d). *Nature (London)* **223**, 1124–1129.

Nass, M. M. K. (1969e). *Science* **165**, 1128–1131.

Nass, M. M. K. (1970a). *Proc. Nat. Acad. Sci. U.S.* **67**, 1926–1933.

Nass, M. M. K. (1970b). *J. Cell Biol.* **47**, 147a.

Nass, M. M. K. (1972). *Exp. Cell Res.* **72**, 211–222.

Nass, M. M. K. (1973a). *J. Mol. Biol.* **80**, 155–175.

Nass, M. M. K. (1973b). *Proc. Nat. Acad. Sci. U.S.* **70**, 3739–3743.

Nass, M. M. K., and Ben-Shaul, Y. (1972). *Biochim. Biophys. Acta* **272**, 130–136.

Nass, M. M. K., and Buck, C. A. (3969). *Proc. Nat. Acad. Sci. U.S.* **62**, 506–513.

Nass, M. M. K., and Buck, C. A. (1970). *J. Mol. Bi ol.* **54**, 187–198.

Nass, M. M. K., and Nass, S. (1962). *Exp. Cell Res.* **26**, 424–427.

Nass, M. M. K., and Nass, S. (1963). *J. Cell Biol.* **19**, 593–611.

Nass, M. M. K., Nass, S., and Afzelius, B. A. (1965). *Exp. Cell Res.* **37**, 516–539.

Nass, S., and Nass, M. M. K. (1963). *J. Cell Biol.* **19**, 613–629.

Nass, S., and Nass, M. M. K. (1964). *J. Nat. Cancer Inst.* **33**, 777–798.

Neubert, D., and Morris, H. P. (1966). *Naunyn-Schmiedebergs Arch. Pharmakol. Exp. Pathol.* **255**, 51–52.

Nussdorfer, G. G., and Mazzocchi, G. (1971a). *Steroidologia* **2**, 244–256.

Nussdorfer, G. G., and Mazzocchi, G. (1971b). *Z. Zellforsch. Mikrosk. Anat.* **118**, 35–48.

O'Brian, T. W. (1971). *J. Biol. Chem.* **246**, 3409–3417.

Ohe, K., Morris, H. P., and Weinhouse, S. (1967). *Cancer Res.* **27**, 1360–1371.

Paoletti, C., and Riou, G. (1970). *Bull. Cancer* **57**, 301–334.

Paoletti, C., and Riou, G., and Pairault, J. (1972). *Proc. Nat. Acad. Sci. U.S.* **69**, 847–850.

Partin, J. C., Schubert, W. K., and Partin, J. S. (1971). *N. Engl. J. Med.* **285**, 1339–1343.

Perlman, P. S., and Mahler, H. R. (1971). *Biochem. Biophys. Res. Commun.* **44**, 261–267.

Perlman, S., Abelson, H. T., and Penman, S. (1973). *Proc. Nat. Acad. Sci. U.S.* **70**, 350–353.

Pica-Mattoccia, L., and Attardi, G. (1972). *J. Mol. Biol.* **64**, 465–484.

Pikó, L., Blair, D. G., Tyler, A., and Vinograd, J. (1968). *Proc. Nat. Acad. Sci. U.S.* **59**, 838–845.

Prescott, D. M., Kates, J., and Kirkpatrick, J. B. (1971). *J. Mol. Biol.* **59**, 505–508.

Radloff, R., Baner, W., and Vinograd, J. (1967). *Proc. Nat. Acad. Sci. U.S.* **57**, 1514–1521.

Radsak, K. D., and Freise, H. W. (1972). *Life Sci., Part II* **11**, 717–724.

Raff, R. A., and Mahler, H. R. (1972). *Science* **177**, 575–582.

Renger, H. C., and Wolstenholme, D. R. (1970). *J. Cell Biol.* **47**, 689–702.

Richert, N. J., and Hare, J. D. (1972). *Biochem. Biophys. Res. Commun.* **46**, 5–10.

Rifkin, M. R., and Luck, D. J. L. (1971). *Proc. Nat. Acad. Sci. U.S.* **68**, 287–290.

Riou, G. (1967). *C. R. Acad. Sci.* **265**, 2004–2007.

Riou, G. (1968). *C. R. Acad. Sci.* **266**, 250–252.

Riou, G., and Lacour, F. (1971). *Biochimie* **53**, 47–49.

Robberson, D. L., Kasamatsu, H., and Vinograd, J. (1972). *Proc. Nat. Acad. Sci. U.S.* **69**, 737–741.

Roberts, S., Creange, J. E., and Fowler, J. D. (1964). *Nature (London)* **203**, 759–761.

Sambrook, J., Westphal, H., Srinivasan, P. R., and Dulbecco, R. (1968). *Proc. Nat. Acad. Sci. U.S.* **60**, 1288–1295.

Schatz, G., Groot, G. S. P., Mason, T., Rouslin, W., Wharton, D. C., and Saltzgraber, J. (1972). *Fed. Proc., Fed. Amer. Soc. Exp. Biol.* **31**, 21–29.

Schimmer, B. P. (1969). *J. Cell. Physiol.* **74**, 115–122.

Shafig, S. A., Milhorat, A. T., and Gorycki, M. A. (1967). *Arch. Neurol. (Chicago)* **17**, 666–671.

Shipman, C., Jr., Smith, S. H., and Drach, J. (1972). *Proc. Nat. Acad. Sci. U.S.* **69**, 1753–1757.

Shy, G. M., Conatas, N. K., and Perez, M. (1966). *Brain* **89**, 133–158.

Sinclair, J. H., and Stevens, D. J. (1966). *Proc. Nat. Acad. Sci. U.S.* **56**, 508–514.

Slonimski, P. P., Perrodin, G., and Croft, J. H. (1968). *Biochem. Biophys. Res. Commun.* **30**, 232–239.

Smith, A. E., and Marcker, K. A. (1968). *J. Mol. Biol.* **38**, 241–243.

Smith, C. A., Jordan, J. M., and Vinograd, J. (1971). *J. Mol. Biol.* **59**, 255–272.

Smith, U., Smith D. C., and Yunis, A. (1970). *J. Cell. Science* **7**, 501–521.

Sneider, T. W., and Potter, V. R. (1969). *J. Mol. Biol.* **42**, 271–284.

Soslau, G., and Nass, M. M. K. (1971). *J. Cell Biol.* **51**, 514–524.

Soslau, G., Fuhrer, J. P., Nass, M. M. K., and Warren, L. (1974). *J. Biol. Chem.* (in press).

Ter Schegget, J., Flavell, R. A., and Borst, P. (1971). *Biochim. Biophys. Acta* **254**, 1–14.

Tschiersch, B., and Graffi, A. (1970). *Arch. Geschwulstforsch.* **35**, 217–226.

Tzagoloff, A., and Akai, A. (1972). *J. Biol. Chem.* **247**, 6517–6523.

Tzagoloff, A., and Meagher, P. (1972). *J. Biol. Chem.* **247**, 594–603.

Van Bruggen, E. F. J., Borst, P., Ruttenberg, G. J. C. M., Gruber, M., and Kroon, A. M. (1966). *Biochim. Biophys. Acta* **119**, 437–439.

Van Tuyle, G. C., and Kalf, G. F. (1972). *Arch. Biochem. Biophys.* **149**, 425–434.

Vesco, C., and Basilico, C. (1971). *Nature (London)* **229**, 336–338.

Vesco, C., and Penman, S. (1969). *Nature (London)* **224**, 1021–1023.

Waring, M. J. (1968). *Nature (London)* **219**, 1320–1325.

War ren, L., Fuhrer, J. P., and Buck , C. A. (1973). *Fed. Proc., Fed. Amer. Soc. Exp. Biol.* **32**, 80–85.

Weinhouse, S. (1955). *Advan. Cancer Res.* **3**, 269–325.

Weinhouse, S. (1972) *Cancer Res.* **32**, 2007–2016.

Weiss, H. (1972). *Eur. J. Biochem.* **30**, 469–478.

Wintersberger, U., and Wintersberger, E. (1970). *Eur. J. Biochem.* **13**, 20–27.

Wolstenholme, D. R., Koike, K., and Cochran-Fouts, P. (1973). *J. Cell Biol.* **56**, 230–245.

Wu, M., Davidson, N., Attardi, G., and Aloni, Y. (1972). *J. Mol. Biol.* **71**, 81–93.

Wunderlich, V. (1971). *Pharmazie* **5**, 257–271.

Wunderlich, V., Schütt, M., and Graffi, A. (1966). *Acta Biol. Med. Ger.* **17**, 1227–32.

Yasumura, Y., Buonassisi, V., and Sata, G. (1966). *Cancer-Res.* **26**, 529–535.

Yu, F. L., and Feigelson, P. (1972). *Biochim. Biophys. Acta* **213**, 134–141.

Zylber, E., Vesco, C., and Penman, S. (1969). *J. Mol. Biol.* **44**, 195–204.

CHAPTER X

ABNORMAL HORMONAL CONTROL IN THE NEOPLASTIC ADRENAL CORTEX

HOWARD T. HINSHAW AND ROBERT L. NEY

I. Introduction*

The understanding of the control of adrenocortical function has advanced rapidly in recent years. The pituitary hormone ACTH exerts a profound regulatory influence over the normal adrenal cortex. This influence is not limited to stimulation of corticosteroid synthesis, but includes as well the maintenance of tissue integrity. Both of these functions of ACTH appear to be mediated by intracellular cyclic AMP.

The relationship of cyclic AMP to ACTH and to adrenal steroidogenesis was first proposed by Haynes who demonstrated that ACTH increases the accumulation of cyclic AMP in the adrenal cortex (Haynes, 1958) and subsequently, that cyclic AMP in turn is capable of stimulating adrenal steroid hormone production (Haynes et al., 1959). The concept of cyclic AMP as the intracellular mediator of ACTH action in the adrenal cortex was formulated by Sutherland (1961) and has been substantiated by subsequent work (Grahame-Smith et al., 1967). The initial event in ACTH action appears to be the reversible binding of ACTH with a specific receptor which is located in the plasma membrane of the adrenocortical cell (Lefkowitz et al., 1970; Schimmer et al., 1968). With the binding of ACTH the membrane-bound adenylate cyclase system is activated. The current model of the adenylate cyclase system includes a receptor subunit oriented

---

* The abbreviations used are ACTH, adrenocorticotrophic hormone; TSH, thyroid stimulating hormone; LH, luteinizing hormone; FSH, follicle stimulating hormone; cyclic AMP, adenosine $3',5'$-cyclic monophosphate; PGE_1 and PGE_2, prostaglandins E_1 and E_2, respectively.

toward the cell surface and a catalytic subunit oriented toward the cell interior (Robison *et al.*, 1967). The catalytic unit, after activation by the hormone-receptor subunit complex, acts to increase the formation within the cell of cyclic AMP from ATP. The intracellular cyclic AMP thus formed mediates the observed actions of ACTH on the adrenal. The levels of cyclic AMP which accumulate in the cell depend not only on its rate of formation, but also on the rate of its degradation to 5′-AMP by the enzyme 3′, 5′-nucleotide phosphodiesterase. While the inhibition of this enzyme by ACTH would have the same effect on intracellular cyclic AMP levels as does the stimulation of adenylate cyclase, no such effect of ACTH on cyclic AMP degradation has been found (Taunton *et al.*, 1967).

ACTH is the only hormone known to influence cyclic AMP levels in the normal adrenal cortex (Haynes, 1958). Recently this specificity was noted to be altered in an adrenocortical carcinoma (Schorr and Ney, 1971; Schorr *et al.*, 1971). In subsequent sections we will review work that deals with the control of adenylate cyclase activity and cyclic AMP levels in normal adrenal tissue and in adrenocortical tumor cells.

A. *Adenylate Cyclase*

TABLE I

Adenylate Cyclase Activity in Normal Rat Adrenals and in a Rat Adrenocortical Tumor[a]

	Adenylate cyclase activity [pmoles cyclic AMP/mg protein/20 min] (Mean ± SEM)			
	Adrenal		Tumor	
Tissue fraction	Basal	ACTH	Basal	ACTH
Whole homogenate	463 ± 88 (17)	1218 ± 95 (10)	457 ± 46 (17)	1558 ± 223 (10)
1000 g particles	300 ± 29 (14)	1213 ± 148 (7)	513 ± 57 (15)	3144 ± 514 (9)
10,000 g particles	256 ± 29 (11)	990 ± 251 (6)	281 ± 52 (12)	1387 ± 492 (7)
105,000 g particles	39 ± 5 (12)	100 ± 21 (6)	26 ± 6 (12)	70 ± 17 (7)

[a] Enzyme activity was assayed either in whole homogenates or in particulate fractions derived from them by successive centrifugation. ACTH was added at a final concentration of $0.5 \times 10^{-5}\ M$. Numbers in parentheses are the number of determinations. From Schorr and Ney (1971).

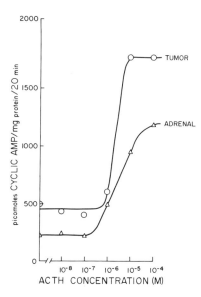

Fig. 1. Effect of ACTH on adenylate cyclase activity of normal rat adrenals and a rat adrenocortical carcinoma. The enzyme assay was performed using particles sedimenting at 1000 g derived from tissue homogenates. (From Schorr and Ney, 1971.)

II. Hormonal Control in the Normal Adrenal Cortex

Studies of the hormonal regulation of cell free preparations of normal adrenal adenylate cyclase have been limited. A stimulatory effect of ACTH on cyclic AMP accumulation in rat adrenal homogenates was noted by Grahame-Smith *et al.* (1967). Further work with rat adrenal homogenates has shown that the enzyme activity is largely associated with particulate fractions derived from crude adrenal homogenates (Table I). The maximal response is in the low speed fractions, a finding which is consistent with the presumed primary localization of the enzyme in the plasma membrane. The effect of ACTH is dose related with the maximal responses noted at an ACTH concentration of 10^{-4} M (Fig. 1). Other peptide hormones including insulin, glucagon, TSH, LH, and epinephrine are without effect (Table II). PGE_1 has a minimal effect in activating the cyclase (Table III).

The adenylate cyclase of bovine adrenal homogenates has reacted similarly to stimulation by ACTH. The majority of the adenylate cyclase activity has been found in the 2000 g fraction, again compatible with its localization being primarily in the plasma membrane (Kelly and Koritz,

TABLE II

Effects of Various Hormones on the Adenylate Cyclase Activity of Normal Rat Adrenals and a Rat Adrenal Tumor[a]

Hormone	Adenylate cyclase activity ($\%$ of basal activity)	
	Adrenals	Tumor
Basal	100	100
Epinephrine (10^{-4} M)	89	388[b]
Norepinephrine (10^{-4} M)	91	514[b]
TSH (10^{-5} M)	92	214[b]
FSH (10^{-6} M)	92	188[b]
LH (10^{-5} M)	91	138[b]
Glucagon (10^{-4} M)	72	101
Parathyroid hormone (10^{-5} M)	69	84
Thyrocalcitonin (10^{-4} M)	88	103
Insulin (10^{-4} M)	75	102
Growth hormone (10^{-4} M)	106	97

[a] Enzyme activity assayed using 1000 g particles derived from tissue homogenate. From Schorr and Ney (1971).
[b] Significant at $P < 0.05$.

TABLE III

Effects of PGE$_1$ and ACTH on the Adenylate Cyclase Activity of Normal Rat Adrenals and a Rat Adrenocortical Tumor[a]

	Adenylate cyclase activity (pmoles cyclic AMP/mg protein/20 min)	
	Adrenals	Tumor
Basal	104	223
PGE$_1$ 10^{-4} M	135	387
ACTH 10^{-4} M	213	1456

[a] Enzyme activity assayed using whole tissue homogenates and method described by Schorr et al. (1972). The results are the means of two experiments (adrenals) and 4 experiments (tumor).

1971). In contrast to the cyclases of rat and human adrenals a small and inconsistent activation by epinephrine has been noted in beef adrenals (Hechter *et al.*, 1969).

Human adrenal homogenates possess a cyclase system responsive to ACTH and to NaF. Other polypeptide hormones including epinephrine fail to reproducibly stimulate the adenylate cyclase (Table IV).

B. Regulation of Cyclic AMP Levels and Steroidogenesis

When quartered rat adrenals are incubated *in vitro*, cyclic AMP levels are relatively stable at 1 nmole per gram of tissue. With the addition of ACTH, cyclic AMP levels rise within one minute. This increase precedes any stimulation of corticosterone production (Fig. 2). The same relationship is noted in *in vivo* studies using acutely hypophysectomized rats. The administration of ACTH intravenously in increasing dosage over the range of 0.1 to 1.0 milliunits (mU) results in progressive increases in the levels of adrenal cyclic AMP measured three minutes after the ACTH is given. This is accompanied by progressive increases in corticosterone production

TABLE IV

Adenylate Cyclase Hormone Responses of Two Human Adrenal Glands[a]

Hormone	Adenylate cyclase activity (pmoles cyclic AMP/mg protein/20 min)	
	Case I[b]	Case II[b]
Basal	121	118
ACTH 10^{-4} M	222	206
Epinephrine 10^{-4} M	120	107
TSH 10^{-5} M	147	123
LH 10^{-5} M	165	—[c]
NaF 10 mM	488	311

[a] Enzyme activity was determined in whole tissue homogenates using methods described previously (Schorr *et al.*, 1972).

[b] Tissue in case I was obtained at the time of adrenalectomy for breast carcinoma. Tissue in case II was obtained at surgery for Cushing's Disease of pituitary origin.

[c] Hormone not tested.

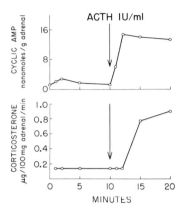

Fig. 2. Time course of the effect of ACTH on cyclic AMP levels and corticosterone production by normal rat adrenals incubated at 37°C in Krebs-Ringer bicarbonate buffer containing 200 mg% glucose in an atmosphere of 95% O_2–5% CO_2. (From Grahame-Smith *et al.*, 1967.)

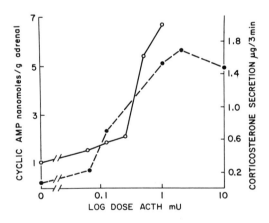

Fig. 3. Relationship among the dose of ACTH (given as an i.v. pulse), the adrenal concentration of cyclic AMP measured 3 minutes after the ACTH pulse, and the corticosterone content of adrenal venous blood collected from 7 to 10 minutes after the ACTH injection in normal rats hypophysectomized 2 hours previously. O———O, cyclic AMP; ●-----●, corticosterone. (From Grahame-Smith *et al.*, 1967.)

measured seven to ten minutes after the ACTH administration (Fig. 3). Doses of ACTH beyond 1 mU produce no further increase in steroid production but cyclic AMP levels continue to rise in a dose-related manner until ACTH levels of 100 mU are reached (Fig. 4). Thus, the maximal level of steroidogenesis that the adrenal can achieve seems not to be limited by the levels of cyclic AMP which can be generated but by limiting factors in the steroidogenic mechanisms. Nucleotide concentrations can occur which are far in excess of those necessary for maximal steroidogenesis.

Since ACTH is capable of increasing cyclic AMP levels beyond those needed for steroidogenesis and since ACTH is associated with functions other than steroidogenesis, the question is raised whether these high cyclic AMP levels have a biological role. Ney (1969) has shown that dibutyryl cyclic AMP partially maintains adrenal weight and the steroidogenic capacity in hypophysectomized rats. In another study it was found that the steroidogenic response of the hypophysectomized rat to intravenous pulses of ACTH progressively decreases so that by four days after hypophysectomy the response is essentially lost (Fig. 5). The capacity of the adrenal to accumulate cyclic AMP, however, is unchanged as long as nine days following hypophysectomy (Grahame-Smith et al., 1967). Thus the ability to generate cyclic AMP is maintained even when the steroidogenic capacity is lost. Recently it has been shown that the cyclic AMP levels beyond those

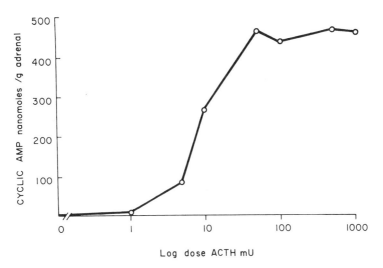

Fig. 4.   Relationship between the intravenous dose of ACTH over a wide dosage range and the adrenal concentration of cycle AMP 3 minutes after the ACTH pulse in normal rats hypophysectomized 2 hours before. (From Grahame-Smith et al., 1967.)

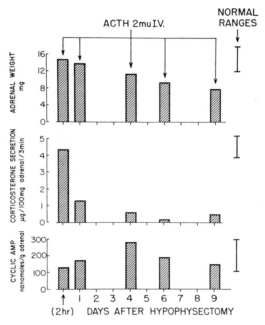

Fig. 5. Effect of chronic hypophysectomy on the response of rat adrenals to an intravenous pulse of 2 mU of ACTH. Adrenal cyclic AMP was measured 3 minutes after the pulse, and corticosterone was measured in the adrenal venous effluent collected 7 to 10 minutes after the injection. (From Grahame-Smith *et al.*, 1967.)

needed for maximal steroidogenesis generated in response to large doses of ACTH are accompanied by proportional elevations in the activity of adrenal ornithine decarboxylase, an enzyme which parallels rates of tissue growth in other systems (Dobbins *et al.*, 1972).

The specificity of the cyclic AMP and steroidogenic responses parallel, as would be expected, the specificity of adenylate cyclase activation. Haynes (1958) demonstrated that polypeptide hormones other than ACTH have no effect on adrenal cyclic AMP accumulation and have no steroidogenic effect. This specificity has been demonstrated further by studies (Grahame-Smith *et al.*, 1967) which show that structural analogs of ACTH possessing varying steroidogenic properties have similar potencies in producing elevations in cyclic AMP. Epinephrine, which has shown inconsistent activation of adrenal adenylate cyclase, does not lead to detectable steroidogenesis (Wilson and Kitabchi, 1971).

The role of the prostaglandins in regulating adrenal cyclic AMP and steroidogenesis is not clear. In studies using superfused adrenal glands from hypophysectomized rats, increases in both cyclic AMP accumulation and steroidogenesis have occurred in response to stimulation with PGE_2 (Flack *et al.*, 1969; Flack and Ramwell, 1972). In bovine adrenal slices both PGE_1 and PGE_2 induce both increased levels of cyclic AMP and increased steroidogenesis (Saruta and Kaplan, 1972).

Thus in summary, ACTH appears to bind to a specific receptor, resulting in the activation of the catalytic unit of the adenylate cyclase system. The resulting accumulation of cyclic AMP then mediates the effects of ACTH on steroidogenesis and most likely on the maintenance of the structural integrity of the gland. Some of the prostaglandins appear to play a role in activating the system but the mechanism and physiological significance are uncertain.

III. Hormonal Control in Adrenocortical Tumors

Adrenocortical tumors exhibit functional disturbances that distinguish them from the normal parent gland. The rate of growth is autonomous or at least is under no recognized control. Similarly, steroidogenesis appears to proceed without regulatory control. Unlike the parent gland the tumor is not under ACTH regulation (Lipsett *et al.*, 1963). Tumor steroidogenesis continues in spite of the fact that host ACTH secretion is suppressed by the glucocorticoids which are produced by the tumor. In most cases, exogenous

TABLE V

Effects of ACTH and MSH Analogs on the Adenylate
Cyclase Activity of Normal Rat Adrenals and a Rat
Adrenocortical Tumor[a]

Hormone ($10^{-4}\ M$)	Adenylate cyclase activity ($\%$ of basal activity)	
	Adrenals	Tumor
ACTH	242	255
α^{1-24}-ACTH	791	322
α^{25-39}-ACTH	107	115
α^{17-39}-ACTH	113	93
α^{11-24}-ACTH	103	110
$\alpha^{1-16\ NH_2}$-ACTH	91	85
α-MSH	114	117
Bovine β-MSH	93	96

[a] From Schorr *et al.* (1971).

ACTH even when given in large quantities produces little or no stimulation of steroidogenesis, in contrast to the stimulation by ACTH noted in normal adrenal glands (Ney *et al.*, 1969). The following sections review investigations into some of these abnormal control mechanisms in certain adrenocortical tumors.

A. A Rat Adrenocortical Carcinoma

1. Adenylate Cyclase

The characteristics of the adenylate cyclase system of a rat transplantable, corticosterone-producing adrenocortical carcinoma described by Snell and Stewart (1959) have been studied and compared to the characteristics of normal rat adrenal cyclase (Ney *et al.*, 1969; Schorr and Ney, 1971; Schorr *et al.*, 1971). ACTH stimulates the adenylate cyclase in a dose-related manner which is similar in character to the stimulation noted in the normal adrenal (Fig. 1). As in the normal adrenal, the cyclase activity is greatest in the whole tissue homogenate and in the 1000 *g* fraction (Table I). The responses of the tumor are generally greater to a given stimulatory concentration of ACTH than are those of the parent adrenal (Fig. 1). The lowest effective concentration of ACTH in each is 10^{-6} moles/liter. ACTH analogs are similar in their stimulatory effects on the cyclases of both the parent adrenal and the tumor (Table V).

In contrast to the adenylate cyclase response of the normal adrenal, the tumor cyclase is stimulated by hormones other than ACTH. TSH produces

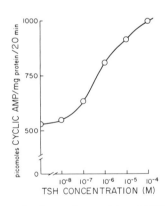

Fig. 6. Effect of TSH on adenylate cyclase activity of 1000 *g* particles derived from a rat adrenocortical carcinoma. TSH had no effect on normal adrenal adenylate cyclase. (From Schorr and Ney, 1971.)

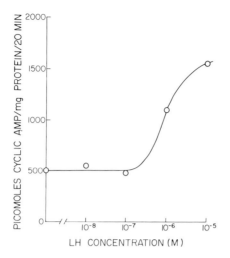

Fig. 7. Effect of highly purified human pituitary LH on adenylate cyclase activity of 1000 g particles from a rat adrenocortical carcinoma. The hormone preparation had no effect on normal adrenal adenylate cyclase. (From Schorr *et al.*, 1971.)

a dose-related response as shown in Fig. 6. LH and FSH also stimulate the tumor cyclase (Figs. 7 and 8). The catecholamines show varying degrees of stimulation of the tumor cyclase (Fig. 9). Propranolol blocks the stimulatory effects of epinephrine and norepinephrine but not those of the other hormones (Fig. 10). Phentolamine in equivalent concentrations does not in-

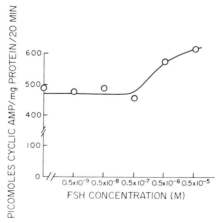

Fig. 8. Effect of highly purified human pituitary FSH on adenylate cyclase activity of 1000 g particles from a rat adrenocortical carcinoma. The hormone had no effect on normal adrenal cyclase. (From Schorr *et al.*, 1971.)

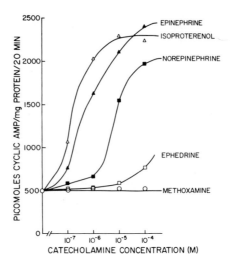

Fig. 9.   Effects of catecholamines on adenylate cyclase of 1000 *g* particles from a rat adrenocortical carcinoma. The compounds had no effect on normal adrenal cyclase. (From Schorr *et al.*, 1971.)

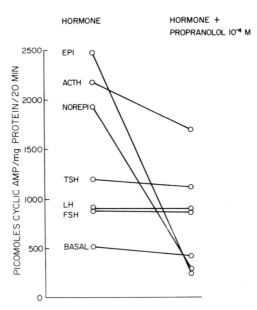

Fig. 10.   Effects of propranolol on the hormonal stimulation of rat adrenocortical tumor adenylate cyclase. Hormones and propranolol were added at 10^{-4} *M* concentrations. (From Schorr, *et al.*, 1971.)

hibit the stimulatory effects of the catecholamines. A variety of other polypeptide hormones including glucagon, insulin, vasopressin, parathyroid hormone, and thyrocalcitonin have no stimulatory effects on the tumor cyclase (Table II). PGE_1 has a minimal effect on the tumor cyclase (Table III). Thus, the tumor adenylate cyclase shows "inappropriate" responses to TSH, LH, FSH, and to the catecholamines, the effects of the latter being blocked by β-adrenergic inhibitors.

Several possible mechanisms can be considered to explain the responses of the tumor to multiple hormones. Does the tumor possess specific receptor sites for multiple hormones, each then activating separate catalytic subunits of the cyclase system? Do separate specific receptor subunits activate a common catalytic unit? Or does the tumor possess an ACTH receptor which is altered and responds nonspecifically to multiple hormones? There are suggestions that the tumor has specific receptors for several hormones, and that these activate a common cyclase catalytic unit. First, at maximally stimulatory concentrations of each hormone there are no additive effects apparent (Table VI). Second, propranolol abolishes the effects of the catecholamines but does not significantly affect the stimulatory effects of the other hormones. This, together with the lack of inhibition by α-blockers and a pattern of stimulation by the catecholamines

TABLE VI

Effects of Hormones Alone and in Combination on the Adenylate Cyclase of a Rat Adrenocortical Tumor[a]

Hormone	Adenylate cyclase activity pmoles cyclic AMP/mg protein/20 min)	
	Experiment 1	Experiment 2
Basal	692	220
ACTH ($10^{-5}\ M$)	2254	536
TSH ($10^{-5}\ M$)	1593	444
Epinephrine ($10^{-4}\ M$)	2230	707
ACTH + TSH	2226	452
TSH + epinephrine	2094	519
ACTH + epinephrine	2538	538
ACTH + TSH + epinephrine	2287	457

[a] Enzyme activity assayed using 1000 g particles derived from homogenate of tumor tissue. From Schorr and Ney (1971).

which parallels their β-adrenergic stimulatory activity in other tissues, suggests an intact specific β-adrenergic receptor. Third, the ACTH receptor in terms of its responsiveness to specific portions of the ACTH molecule is as intact and specific as that of the normal adrenal (Table V). These observations are most compatible with the concept that the adrenal tumor possesses multiple specific receptor subunits and that when the hormone is present, these activate a common catalytic subunit.

2. Tissue Cyclic AMP Levels and Steroidogenesis

The adenylate cyclase of the rat adrenocortical tumor is stimulated by a variety of hormones other than ACTH, but the question remained whether the increased cyclase activity is associated with a concomitant increase in tissue cyclic AMP and steroidogenesis. Basal cyclic AMP levels and phosphodiesterase levels are similar in tumorous and nontumorous adrenal tissue (Ney et al., 1969). ACTH produces only a slight increase in the accumulation of cyclic AMP when incubated in vitro with tumor slices. However, with the addition of the phosphodiesterase inhibitor theophylline, the effect of ACTH is more pronounced. Similar results are noted with TSH and with epinephrine (Table VII).

TABLE VII

Effects of Hormones and Theophylline on Rat
Adrenocortical Tumor Cyclic AMP Levels[a]

Addition	Cyclic AMP accumulation (pmoles/mg protein)[b]
None	48
Theophylline 10 mM	64
ACTH 10^{-4} M	54
ACTH + theophylline	126
TSH 10^{-5} M	60
TSH + theophylline	104
Epinephrine 10^{-4} M	51
Epinephrine + theophylline	71

[a] Tumor slices were incubated for 10 minutes at 37°C in Krebs-Ringer bicarbonate buffer with glucose (200 mg%) with additions as shown.
[b] Cyclic AMP was measured by the method of Gilman (1970).

In intact tumor-bearing rats no increase in corticosterone production is noted following the acute administration of ACTH (Ney *et al.*, 1969). Further, even when tumor cyclic AMP levels in tissue slices are increased by the addition of exogenous cyclic AMP or by the addition of hormone in the presence of a phosphodiesterase inhibitor, only minimal increases in steroidogenesis occur. The tumor tissue is inefficient in corticosterone production compared to normal adrenal tissue. Thus, during incubation of tissue slices, tumor hormone production is approximately 10% that of stimulated normal adrenal tissue per unit of tissue weight (Ney *et al.*, 1969). It appears then that the impaired response in steroidogenesis to hormonal stimulation is due to quantitative limitations in reactions regulated by cyclic AMP rather than to the inability of the tumor to generate sufficient cyclic AMP in response to hormonal activation of adenylate cyclase.

B. Other Animal Tumors

The adenylate cyclase hormone responses of a steroid-producing mouse adrenocortical tumor have been described (Taunton *et al.*, 1967, 1969). The tumor cyclase is stimulated by ACTH in a dose-related manner. Other hormones including epinephrine, parathyroid hormone, insulin, glucagon, and TSH are without stimulatory effects on the tumor cyclase. Prostaglandin E_1 also exhibited no stimulatory effects.

Schimmer (1972) has studied the adenylate cyclase activity in several mouse adrenal tumor cell lines maintained in tissue culture. The cell line which exhibited ACTH-stimulated steroidogenesis possessed an ACTH-responsive cyclase system. Those mutant cell lines which did not demonstrate ACTH-responsive steroidogenesis did not possess ACTH-responsive cyclase systems. That the non-ACTH-responsive cell lines maintained steroidogenic capacity however was demonstrated by the increase in steroidogenesis in the presence of exogenous cyclic AMP. Thus the defect in the mutant cell lines leading to the loss of ACTH-responsive steroidogenesis is the loss of the adenylate cyclase response to ACTH. Hormones other than ACTH were not tested with these tumors.

C. Human Adrenocortical Tumors

The control mechanisms of human adrenocortical tumors have not previously been investigated insofar as the properties of their adenylate cyclase are concerned. However, the behavior of these tumors is similar to that of the animal models in the sense that tumor growth and hormone production appear "autonomous."

The adenylate cyclase hormone responses of four human adrenocortical tumors have been studied (Table VIII). One of these tumors was a carcinoma which resulted in virilization (case 1). The other tumors produced excess quantities of glucocorticoids resulting in Cushing's Syndrome. Tumor tissue was obtained at the time of surgery, and the adenylate cyclase activity determined using methods previously described (Schorr et al., 1972). The cyclase in case 1 was activated by both ACTH and TSH. The lesser response to LH was consistent with the degree of TSH contamination in the impure LH preparation. The cyclase in cases 2 and 3 showed no response to any of the hormones used; however, responses to NaF were evident. The adenylate cyclase in case 4 was activated to a small extent by ACTH and TSH. This patient (case 4) was studied briefly prior to removal of the tumor. On a dosage of triiodothyronine considered sufficient to suppress endogenous TSH, urinary 17-hydroxysteroid excretion diminished by approximately 40% (Fig. 11). Other concomitant measures of tumor steroid secretion such as plasma cortisol levels were not obtained.

IV. Conclusions and Prospects

The studies which have been reviewed provide some initial insight into the regulatory mechanisms operative in tumorous endocrine tissue and into

TABLE VIII

Adenylate Cyclase Hormone Responses of Human Adrenocortical Tumors[a]

Hormone	Adenylate cyclase activity (pmoles cyclic AMP/mg protein/20 min)			
	Case 1 carcinoma	Case 2 adenoma	Case 3 carcinoma	Case 4 adenoma
Basal	371	145	201	98
ACTH ($10^{-4}\,M$)	659	167	162	155
Epinephrine ($10^{-4}\,M$)	299	163	208	92
TSH ($10^{-5}\,M$)	831	125	173	130
LH ($10^{-5}\,M$)	557	127	131	83
Glucagon ($10^{-4}\,M$)	423	173	118	—[b]
NaF 10 mM	3270	508	506	470

[a] Enzyme assayed using whole tissue homogenate and method described by Schorr et al. (1972).

[b] Indicates hormone not tested.

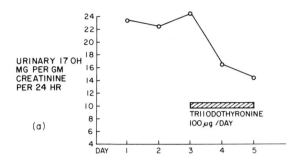

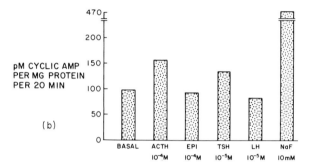

Fig. 11. Responses of a human adrenocortical tumor (case 4, Table VIII). (a) Urinary 17-hydroxysteroid excretion with the administration of triiodothyronine prior to removal of the tumor. (b) *In vitro* adenylate cyclase responses to hormones. The enzyme was measured using methods previously described. (Schorr *et al.*, 1972.)

the etiologies of the functional disturbances which distinguish these from the normal parent tissues. The rat adrenocortical carcinoma which has been described appears to have receptors for "inappropriate" stimulatory hormones. These inappropriate hormones are capable of activating adenylate cyclase and leading to an increase in tissue cyclic AMP levels. Although ACTH is suppressed by tumor corticosterone, the inappropriate endogenous hormones may maintain tumor steroidogenesis at its maximal, although inefficient level. Figure 12 summarizes the functional relationships which are postulated for the tumor-bearing rat.

These inappropriate adenylate cyclase responses are clearly not a general phenomenon. As mentioned previously, the cyclase of a mouse adrenocortical tumor was entirely appropriate in its responses to the hormones tested. Neither is this phenomenon isolated to adrenocortical tumors. Studies of the adenylate cyclase responses in a wide variety of other human

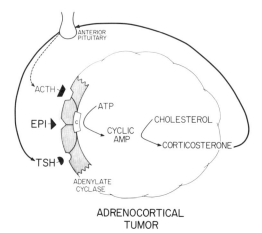

ADRENOCORTICAL
TUMOR

Fig. 12. Postulated functional relationships in the tumor-bearing rat. ACTH levels are suppressed by tumor corticoids.

endocrine tumors have revealed some inappropriate responses (Schorr *et al.,* 1972). Three of 9 pheochromocytomas possessed a glucagon-response cyclase, while the normal adrenal medulla is unresponsive to this hormone.

At present the physiological significance of these aberrant tumor responses is uncertain, and their relationship to tumor function has to remain speculative. However, it is possible that in some cases the "autonomous" behavior of endocrine tumors may be more apparent than real, and that this behavior is the result of stimulation of the tumor by hormones other than the appropriate ones for the parent gland.

ACKNOWLEDGMENTS

These studies were supported by grants AM 05530 and CA 10408 from the National Institutes of Health and grant BC-19B from the American Cancer Society.

REFERENCES

Dobbins, C., Richman, R., Underwood, L., Voina, S., Van Wyk, J., and Ney, R. L. (1972). *Clin. Res.* **20,** 425.

Flack, J. D., and Ramwell, P. W. (1972). *Endocrinology* **90,** 371–377.

Flack, J. D., Jessup, R., and Ramwell, P. W. (1969). *Science* **163,** 691–692.

Gilman, A. G. (1970). *Proc. Nat. Acad. Sci. U.S.* **67,** 305–312.

Grahame-Smith, D. G., Butcher, R. W., Ney, R. L., and Sutherland, E. W. (1967). *J. Biol. Chem.* **242,** 5535–5541.

Haynes, R. C., Jr. (1958). J. Biol. Chem. **233,** 1220–1222.

Haynes, R. C., Jr., Koritz, S. B., and Peron, F. G. (1959). *J. Biol. Chem.* **234,** 1421–1423.

Hechter, O., Bär, H. P., Matsuba, M., and Soifer, D. (1969). *Life Sci., Part I* **8,** 935–942.

Kelly, L. A., and Koritz, S. B. (1971). *Biochim. Biophys. Acta* **237,** 141–155.

Lefkowitz, R. J., Roth, J., Pricer, W., and Pastan, I. (1970). *Proc. Nat. Acad. Sci. U.S.* **65,** 745–752.

Lipsett, M. B., Hertz, R., and Ross, G. T. (1963). *Amer. J. Med.* **35,** 374–383.

Ney, R. L. (1969). *Endocrinology* **84,** 168–170.

Ney, R. L., Hochella, N. J., Grahame-Smith, D. G., Dexter, R. N., and Butcher, R. W. (1969). *J. Clin. Invest.* **48,** 1733–1739.

Robison, G. A., Butcher, R. W., and Sutherland, E. W. (1967) . *Ann. N. Y. Acad. Sci.* **139,** 703–723.

Saruta, T., and Kaplan, N. M. (1972). *J. Clin. Invest.* **51,** 2246–2251.

Schimmer, B. P. (1972). *J. Biol. Chem.* **247,** 3134–3138.

Schimmer, B. P., Veda, K., and Sato, G. H. (1968). *Biochem. Biophys. Res. Commun.* **32,** 806–810.

Schorr, I., and Ney, R. L. (1971). *J. Clin. Invest.* **50,** 1295–1300.

Schorr, I., Rathnam, P., Saxena, B. B., and Ney, R. L. (1971). *J. Biol. Chem.* **246,** 5806–5811.

Schorr, I., Hinshaw, H. T., Cooper, M. A., Mahaffee, D., and Ney, R. L. (1972). *J. Clin. Endocrinol. Metab.* **36,** 447–451.

Snell, K. C., and Stewart, H. L. (1959). *J. Nat. Cancer Inst.* **22,** 1119–1156.

Sutherland, E. W. (1961). *Harvey Lec.* **57,** 17–33.

Taunton, O. D., Roth, J., and Pastan, I. (1967). *Biochem. Biophys. Res. Commun.* **29,** 1–7.

Taunton, O. D., Roth, J., and Pastan, I. (1969). *J. Biol. Chem.* **244,** 247–253.

Wilson, D. B., and Kitabchi, A. E. (1971). *Clin. Res.* **19,** 654.

CHAPTER XI

STEROID-SECRETING TUMORS AS MODELS IN ENDOCRINOLOGY

WILLIAM R. MOYLE AND ROY O. GREEP

The importance of steroid hormones as regulators of homeostasis and reproduction has encouraged studies into the mechanisms controlling steroid synthesis in adrenals and gonads. Since it is clear that steroidogenesis in these organs is dependent on the presence of ACTH or LH, a large effort has been directed toward learning how these hormones stimulate the synthesis of corticoids, progestins, androgens, and estrogens. Recently, much of our knowledge of this process has come from studies utilizing neoplastic adrenal and gonadal tissues which synthesize steroids in response to ACTH or LH stimulation. This article proposes to explore the potential and realized benefits of employing the neoplastic tissues as models to study steroidogenesis. The results derived from these studies should prove valuable for scientists interested in the carcinogenic rather than steroidogenic aspects of these tissues as well.

The review is divided into four principal sections. In the first we discuss the properties of the tumors which make them a unique model system. Second, we catalog the types of tumors available to study. Next, we compare the results obtained utilizing the tumors with what is known and hypothesized about the mechanism of action of ACTH and LH upon steroidogenesis, and finally we suggest alternatives for future consideration. Where possible the material considered in this review has been limited to transplanted lines. Unfortunately, this eliminates much human material. The recent attempts at growing human cancers as transplanted tumors in laboratory animals offer the hope that human material may become more available in the future (Evgenjeva, 1970; Trelford, 1970).

I. Characteristic Features of Steroid-Secreting Neoplasms

Anyone who has ever seen a 25-gm mouse sporting a subcutaneous adrenal or gonadal tumor as large as a human thumb can well appreciate that the tumors offer an abundance of tissue for study. For studies of steroidogenesis in small laboratory animals where the supply of tissue is limited, the mere size of the tumor may provide a source of adrenal or gonadal tissue otherwise hard to obtain. Furthermore, the tumor may offer a convenient source of cells free from endocrine "contamination." As an example, consider the fact that testosterone-secreting cells comprise less than 10% of the total cells in the testes of most common laboratory species (Bascom and Osterud, 1925). These cells are distributed throughout the testes in a fashion precluding their separation from the germinal cells. Testicular tumors composed of testosterone producing Leydig cells have been found to be a useful model for studying the mechanism by which LH stimulates testicular steroidogenesis (Moyle and Armstrong, 1970).

By definition, neoplastic cells display an unusual ability to grow relative to the cells of their origin. As a result of this growth potential the tumor cells have been utilized successfully in long-term culture experiments. Thus Sato's laboratory has developed adrenal and gonadal steroid-secreting lines adapted to culture (Sato et al., 1970, 1971). The clonal lines developed from these studies have added enormously to our knowledge of steroidogenesis.

In spite of these desirable characteristics offered by the neoplasms, their use as models to study steroidogenesis has only recently become fashionable. This may stem from the fact that even though the tumors secrete steroids and respond to ACTH or LH, they are, nonetheless, abnormal tissues. We often hear the argument that steroidogenesis in neoplastic cells may be regulated differently from that in normal adrenal and gonadal tissues. Although this problem can be minimized by studying tumors which are as nearly identical to the original tissue as possible (minimal deviation tumors), without knowing the exact steps in steroidogenesis in any tissue, we cannot rule out the possibility that differences do occur. It should be emphasized that similar considerations arise when comparing steroidogenesis in adrenals or gonads between species. Steroidogenesis in human corpora lutea may be controlled quite differently than it is in rabbit corpora lutea. Comparative endocrinology has demonstrated the value of using one model system to study another. Thus studies of rabbit corpora lutea may help to understand the function of the human corpus luteum. Likewise the tumor provides a complementary model for studying the mechanism of steroidogenesis relative to the cells of its origin.

Perhaps the most noteworthy feature of steroid secreting tumors is their "instability." After a period of transplantation, changes in the steroid excretion pattern (Bloch and Cohen, 1960; Moyle et al., 1971; Ueda et al., 1971), hormonal dependence (Huseby, 1958, 1960; Mühlbock et al., 1958), and responsiveness (Moyle and Armstrong, 1970) often occur. Thus a transplanted Leydig cell tumor in one generation may produce testosterone in vitro when stimulated by LH, whereas subsequent tumors fail in this respect, either because they are not producing steroids or are not responding to LH (Moyle and Armstrong, 1970). Heterogeneity of the tumor cells has been thought to be the cause of instability during serial passage or culture. Loss of function might occur because the nonfunctional cells grow rapidly and replace functional ones. Yasumura et al. (1966) noted that an adrenal tumor line was composed of 2 morphological cell types after it had lost its ability to respond to ACTH in culture. Clonal selection of an epithelial cell type produced a stable line which retained the ability to respond to ACTH. Heterogeneity has also been noted in a gonadotropin-induced rat Leydig cell tumor (Rivière et al., 1967). Although rat cells normally contain 42 chromosomes, the karyotype of the tumors varied considerably, indicating that several cells lost or gained chromosomes. The rat Leydig cell tumor produced androgens, however, it grew in the absence of gonadotropin stimulation. Most likely the cells able to grow in the absence of stimulation grew rapidly and eventually dominated the tumor population. Stephens et al. (1968) observed ultrastructural differences between 4 cell types in another mouse testicular tumor. One cell type contained type A virus particles. In addition Huseby (196) noted morphological heterogeneity in estrogen-induced mouse Leydig cell tumors. Biochemical confirmation of this morphological heterogeneity was obtained by Dominquez and Huseby (1968) who found that the rates of steroid metabolism differed between small fragments in individual tumors. Several enzyme systems, in particular 17α-hydroxylation and 21-hydroxylation, declined from the levels in normal tissue apparently at random while the reduction of the ketone at C-20 increased. These differences were even more pronounced after transplantation indicating that changes in enzyme activities probably occurred as a result of selective growth.

The causes of heterogeneity are not well understood. Clearly it can be created by mutation as reflected in the karyotype. Bunker (1966) noted that the Y chromosome was lost in certain testicular tumors after transplantation. Schimmer (1969) showed that subclones of the Y-1 adrenal tumor cell line contained a metacentric chromosome not present in the initial line (Yasumura *et al.*, 1966). Heterogeneity can also be the result of multifocal tumorification (Huseby, 1960; Dominquez and Huseby, 1968), leading to the presence of several cell types in the tumor from its beginning. Lipschutz (1968) suggests that granulosa and luteal cell tumors induced by a variety of methods undergo an evolutionary pattern caused by differential growth of at least two cell types. The luteal cell tumors are the first to develop following ovarian transplantation or X-irradiation. Granulosa cell tumors develop from stromal cells in these ovaries following a variable latent period. Thus ovarian tumors are often composed of mixtures of the two cell types. Multifocal tumors have also been noted in DMBA-treated ovaries (Marchant, 1961; Jull, 1969; Krarup, 1970). However, many of these foci disappear leaving one large unilateral tumor. Even tumors which arise spontaneously are multifocal as evidenced by the bilateral nature of testicular neoplasms in aged Fischer rats (Jacobs and Huseby, 1967). Thus it seems likely that heterogeneity may arise as the result of transformation of more than one cell and more than one cell type.

Although instability may result from differential growth rates of heterogeneous cell populations, evidence is accumulating that homogeneous tumor cells may be functionally unstable. Schimmer's (1969) studies with the Y-1 adrenal cells seem to be an excellent source of such evidence. Schimmer isolated a subclonal line (designated OS-3) from the Y-1 adrenal cells and found it lacked the ability to synthesize steroids when stimulated by ACTH. If this cell line were grown as tumors in LAF_1 but not CD-1 mice, it reacquired the ability to respond to ACTH. The karyotype of the OS-3 cells was unchanged by passage *in vivo*. Thus, selection of the functional parental cell type as had been proposed originally (Stollar *et al.*, 1964) could not account for the reacquisition of function. It appears as if the nonfunctional cells were "redifferentiating." Recent evidence obtained in other experiments suggests the possibility that the hormonal environment of the animal may be important for the restoration of tumor function. Kowal (1969) has shown that prolonged treatment of the adrenal tumor cells with ACTH leads to increased levels of 11β-hydroxylase. It is doubtful that ACTH was responsible for restoration of its own ability to stimulate the nonfunctional OS-3 line in Schimmer's experiment (1969), however, the fact that hormone treatment of tumor cells can lead to alterations in phenotype may mean that maintenance of a balanced endocrine environment is important for maintenance of differentiated characteristics.

Further evidence that the hormonal state of the animal can influence the ability of transplanted tumors to synthesize steroids arises from another source. One of us (WRM) has noted that Leydig cell tumor M5480 which had apparently lost the ability to synthesize testosterone following passage in male C57BL/6J mice for three years regained that function after transplantation to female C57BL/6J mice. It is interesting that although the tumors grown in males did not produce testosterone or other ultraviolet-absorbing steroids, they retained the ability to synthesize large amounts of cyclic AMP when exposed to LH or HCG. In studies of this same tumor line in its sixty-seventh generation of growth in male C57BL/6J mice, Neaves (1973) showed that the Leydig cells had lost the morphological appearance associated with steroid secretion. Stimulation with HCG restored the smooth endoplasmic reticulum expected of steroid secreting-Leydig cells. Thus the hormonal environment of the cells may be important for maintenance of the functional state. Although the possibility that reacquisition of function by the M5480 cells occurred as a result of selection cannot be ruled out, the fact that biochemical function and morphological appearance were altered within one generation argue against this explanation.

Changes in the cellular function due to a lack of nutrients have also been thought to occur. Growth in medium deficient in glutamine, certain amino acids (Sato et al., 1965) and vitamins (Gardner et al., 1972) have led to loss of steroid function. These losses appear to be reversible.

Steroid-secreting tumors often lose their hormone dependence following continued transplantation. Thus, although LH stimulation is required to induce granulosa and luteal cell tumors, the tumors are seldom dependent on continued hormonal stimulation during subsequent transplantation. This loss in dependence is probably due to preferential growth of cells which have become independent of LH stimulation. Recently, after considerable effort, Clark et al. (1972) were able to establish an ovarian cell line in vitro which required hormonal stimulation for growth. Some confusion still remains about the identity of the hormonal factor which was originally postulated to be LH. LH obtained from the National Institutes of Health (NIH) was capable of stimulating cell growth but highly purified material failed unexpectedly. NIH-LH seems to contain an unidentified growth factor. Jacobs and Huseby (1972) noted that estradiol dependence in vivo was maintained in vitro, at least for a limited time.

Clearly the steroid secreting tumors offer the endocrinologist unique models for studying hormone action. Although we do not understand the causes of "instability" in the tumor cells, this characteristic has not precluded the usefulness of the tumors as model systems. On the contrary the results of Schimmer (1972) indicate that the instability associated with tumor cells will eventually provide endocrinologists with altered cell types facilitating the study of molecular biology in differentiated mammalian cells. Indeed we foresee the time when induced neoplastic transformation of adrenal and gonadal cells will be a preliminary step in preparing tissues for studying steroid secretion. With the proper choice of carcinogenic procedures—many of which are well known at present—researchers will initiate adrenal and gonadal tumors having limited deficiencies which prevent the tumors from producing steroids in response to hormonal stimulation. Tumor cells having altered hormone-binding sites, altered ability to translate binding into function, or altered capacity to synthesize steroids in response to hormonal stimulation may be produced. Observation of the biochemical differences among the various cell types will facilitate identification of the predetermined limiting mechanisms giving rise to the hormonal requirements of steroidogenesis. Developments in cell culture should provide the technology to select for cells based on the appearance of lesions as well as to maintain lines of altered cells. With a bit of luck, hormonally active tumors will become the *Escherichia coli* of endocrinology.

II. Sources of Transplantable Tumors Available for Study of ACTH and LH Response

This topic has been the subject of several excellent articles and is included here only to provide a compilation of those tumors which have been used *in vitro* to study the mechanism of ACTH or LH action. Valuable methods for inducing tumor formation are reviewed by Russfield (1966), Lacassagne (1971), and Lipschutz (1968). The annual bibliography "Research Using Transplanted Tumors of Laboratory Animals: A Cross-Referenced Bibliography" edited by Roberts serves as an excellent source of information. In addition, the twelfth volume of the Ciba Foundation Colloquim in Endocrinology provides details of the earlier studies in this field. We have limited the data in Table I to those transplanted tumors which have been used specifically to study the mechanisms of action of ACTH or LH to keep the table manageable in size.

A. *Gonadal Tumors*

Spontaneous tumors are found in older animals depending on the species, strain, and sex (Russfield, 1966). Often transplantable, these tumors may produce steroids and a few have been shown to be hormone responsive. They are not likely to be hormone dependent. Gonadal tumors can be induced by several methods which depend on destroying the ger-

TABLE I

Transplanted Tumors Used To Study the Mechanism of Action of LH or ACTH

Type	Species	Strain	Origin	Tumor	Cultured	Steroids[a]	Growth dependence	Steroidogenic response	References
Leydig	Mouse	C57B1/6	Spontaneous	M5480	No	A, P	None	HCG, LH, cAMP	b
Leydig	Mouse	BALB/C	Spontaneous	H10119	Yes	P	None	cAMP	c
Leydig	Rat	Fisher	Spontaneous		Yes	A, P	Some		d
Granulosa	Rat		Spleen transplant		Yes		LH		e
Luteoma	Mouse	BALB/C			No	P, C, A	None	Bound LH, no steroidogenesis	f
Adrenal	Rat	Osborne Mendel	Spontaneous	Snell 494	No	C, E, A	None	Not LH Not cAMP	g
Adrenal	Mouse	LAF₁	Spontaneous (X-rays?)	Y–1 LCT Y–6 OS–3	Yes	P	None	ACTH, CAMP	h

[a] A, Androgens; C, corticoids; P, progestins; E, estrogens.

[b] Moyle and Armstrong, 1970; Moudgal et al., 1971; Moyle et al., 1971, 1973a,b; Pokel et al., 1972; Moyle and Ramachandran, 1973; Neaves, 1973.

[c] Shin, 1967; S. I. Shin, personal communication, 1968; Trelford, 1970; Shin and Sato, 1971.

[d] Jacobs and Huseby, 1967, 1968; Roth et al., 1970.

[e] Clark et al., 1972.

[f] Roth et al., 1972.

[g] Snell and Stewart, 1959; Ney et al., 1969; McMillan et al., 1971; Schorr and Ney, 1971; Schorr et al., 1971; Maynard and Cameron, 1972; Sharma, 1972; Sharma and Hashimoto, 1972.

[h] Woolley, 1950; Cohen et al., 1957; Bloch and Cohen, 1960; Stollar et al., 1964; Sato et al., 1965; Sato and Yasumura, 1966; Pierson, 1967; Taunton et al., 1967, 1969; Fiala and Fiala, 1968; Kowal and Fiedler, 1968, 1969; Schimmer et al., 1968; Kowal, 1969a,b,c, 1970a,b,c, 1971, 1972; Rouiller et al., 1969; Schimmer, 1969, 1972; Grower and Bransome, 1970; Lefkowitz et al., 1970a,b, 1971; Pastan et al., 1970; Sato et al., 1970, 1971; Masui and Garren, 1971; Gardner et al., 1972; Kowal et al., 1972; G. Rouiller, B. Schimmer, and A. L. Jones, personal communication, 1973; Temple and Wolff, 1973.

minal cells and/or promoting increases in the levels of circulating gonadotropins. Tumors have been induced by transplantation of the gonads to the spleen (Biskind and Biskind, 1944, 1945), X-irradiation of the gonads (Furth and Furth, 1936; Lindsay *et al.*, 1969), ligation of the gonadal vasculature, and treatment with progestins and estrogens (Lipschutz, 1968), [including DES (Baroni *et al.*, 1966)], carcinogens [particularly DMBA (Marchant, 1961)], Cd salts (Gunn *et al.*, 1965), lead salts (Zawirsha and Medas,1972), or gonadotropins. Not all the tumors induced produce steroids or can be transplanted. Several are hormone dependent. Many gonadal tumors produce corticoids in addition to the expected progestins, androgens, and estrogens.

B. Adrenal Tumors

Adrenal tumors arise spontaneously in older animals depending on the sex, species, and strain of the animals. Several methods have been used to induce the tumors. Among these are castration (Woolley, 1950) and treatment with carcinogens (Mody, 1969) or estrogens (Dunning *et al.*, 1953; Mobbs, 1970). Induction of adrenal tumors by castration apparently depends on the secretion of gonadotropins by the pituitary; tumor induction is inhibited by treatment with estradiol but not corticosterone. It is surprising that an estrogen-dependent adrenal tumor has been found which does not bind estradiol (Mobbs, 1970).

III.   Studies of the Action of ACTH and LH in the Tumors

A. Binding of the Hormones to the Cells and Activation of Adenyl Cyclase

The first step in the interaction of ACTH or LH with adrenal or gonadal cells appears to be the noncovalent binding of the hormone to the cells. Presumably this attachment occurs between the hormones and the "receptor" complex on the cell surface. The strict specificity and high affinity of the hormone–receptor interaction suggests that the complex is similar to that formed by antibodies and antigens or enzymes and substrates. Once formed the hormone receptor unit promotes the stimulation of adenyl cyclase activity leading to synthesis of cyclic AMP. The mechanism by which the hormone receptor unit interacts with the adenyl cyclase remains mysterious.

ACTH-binding sites have been demonstrated in adrenal tumor cells by Lefkowitz *et al.* (1970a,b) who showed that [^{125}I]ACTH was bound reversibly to a "soluble" particle derived from the Y-1 cells. In addition, derivatives of ACTH having hormonal activity displaced [^{125}I]ACTH from the receptor. Peptides which lacked the ability to stimulate adenyl cyclase failed to displace the $[^{125}I]$ACTH suggesting that the inability to stimulate adenyl cyclase was due to lack of binding. Two receptor sites with binding constants of 10^{-12} M and 3×10^{-8} M for ACTH were present in the soluble preparations derived from the Y-1 cells (Lefkowitz *et al.*, 1971). By estimation, Lefkowitz *et al.* (1971) calculated that roughly 60 high affinity and 360,000 low affinity sites were present on each cell. The low affinity site may have been the one coupled with measurable adenyl cyclase activity as evidenced by the observation that the ACTH concentration required to stimulate the cyclase enzyme half-maximally in the Y-1 cells was roughly 10^{-7} M (Taunton *et al.*, 1967, 1969). The site with high affinity for ACTH seemed responsible for stimulation of steroidogenesis in view of the observation made by Kowal and Fiedler (1968) that the amount of ACTH required to stimulate steroidogenesis half-maximally in Y-1 cells was only 2 $\times 10^{-11}$ M.

Shorr *et al.* (1971) and Shorr and Ney (1971) were able to show that the Snell 494 adrenal tumor was capable of binding ACTH, LH, TSH, FSH, epinephrine, and norepinephrine. The ability of the various hormones to activate the adenyl cyclase was utilized as an index of binding. It remains to be seen whether the lack of specificity was due to the presence of several cell types within the tumor or whether it was due to multiple binding sites on the tumor cell. This question could be best resolved by cloning the tumor cells. The responses to LH, TSH, and FSH are not additive suggesting that they interact with one site possibly through the common (α) subunit. Surprisingly, the purified α subunit appeared to inhibit the cyclase. Although the observation that glycoprotein and ACTH receptors could be found in adrenal tissue was unusual, it was not altogether unexpected. Inasmuch as ovariectomy can induce adrenal tumorgenesis in some species, and since the efficacious agent is probably the elevated levels of gonadotropins, one might expect to find an influence of gonadotropins on some adrenal tumors. ACTH does not increase cyclic AMP levels or stimulate steroidogenesis in intact Snell 494 cells (Ney *et al.*, 1969). Failure of ACTH to elevate cyclic AMP levels in the intact cells could not be explained by effects of ACTH on the activity of phosphodiesterase in the tumor (Sharma, 1972). Guanyl cyclase activity present in the tumor cells was not altered by ACTH stimulation (McMillan *et al.*, 1971).

ACTH receptors have been thought to lie on the surface of the plasmalemma primarily because the adenyl cyclase has been associated with this membrane. This location of adenyl cyclase favored the concept that ACTH might stimulate steroidogenesis without entering the cell. Experimental evidence supporting this idea was described by Schimmer *et al.* (1968) who observed that particles composed of an ACTH octadecapeptide covalently bound to cellulose had the ability to stimulate steroidogenesis in the Y-1 adrenal cells. The N-terminal octadecapeptide of ACTH was chosen for use in these experiments to reduce the possiblity that hormonal activity of the cellulose-ACTH particles could have been due to solubilization of active ACTH fragments. Perhaps a better control to eliminate the possibility that ACTH activity was being solubilized in these experiments would consist of labeling the peptide with [^{125}I] (Lefkowitz et al., 1970b) and coupling the radioiodinated peptide to the resin as before. If ACTH was being released into the medium it would be readily detectable.

The obligatory role of cyclic AMP as a second messenger has been questioned recently by the finding that little of the cyclic AMP measured in response to ACTH stimulation is required for maximal steroidogenesis (Moyle et al., 1973c). It seems possible that the amounts of cyclic AMP required for transmission of the ACTH message are too small for accurate measurement. Recently, a clone (OS-3) of Y-1 mutant cells was obtained by Schimmer (1972). These cells lacked the ability to synthesize cyclic AMP and steroids in response to ACTH stimulation although cyclic AMP stimulated OS-3 steroidogenesis. Thus the failure of ACTH to stimulate steroidogenesis was attributed to failure of the hormone to stimulate cyclic AMP synthesis suggesting that formation of cyclic AMP was required for hormonal activity. Although the exact nature of the biochemical lesion in the OS-3 cells is still uncertain, Schimmer (1972) postulated that it might be associated with binding of ACTH to the receptor or interaction of the hormone-receptor complex with the adenyl cyclase. These cells provide exciting possibilities for identifying the ACTH receptor and/or the hormone-receptor–adenyl cyclase coupling factor.

The requirement for calcium ions in adrenal steroidogenesis has been known for more than two decades (Birmingham et al., 1953). Utilizing the partially purified adenyl cyclase from the Y-1 tumor cells Lefkowitz et al. (1970a) have shown that Ca^{2+} is essential for the stimulation of cyclic AMP synthesis by ACTH in an isolated adenyl cyclase preparation (Pastan et al., 1970). Binding of ACTH to the receptor was undiminished in the absence of the cation. Apparently the interaction of the ACTH-receptor complex with the adenyl cyclase requires the calcium.

LH has been shown to bind to M5480 Leydig tumor cell suspensions (Moyle et al., 1971; Moudgal et al., 1971). Bound hormone was detected in plasma membrane fractions by means of a sensitive LH-radioimmunoassay capable of detecting subnanogram quantities of the gonadotropin. [^{125}I]LH was not utilized in these studies as it did not bind to gonadal cells. Removal of the nonbound hormone from the cells by changing the incubation medium was ineffective in removing the tightly bound LH from the cells (Fig. 1) and was also ineffective in terminating steroidogenesis (Table II).

Steroidogenesis was halted only when antiserum to LH was added to the cells. The fact that antiserum could terminate steroidogenesis suggested that the effective hormone was attached to the surface of the cell in a manner which permitted immunological recognition. Moudgal *et al.* (1971) reported that tight binding of LH to the M5480 cells paralleled the ability of the hormone to stimulate tumor steroidogenesis. Concentrations of LH which exceeded those required to elicit maximal steroidogenesis did not produce further binding of the hormone to the cells (Fig. 2). We were surprised to observe (Moyle and Ramachandran, 1973) that the amount of LH required to stimulate cyclic AMP synthesis was at least 10-fold that required to stimulate testosterone biosynthesis (Fig. 3). Could LH have stimulated cyclic AMP accumulation without being bound to the cells? The apparent dilemma was resolved by the realization that our measurements of bound LH would recognize only that hormone which remained associated with the cells during the lengthy process used to separate free and unbound hormone. We reasoned that LH bound to a receptor with lower affinity might be more readily dissociated than that bound to the

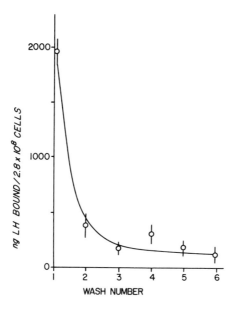

Fig. 1. Binding of LH to M5480 Leydig tumor cells. Following incubation of a Leydig cell suspension with LH, the free and unbound LH were separated by replacing the buffer containing the cells 6 times. Each successive buffer change should have produced a 10-fold drop in nonbound LH. Methodology of incubation and LH assay was described by Moudgal *et al.* (1971).

TABLE II

Steroid Production after Incubation with LH and Removal of Latter by
Washing with Hormone-Free Buffer

Experiment	Prior incubation[a] (μg/ml)	Incubation[b]	Steroid per flask[c] (μg)
1	1	NaCl solution	3.07 ± 0.276
	1	1 μg of LH per ml	3.68 ± 0.496
	1	LH antiserum[d]	1.88 ± 0.266[e]
	1	LH antiserum + LH[f]	4.02 ± 0.187
	0.01	0.01 μg of LH per ml	0.37 ± 0.076[e]
2	0.5	NaCl solution	0.82 ± 0.10
	0.5	0.5 μg of LH per ml	0.69 ± 0.07
	0.5	LH antiserum[d]	0.42 ± 0.09[e]
	0.5	LH antiserum + LH[f]	0.80 ± 0.17
	0.005	0.005 μg of LH per ml	0.09 ± 0.01[e]
	0.5	Not incubated	0.10 ± 0.02[e]

[a] Prior incubation period with LH was 15 minutes, after which all cells were washed.

[b] Incubation time, 1 hour.

[c] Tumors used in the first experiment synthesized testosterone as the major steroid, whereas those in the second experiment made progesterone primarily. Consequently, the steroids measured in experiments 1 and 2 were testosterone and progesterone, respectively.

[d] LH antiserum neutralized 5 μg of LH.

[e] Significantly different from the control at $P < 0.05$.

[f] LH added again at 10 μg per flask.

high affinity receptors. To test this possibility we repeated the experiment described in Table II taking care to measure cyclic AMP synthesis as well as steroidogenesis. Indeed, removal of the excess LH by changing the buffer was sufficient to terminate the hormonal effect on cyclic AMP accumulation but not on steroidogenesis (Fig. 4). We concluded that LH bound to two receptors as did ACTH. Binding to a high affinity receptor led to increased steroidogenesis while binding to a lower affinity receptor was required for detectable cyclic AMP production. We again emphasize that this result did not disprove the role of cyclic AMP as a mediator of steroidogenesis. Functional cyclic AMP levels may be unmeasurable by present techniques. In fact much of the cyclic AMP formed after LH stimulation of the tumor cells was found extracellularly.

Gonadotropin binding to ovarian tumors has been demonstrated.

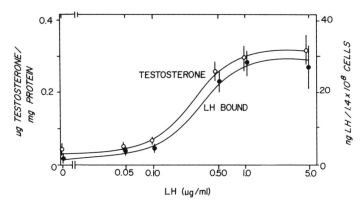

Fig. 2. Comparison of tight binding and stimulation of testosterone synthesis in M5480 Leydig tumor cells. Varying concentrations of NIH-LH-S-16 were incubated with the tumor cells. Steroidogenesis was measured as described by Moyle and Armstrong (1970) and the LH binding was measured as described by Moudgal *et al.* (1971).

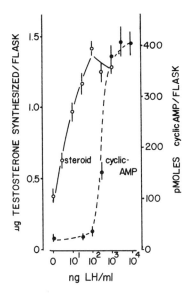

Fig. 3. Stimulation of steroidogenesis and cyclic AMP synthesis by highly purified LH preparations in M5480 Leydig tumor cells. Leydig tumor cells were incubated with LH which had approximately 2.5 times the potency of NIH-LH-S-1. Steroidogenesis and cyclic AMP accumulation were measured as described by Moyle and Ramachandran (1973).

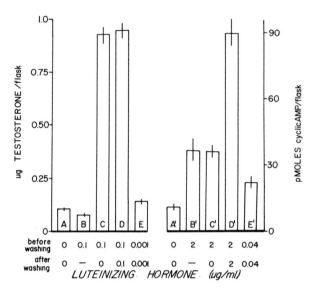

Fig. 4.   Effect of removal of LH on steroidogenesis and cyclic AMP accumulation. LH was added to the M5480 cells for 5 minutes and removed as described in Table II. The numbers below each bar represent the concentration of LH added during each incubation. Measurements of cyclic AMP were made 15 minutes following reincubation in treatments A, C, D, and E. Treatment B was not reincubated. If cyclic AMP synthesis continued after washing then the value of C′ should be equal to that of D′ rather than B′. Thus LH was not tightly bound to the receptors responsible for cyclic AMP accumulation. Steroidogenesis continued after washing treatment and C equaled treatment D as expected from previous results. Thus LH remained bound to the receptors responsible for steroidogenesis after the free LH had been removed by the washing procedure. The concentrations of LH used in flasks E and E′ represent those which would have been present after the dilution procedure.

Mizejewski *et al.* (1972), Mizejewski (1972), and Carlson *et al.* (1972) have shown that ovarian tumors bind [^{125}I]HCG. Thecal cell tumors but not granulosa cell tumors bind the iodinated glycoprotein. Prolactin is not accumulated by the cells. Roth *et al.* (1972) have found [^{125}I]hLH-binding sites in a BALB/C mouse ovarian tumor consisting of luteinized stromal cells. LH did not stimulate steroidogenesis in this luteoma.

B. Stimulation of Steroidogenesis by Cyclic AMP

According to the second messenger concept ACTH and LH act to induce the formation of cyclic AMP which in turn stimulates steroidogenesis (Robison *et al.*, 1971). Addition of cyclic AMP to the cells should stimulate steroidogenesis in the same manner as ACTH. In 1964 Stollar *et al.* observed that cyclic AMP stimulated steroidogenesis in the Y-1 adrenal cell line. 5′-AMP had little or no measurable effect on steroid synthesis. Five years later Kowal and Fiedler (1969) reported that the apparent specificity for cyclic AMP had been lost. Other nucleotides, notably those containing adenine (5′ATP, 5′ADP, 5′AMP, adenosine), UMP, and CTP, were also able to stimulate steroidogenesis. The loss in specificity was not explained but could have been due to several factors including stimulation of endogenous cyclic AMP synthesis. Another cell line (LCT) derived from the same tumor responded only to cyclic AMP and its dibutyryl derivative (Kowal, 1970b). Stimulation of the LCT line by cyclic AMP was never equal to that due to ACTH presumably because the nucleotide did not readily enter the cell. Comparison of the adenyl cyclases, protein kinases, and phosphodiesterases of the Y-1 cells with those in LCT cells may indicate which factors are required to insure specificity of the nucleotide response. The Snell adrenal tumor 494 did not synthesize increased amounts of corticosterone in response to cyclic AMP (Sharma and Hashimoto, 1972).

Shin (1967) has shown that Leydig tumor cells in tissue culture will synthesize progestins (progesterone and 20α-dihydroprogesterone) following cyclic AMP treatment. It is interesting that the original tumor line may have produced androgens and estrogens (Ueda et al., 1971). LH did not initiate steroidogenesis in the cultured cells presumably because it did not stimulate the adenyl cyclase. After growing in vitro for prolonged periods the cells lost their ability to respond to cyclic AMP. Restoration of this response was observed if the cells were grown as tumors. Growth of the cells in vivo did not restore the ability of LH to stimulate steroidogenesis. As with the Y-1 cells these Leydig tumor cells acquired the ability to respond to other nucleotides (S. I. Shin, personal communications, 1968). Inasmuch as this is the second cell type observed to respond to non-cyclic AMP nucleotides, it seems that studies to determine how specificity is maintained would be very useful.

Cyclic AMP has been shown to stimulate testosterone biosynthesis in the M5480 Leydig tumor cells (Moyle et al., 1971). The continued presence of the nucleotide was required for prolonged elevation of steroidogenesis.

Thus far it is not known how cyclic AMP stimulates steroidogenesis in the tumor cells. Activation of protein kinases may be a key step in this mechanism (Garren et al., 1971). The tumors should provide excellent models for studying the effects of cyclic AMP on the kinases.

C. Role of Cholesterol Metabolism in Steroidogenesis

Activation of the conversion of cholesterol to steroids was first shown to be a key factor in the stimulation of steroidogenesis 20 years ago (Stone and Hechter, 1954). Kowal (1969a,b) showed that ACTH increased the conversion of cholesterol to steroids in the Y-1 adrenal cells. Studies with aminoglutethimide showed that the side chain cleavage of cholesterol, not cholesterol synthesis, appeared to be the limiting step in steroidogenesis. Temple and Wolff (1973) suggest that transport of cholesterol into mitochondria may stimulate steroidogenesis. Yasumura *et al.* (1966) have noted that the presence of cholesterol in the medium may be beneficial for steroidogenesis following prolonged cultivation.

In the Leydig tumor cells, Shin (1967) found that cyclic AMP induced the conversion of cholesterol to progestins. The nucleotide did not stimulate the conversion of pregnenolone to progesterone indicating that the rate-limiting step might be the side chain cleavage of cholesterol. Moyle *et al.* (1973a,b) showed that LH and cyclic AMP stimulated the hydrolysis of cholesterol esters *in vitro* in the M5480 Leydig cell tumor. The response could be observed within 10 minutes provided the cellular levels of choles-terol were depleted by prior incubation of the cells in fetal calf serum (Fig. 5). The hydrolysis of the cholesterol esters was thought to provide the sterol for side chain cleavage. Esterified cholesterol was not oxidized to steroids by the tumor mitochondria unless it were first hydrolyzed to free choles-

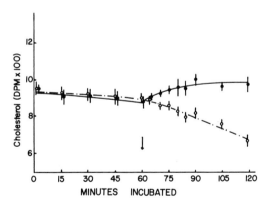

Fig. 5. Effect of LH on M5480 Leydig cell cholesterols. [1,2-³H]Cholesterol (50 μCi) was injected intravenously into a tumor-bearing C57B1/6J mouse. Five days after injection the tumor was excised and a cell suspension in fetal calf serum prepared as by Moyle *et al.* (1973a). The suspension was incubated in quadruplicate flasks, 1-ml portions being removed from each for analysis at the times indicated on the abscissa. Change in radioactivity ——, cholesterol; – · –, esterified cholesterol. LH (5 μg/ml) was added (vertical arrow) after 1 hour of incubation. Vertical bars represent the SEM. When LH was not added the rate of loss of both cholesterol and esterified cholesterol continued as during the first hour (results not shown).

TABLE III

Conversion of Cholesteryl Palmitate and Cholesterol and Steroids by
M5480 Mitochondria[a]

	Rate of conversion (dpm/hour)		
Treatment	[³H]Cholesteryl palmitate to [³H]cholesterol	[³H]Cholesteryl palmitate to ³H-labeled steroids	[³H]Cholesterol to ³H-labeled steroids
None	3861 ± 282	157 ± 24	361 ± 10.0
Frozen–thawed	2170 ± 96	63 ± 24	552 ± 44.1
Sonication	264 ± 46	35 ± 30	938 ± 105.2
Tween (0.5 mg/ml)	−19 ± 23	13 ± 40	948 ± 97.0

[a] Mitochondria were incubated in 0.25 M sucrose–0.001 M EDTA–0.02 M Tris-HCl, pH7.4, with 0.5 mg of NADPH/ml for 0, 30, 60, and 90 minutes. A fraction of the mitochondria was frozen at −20°C and rapidly thawed in a water bath at 37°C and a fraction was sonicated for 2 minutes at 15-second intervals in an ice bath. [1,2-³H]Cholesteryl palmitate (0.05 μCi; 50 Ci/mmole) was used to evaluate the conversion of cholesteryl palmitate into cholesterol and steroids. [26-¹⁴C]Cholesterol (0.01 μCi) and [1,2-³H]cholesterol (0.01 μCi; 50 Ci/mmole) were used to evaluate the conversion of cholesterol into steroids. No ¹⁴C was isolated in any steroids. Isolation of sterols and steroids is described in Moyle et al. (1973b). Values represent the slope of the line drawn through points representing the dpm of product isolated at each time ± S.D.

terol by an enzyme present in the microsomes (Table III). Although the cells had more free cholesterol than was required to synthesize steroids on a molar basis during incubation, the concentration of cholesterol was low in the vicinity of the inner mitochondrial membrane, the site of the side chain cleaving enzyme (Table IV). The effect of LH or cyclic AMP on the cholesteryl ester hydrolase may have been required to replace the mitochondrial cholesterol oxidized to pregnenolone. Pokel et al. (1972) demonstrated that LH was capable of inducing a depletion in cellular esterified cholesterol levels in vivo which was probably related to the hormones' ability to increase ester hydrolysis. The mechanism by which the metabolism of esterified cholesterol is controlled has yet to be reported for tumor cells. Cholesterol and the cholesterol-binding proteins may serve as regulators of cholesteryl ester levels. The possibility that protein kinases are involved should not be overlooked.

TABLE IV

Submitochondrial Localization of Cholesterol Side Chain-Cleaving Enzyme[a]

Membrane fraction	Protein (% of total)	Monoamine oxidase (% of total)	Succinate dehydrogenase (% of total)	Side chain-cleaving enzyme (% of total)	Cholesterol (% of total)
Outer	15.7 ± 7.5 (3)	43.3 ± 2.2 (3)	9.1 ± 8.7 (5)	7.7 ± 5.0 (3)	34.1 ± 8.8 (3)
Inner	77.3 ± 2.0 (3)	56.1 ± 2.8 (3)	88.0 ± 7.4 (5)	85.3 ± 9.3 (3)	39.4 ± 2.0 (3)

[a] Mitochondrial fractions were isolated at 7000 g_{av} and fractionated as described by Moyle et al. (1973b). Distribution of monoamine oxidase, succinate dehydrogenase, cholesterol side chain-cleaving enzyme, cholesterol, and protein were determined as described in the text. Membrane fragments were incubated in 1 ml of 0.1 M Tris-HCl (pH 7.4), 0.005 M MgCl$_2$ and 0.1 M NaCN. NADPH (1 mg/ml) plus a mixture of [26-^{14}C]cholesterol (0.1 μCi; 50 mCi/mmole) and [7α-^{3}H]cholesterol (0.2 μCi; 10 mCi/mmole) were used as the substrates. Incubation was continued for 60 minutes. No ^{14}C appeared in any of the steroids isolated. Percentages are based on amounts measured in mitochondria immediately after swelling in phosphate buffer. Values are means ± S.D. The number of experiments used to calculate the means is shown in parentheses.

D. Requirement for Protein Synthesis

Induction of steroidogenesis by ACTH or LH apparently involves the synthesis of a rapidly turning over protein. Most antibiotics capable of inhibiting protein synthesis are capable of inhibiting the stimulatory effects of ACTH or LH even when steroidogenesis has already been initiated (Garren, 1968).

Attempts to isolate this rapidly turning over protein have been frustrating. Grower and Bransome (1970) using the Y-1 adrenal cells were able to detect a leucine-containing protein by gel electrophoresis which was synthesized in response to ACTH. The role of this protein in steroidogenesis seems doubtful since it is formed after steroidogenesis has been stimulated. Kowal (1970c) observed that cycloheximide and puromycin inhibited the ACTH stimulation of steroidogenesis in the Y-1 cells, however, these antibiotics also inhibited steroidogenesis in the unstimulated cells. Kowal noted that protein synthesis could be depressed by as much as 60% before effects on steroidogenesis were produced. Apparently the antibiotics inhibit the conversion of cholesterol to pregnenolone.

Shin (1967) reported that cycloheximide inhibited the steroidogenic response induced by cyclic AMP in Leydig tumor cells. Shin and Sato (1971) reported that actinomycin D and puromycin were also effective inhibitors of the response. The role of RNA synthesis in this response as suggested by the inhibitory effects of actinomycin D is controversial. Moyle *et al.* (1971) showed that cycloheximide inhibited testosterone synthesis in the M5480 tumor cells. Inhibition occurred even though the cells had been treated previously with LH.

Clearly a great deal of work has yet to be done in this area with tumor cells. It is conceivable that protein synthesis may not play a major role in the immediate response to the hormones. Inhibitors of protein synthesis may inhibit steroidogenesis by such effects as inhibiting cholesterol transport or protein kinase activation. The rapidly turning over proteins need to be identified and their effects on steroidogenesis in homogenates need to be established.

E. ACTH and Glycolysis

ACTH has been shown to stimulate glycolysis in Y-1 adrenal tumor cells by increasing phosphofructose kinase activity (Kowal, 1969a; Kowal *et al.*, 1972). The effects on glycolysis appeared to be independent of the glucose concentration in the medium ruling out effects of ACTH on glucose entry into the cells. ACTH did not increase the activity of pyruvate decarboxylase.Thus most of the glucose metabolized appeared as lactic acid. Inhibition of steroidogenesis by treating the cells with puromycin or cycloheximide (Kowal, 1970c) did not effect the glycolytic response to ACTH. The Y-1 cell line will grow and respond to ACTH if the glucose of the medium is replaced by xylitol, xylose, pyruvate, or fructose but not galactose. The LCT cultures required glucose (Kowal 1969a) to respond to ACTH. The requirement for NADPH as a cofactor in cholesterol side chain cleavage has led Kowal (1971) to examine the metabolism of glucose through the pentose pathway. Reduction of NADP to NADPH occurs as a consequence of the oxidation of glucose 6-phosphate to 6-phosphogluconolactone in this pathway. ACTH failed to stimulate oxidation of glucose via the pentose pathway. To our knowledge similar studies have not been undertaken with transplantable gonadal tumors during LH stimulation.

F. Effects of ACTH and LH on DNA Synthesis and Cell Growth

ACTH is known to increase the growth of the adrenal gland in hypophysectomized animals. In contrast ACTH appears to inhibit the growth of the

Y-1 adrenal tumor cells when grown as tumors *in vivo* (Fiala and Fiala, 1968) or as isolated cells *in vitro* (Masui and Garren, 1971). The reasons for the unexpected effects of the peptide on tumor growth are not very clear at this time. Masui and Garren (1971) showed that both ACTH and cyclic AMP decreased the incorporation of [³H]thymidine into DNA. Cyclic GMP and cyclic IMP failed to decrease DNA synthesis. Thus the effect of ACTH on cell growth appeared to be mediated by cyclic AMP. Recent studies with fibroblastic cells have shown that cyclic AMP may mediate growth and DNA synthesis in other cell types as well (Otten *et al.*, 1972). Thus it appeared likely that the effects of cyclic AMP on the Y-1 tumor cells may have been caused by the fact that these are tumorous cells rather than by the fact that they are adrenal cells. The fact that these cells contain viruses (G. Rouiller, B. Schimmer, and A. L. Jones, personal communication, 1973) may also contribute to this result. Recent evidence reported by Kowal (1972) suggests that the cyclic AMP inhibition of growth in the Y-1 cells was due to a metabolite of cyclic AMP. Incorporation of [³H]deoxyribose thymidine into DNA was better inhibited by adenosine than cyclic AMP. The role of steroidogenesis as an inhibitor of DNA synthesis was ruled out by the finding that cyclic CMP increased steroidogenesis but did not inhibit DNA synthesis.

Gonadotropins enhance the growth rates of ovarian, adrenal, and testicular tumors. Clark *et al.* (1972) have described an ovarian cell line requiring LH forgrowth *in vitro* which had been developed by the ovarian spleen grafting procedure of Biskind and Biskind (1944). Tumor development in this procedure is dependent on the constant stimulation of the ovary by elevated levels of gonadotropins. Antiserum to LH inhibits tumorigenesis (Ely *et al.*, 1966). Constant stimulation by LH is apparently the cause of adrenal tumors in various strains of ovariectomized mice. Procedures which decrease LH levels such as estrogen administration (Woolley, 1950) prevent tumor formation. Treatments with corticoids which alter ACTH levels do not alter tumorigenesis (Monsen, 1952). LH has also been shown to enhance the growth of testicular tumors by Jacobs and Huseby (1968) who showed that transplanted Leydig cell tumors grew more rapidly in castrated male rats than in intact controls.

Both ACTH and LH are thought to stimulate cell growth by similar mechanisms. Thus it seems strange to learn that LH is carcinogenic whereas ACTH is anticarcinogenic. It is conceivable that the inhibitory effects of ACTH on the Y-1 cells are due to its ability to promote substantial increases in the levels of cyclic AMP in these cells. The elevated cyclic AMP levels may retard cell growth by altering the transformation produced by the viral infection of the Y-1 cells. The reason for the discrepancy between the effects of ACTH and LH on tumor growth will be resolved only by further study. It is highly conceivable that hormonal regulation of adrenal growth is controlled differently than that of ovarian growth.

G. Influence of ACTH and LH on the Fine Structure of Adrenal and Gonadal Tumors

Adrenal and gonadal steroid-secreting cells are characterized by their content of smooth endoplasmic reticulum, lipid droplets, and unusual mitochondria (Fawcett et al., 1969). Steroid-secreting tumors show these characteristic features of normal adrenal and gonadal cells. Sharma and Hashimoto (1972) have examined the fine structure of the Snell 494 adrenal tumor. This tumor actively synthesizes corticosterone from pregnenolone but does not synthesize corticosterone upon stimulation by ACTH or cyclic AMP. The Snell 494 cells had abundant Golgi and smooth endoplasmic reticulum but contained only few lipid droplets and mitochondria. As mitochondria contain the enzymes required for cholesterol side chain cleavage, the relative lack of these organelles may indicate that little cholesterol is being oxidized to pregnenolone in this tumor. Inasmuch as short term treatment with ACTH accelerates cholesterol side chain cleavage and not the steps between pregnenolone and corticosterone, the lack of mitochondria may explain the insensitivity of the Snell 494 tumor to ACTH stimulation. Rouiller et al. (1969; G. Rouiller, B. Schimmer, and A. L. Jones, personal communication, 1973) have noted that the Y-1 adrenal cells contain mitochondria with lamellar cristae which are characteristic of the cells found in the zona glomerulosa of the mouse. The smooth endoplasmic reticulum was not especially prominent in these cells (Fig. 6). As cholesterol side chain cleavage and 11-hydroxylation are found mitochondrially whereas the 21-hydroxylase is located microsomally, lack of abundant smooth endoplasmic reticulum may account for production of 11β-hydroxyprogesterone rather than corticosterone. Although the shape of the Y-1 adrenal cells undergoes a rapid change upon stimulation by ACTH or cyclic AMP (Sato and Yasumura, 1966), the major ultrastructural change noted by Rouiller et al. (1969; G. Rouiller, B. Schimmer, and A. L. Jones, personal communication, 1973) (Fig. 7) was seen to be associated with increased amounts of Golgi rather than with mitochondria. As Kowal (1969c) has demonstrated that prolonged ACTH treatment induces the formation of 11β-hydroxylase it would be interesting to look at the effects of prolonged ACTH stimulation in the Y-1 cells. The reasons for the rapid "rounding up" of the cells described by Sato and Yasumura (1966) have recently been studied by Temple et al. (1972) and Temple and Wolff (1973) who examined the roles of microtubules in the Y-1 cells. It was noted that agents which disrupted microtubular structure (colchicine, vinblastine, or podophyllotoxin) were capable of stimulating steroidogenesis after a 6- to 9-hour lag period. D_2O (^2H_2O), an agent which is kown to stabilize microtubules, was a partial inhibitor of the effects of vinblastine, ACTH, or cyclic AMP. D_2O also inhibited the change in shape induced by

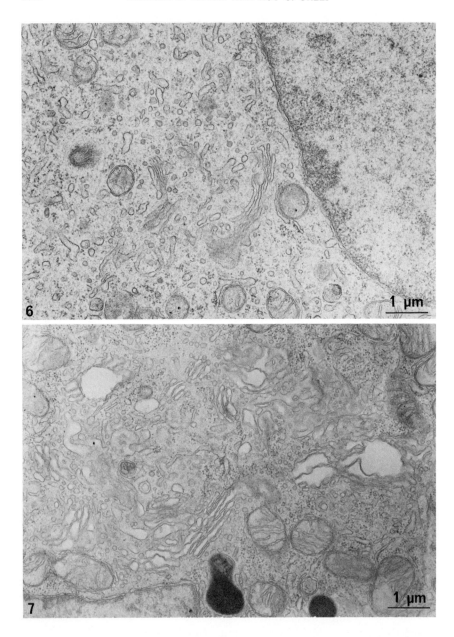

Fig. 6. Ultrastructure of Y-1 adrenal cells: This micrograph illustrates the ultrastructure of the Y-1 adrenal tumor cells prior to ACTH treatment. Note the relative lack of smooth endoplasmic reticulum. From G. Rouiller, B. Schimmer, and A. L. Jones (personal communication, 1973).

cyclic AMP. Nonetheless the role of microtubules in ACTH stimulation of steroidogenesis remains mystifying. Not all cells responding to ACTH display the capacity to round up. Temple and Wolff (1973) suggest that microtubules may increase mitochondrial cholesterol transport.

Roth *et al.* (1972) have studied the ultrastructure of a transplantable mouse luteoma. Morphological analysis indicated that the tumor originated from luteinized stromal cells. This tumor had abundant smooth endoplasmic reticulum and mitochondria with tubular cristae. The tumor produced androstenedione, progesterone, and 21-hydroxyprogesterone. It is interesting that LH did not stimulate steroidogenesis in these cells even though it was bound to cell membranes. This tumor contained type A virus particles. Roth *et al.* (1970) also studied the fine structure of transplantable spontaneous Leydig cell tumors obtained from aged Fischer rats. Those tumors which produced androgens contained cells having smooth endoplasmic reticulum and mitochondria with tubular cristae. Tumors which failed to secrete steroids had almost no smooth endoplasmic reticulum but contained much more rough endoplasmic reticulum. The mitochondria of these nonfunctional tumors contained lamellar cristae. Neaves (1973) showed that treatment of M5480 Leydig cell tumors with HCG promoted the appearance of smooth endoplasmic reticulum, lipid droplets, and a reduction in the nucleocytoplasmic volume (Figs. 8 and 9). Alterations in the structure of the mitochondria were less marked. Thus gonadotropin stimulation can increase cytodifferentiation of tumor cells as well as stimulating tumor formation and growth.

Although treatment with ACTH and LH promotes ultrastructural changes in the adrenal and gonadal tumors, it is unlikely that these morphological alterations are the cause of increased steroidogenesis seen immediately after hormone treatment. Elevation of steroidogenesis occurs within minutes after addition of ACTH or LH to the cells, whereas the ultrastructural changes require hours or even days to become apparent. It is not clear that the steroid secretion and morphological changes seen after hormone treatment are controlled by the same mechanism.

H. Metabolism of Steroids by Adrenal and Gonadal Tumors

Adrenal and gonadal tumors have been shown to metabolize pregnenolone to several different steroids. Many tumors, however, produce steroids which are not synthesized in large amounts by normal adrenal or gonadal

---

Fig. 7. Effect of ACTH on the ultrastructure of Y-1 adrenal cells. Shortly after treatment with ACTH the Golgi complex of the Y-1 cells enlarges strikingly as shown here. From G. Rouiller, B. Schimmer, and A. L. Jones (personal communication, 1973).

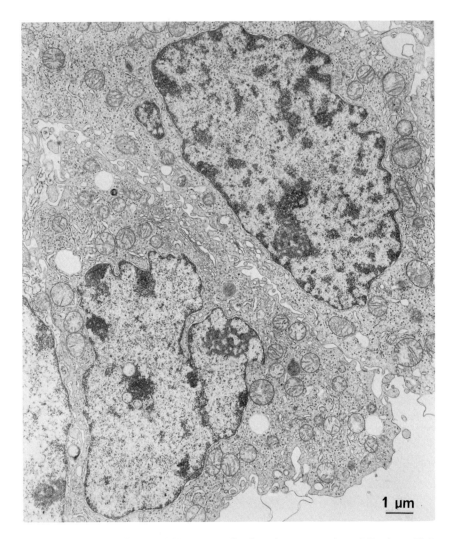

Fig. 8. The cells of tumor M5480 normally show few structural specializations. Their generalized complement of organelles, including polyribosomes, Golgi complex, and spherical mitochondria, is usually seen in relatively undifferentiated cells. Note the paucity of smooth endoplasmic reticulum, an organelle that is particularly active in steroidogenesis. ×7700. (From Neaves, 1973.)

cells. Adrenal tumors often synthesize large amounts of androgens and estrogens while gonadal tumors may synthesize compounds with corticoid activities. The change in metabolism is usually associated with losses of certain enzyme systems accompanied by gains in others. The Y-1 adrenal tumor cells fail to produce corticosterone due to a deficiency in 21-

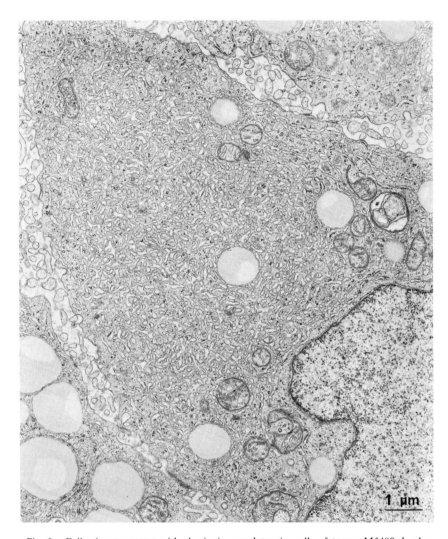

Fig. 9. Following treatment with chorionic gonadotropin, cells of tumor M5480 develop large quantities of smooth endoplasmic reticulum seen here as contorted arrays of branching and anastomosing tubules. Coincident with the proliferation of smooth endoplasmic reticulum is a marked reduction of nucleocytoplasmic ratio in the tumor cells. ×10,500. (From Neaves, 1973.)

hydroxylation and produce 20α-dihydroprogestins due to an increase in the content of 20α-hydroxysteroid dehydrogenase (Pierson, 1967; Kowal and Fiedler, 1968). The alteration in the metabolism of pregnenolone does not interfere with the ability of ACTH to stimulate steroidogenesis in these cells. These changes in steroid synthesis occurred gradually during continuing transplantation (Bloch and Cohen, 1960) and culture (Pierson, 1967). Thus the Y-1 tumor synthesized 11-deoxycorticosterone, corticosterone, 11β-hydroxyprogesterone, 11β-hydroxyandrostenedione, and progesterone in the third generation, it produced 11β-hydroxyandrostenedione, progesterone, and an unidentified metabolite in the eleventh generation while in culture the tumor produced progesterone, 11β-hydroxyprogesterone, 20α-dihydroprogesterone, 11β-hydroxy-20α-dihydroprogesterone, and 11-keto-20α-dihydroprogesterone. From these changes in metabolites, it was thought that the tumor cells progressively lost the 21-hydroxylase, 17α-hydroxylase, and the 17,20-desmolase while they gained the 20α-hydroxysteroid dehydrogenase. Sharma and Hashimoto (1972) observed that the Snell tumor 494 synthesized corticosterone from pregnenolone. This is not in complete agreement with the results of Maynard and Cameron (1972) who noted the conversion of pregnenolone to 11-deoxycorticosterone in this tumor. This latter group also found that the tumor had less 5α-reductase activity than normal rat adrenal tissues. Dominquez and Huseby (1969) observed that an adrenal cortical carcinoma from a BALB/C mouse which had been ovariectomized produced 20α-dihydroprogesterone and 17β-hydroxy-20α-dihydroprogesterone. The enzymes characteristic of adrenal tissues, 21-hydroxylase and 11β-hydroxylase were absent in this tumor. The adrenal tumor steroids had characteristics expected of gonadal secretion. Rosner et al. (1966) observed that adrenal tumors in C3H/EP mice secreted estrogens and androgens. Neville et al. (1968) measured steroid synthesis from adrenal tumors produced by castration of CE mice. They found enzymes capable of converting progesterone to cortisol (i.e., 21-hydroxylase, 17β-hydroxylase, 11β-hydroxylase). They also observed transformation of dehydroepiandrosterone to androstenedione. This tumor retained these enzymes even after culture for 19 days. It is not clear why some adrenal tumors secrete adrenal corticoids and others synthesize sex hormones.

Gonadal tumors, on the other hand, often have enzymes found in adrenal cells. The 21-hydroxylase has been observed in Leydig cell tumors by Lucis and Lucis (1969, 1970), Dominquez and Huseby (1968), Inano et al. (1968, 1972), and Inano and Tamaoki (1969). In addition these tumors made androgens and estrogens. Evidence suggesting the presence of considerable amounts of 20α-dihydroreductase was found in these studies and in those by Moyle et al. (1971), Shin (1967), and Shin et al. (1968). The reason for the appearance of the 20-hydroxysteroid reductase is not known. Possibly its induction results from failure of prolactin to inhibit its synthesis. Prolactin inhibits the appearance of the 20-reductase in ovarian tissues after hypophysectomy (Armstrong, 1968).

Changes in the pattern of steroid synthesis were noted in the gonadal tumors after serial transplantation. Moyle and Armstrong (1970) observed that the M5480 tumor initially produced testosterone and progesterone. After repeated transplantation the pattern of steroid synthesis favored progesterone and 20α-dihydroprogesterone. It is not known whether the enzymes capable of converting pregnenolone to testosterone were absent or whether the reduction at C-20 prevented androgen synthesis in the latter tumors. Inano et al. (1972) noted that an interstitial tumor arising spontaneously in RF mice lost the 21-hydroxylase when grown in culture. Apparently the enzymes for steroidogenesis can be lost independently of one another.

Roth et al. (1972) isolated 11-deoxycorticosterone synthesized from [1-^{14}C]acetate in transplantable luteomas. They also observed the production of androstenedione and small amounts of testosterone. Rice and Segaloff (1967) observed that luteomas produced by spleen grafting were capable of synthesizing progesterone and 20α-dihydroprogesterone. Other metabolites were not found. Granulosa cell tumors did not synthesize labeled hormones from acetate.

IV. Areas for Future Study

As discussed in the previous section the studies of tumor steroidogenesis have complemented and extended our knowledge of the mechanism by which ACTH and LH alter steroidogenesis. Our view of this mechanism is depicted in Fig. 10. LH and ACTH (abbreviated as H) interact with gonadal and adrenal receptors in a complex manner. The possibility that the hormones interact with a single receptor in a one to one ratio can now be ruled out (Moyle et al., 1973c,d). We favor the view that at least two types of receptors with differing affinities for the hormones are present on the cell membrane. Interaction of the hormones with one receptor (R_1) is responsible for the stimulation of steroidogenesis, whereas interaction of higher concentrations of the hormone with the other receptor (R_2) is responsible for the stimulation of adenyl cyclase and accumulation of measurable amounts of cyclic AMP. For completeness we mention a second mechanism for hormone binding which is not depicted in Fig. 10. In this mechanism the cells have one type of receptor, however, this receptor is capable of binding two or more molecules of hormone. This could be visualized in a manner similar to that of oxygen being bound to hemoglobin. Stimulation of steroidogenesis would occur when one hormone molecule had bound to the receptor. Accumulation of cyclic AMP would occur when two or more hormone molecules had bound to the receptor. To our knowledge neither model is favored by experimental evidence, however, we prefer the first as it seems less complex. The existence of two receptors (or

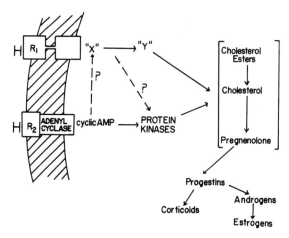

Fig. 10. Mechanism of ACTH and LH stimulation of steroidogenesis. ACTH or LH (H) can bind to more than one receptor (R_1 and R_2) on the plasma membrane of the tumor cells. Interaction with R_1 leads to the production of an unknown second messenger (possibly compartmentalized cyclic AMP) which stimulates the side chain cleavage of cholesterol via effects on protein kinases or unknown enzymes ("Y"). Interaction with R_2 results in the production of cyclic AMP which may stimulate the production of "X" or which may enhance protein kinase activity directly. The significance of R_2 is unknown.

perhaps more) puzzles us, particularly since the binding constants are separated by at least one and probably two or three orders of magnitude. It is doubtful that hormone concentrations reach the high levels required to saturate R_2 *in vivo* since stimulation of R_1 results in steroid secretion which tends to reduce the levels of circulating ACTH or LH. It is conceivable that receptor R_2 serves as a partially formed precursor of R_1. In combination with unknown coupling factors, R_2 might be converted into R_1. Nonetheless, the discovery of multiple receptors reopens discussion as to whether several second messengers are synthesized in response to hormonal stimulation. Could adrenal, ovarian, or testicular growth be controlled through a different receptor than steroidogenesis? The answer to this fundamental question should be available in the near future with the development of chemically modified hormonal molecules which fail to interact with one of the receptors. We also expect that tumor cells lacking one or another receptor should soon be found now that their existence is predicted.

Closely related to this problem of the two receptors is the question of which second messenger is responsible for the stimulation of steroidogenesis by physiological concentrations of ACTH and LH. Clearly, cyclic AMP will stimulate steroidogenesis but that observation alone does not prove its role particularly in light of the fact that very small changes in the levels of cyclic AMP are noted during stimulation of steroidogenesis. We might take the position that the levels of the functional nucleotide are unmeasurable by present techniques. For example, if the functional nucleotide were compartmentalized and represented only 1–5% of the total cyclic AMP pool, our measurements of total cyclic AMP would not provide an accurate estimate of functional cyclic AMP concentration. It is interesting that the concentration of cyclic AMP in the cell is higher than that required to stimulate partially purified protein kinase activity maximally. This enzyme is not fully activated in unstimulated cells. Although several factors may prevent complete activation of the protein kinases such as the presence of substrates (ATP or proteins) or inhibitors, the concentration of cyclic AMP at the site of the enzyme may be much lower than our measurements of total cyclic AMP indicate. Compartmentalization of cyclic AMP would explain this result. An opposing view would consider that cyclic AMP is not directly involved in the stimulation of steroidogenesis. This implies that an alternative messenger which we have designated "X" may be the physiological second messenger of steroidogenesis. Although "X" might be another nucleotide, little evidence supports this view. The stimulation of steroidogenesis seen after cyclic AMP treatment may be related to the ability of cyclic AMP to stimulate the synthesis of "X." We feel that the time has come to reexamine the nature of the second messenger. Is the physiological mediator of steroidogenesis compartmentalized cyclic AMP or is its chemical identity still elusive?

The role of protein kinases in steroidogenesis is even more tenuous than that of cyclic AMP as we indicate in Fig. 10 by providing an alternate pathway ("Y") for hormone action. With the exeption of a few enzymes, histones, and ribosomal proteins, the substrates for kinase activity are not established. We would expect to find effects of protein kinases on enzymes directly related to steroidogenesis such as the cholesteryl ester hydrolase or cholesterol side chain cleaving enzyme. Furthermore, the roles of the kinases cannot be proven unless their activity is shown to be increased during stimulation of steroidogenesis. Since the kinases are activated by cyclic AMP, their physiological relevance must be scrutinized under conditions in which steroidogenesis is stimulated without apparent increase in cyclic AMP concentrations.

We have deliberately avoided diagramming (Fig. 10) the rapidly turning over protein which has been thought to mediate hormone stimulated steroidogenesis. The existence of these proteins depends on the observation that inhibitors of protein synthesis inhibit the effects of ACTH and LH on steroidogeneses. These inhibitors of protein synthesis also inhibit the steroidogenesis measured in the absence of hormonal treatment. Therefore, it seems that inhibitors of protein synthesis block the hormone stimulated steroidogenesis because they block steroidogenesis itself. Future studies should concentrate on isolation of newly synthesized proteins in response to LH and ACTH. These proteins should be isolated and their activities tested. ACTH and LH alter protein synthesis and growth rates of tumor cells, however, it seems doubtful that this is a prerequisite for the effects of the hormones on short-term stimulation of steroidogenesis.

The ultimate effect of hormone stimulation on adrenal and gonadal tumor steroidogenesis increases the side chain cleavage of cholesterol to steroids. Once the six-carbon side chain has been cleaved from cholesterol, the synthesis of the individual steroids continues in the absence of further hormone stimulation. Although it is generally agreed that side chain cleavage of cholesterol is the rate-limiting step in steroidogenesis stimulated by hormonal treatment, the mechanism by which hormones activate this oxidation is still in doubt. We feel that the supply of a substrate, cholesterol, limits side chain cleavage because of the relative paucity of this sterol in the inner mitochondrial membrane where side chain cleavage occurs. Hormonal effects on the cholesteryl ester hydrolase or on cholesterol transport would increase the availability of mitochondrial cholesterol and as a result increase steroidogenesis. It would be interesting to determine whether the cholesteryl ester hydrolase or the cholesterol carrier proteins are substrates for protein kinases.

Finally, we should include mention of the prostaglandins in this review. Very little has been reported concerning the synthesis or effects of prostaglandins in tumor cells. Prostaglandins may be important in controlling steroidogenesis as an alternative second messenger. Could the mysterious second messenger be prostaglandins?

ACKNOWLEDGMENT

We are greatly indebted to Dr. W. B. Neaves and Dr. A. L. Jones for giving us copies of their manuscripts prior to publication and for allowing us to use the electron micrographs in Figs. 6, 7, 8, and 9. This review was supported by The Ford Foundation.

REFERENCES

Armstrong, D. T. (1968). *Recent Progr. Horm. Res.* **24,** 255–319.
Baroni, C., Magrini, U., Martinazzi, M., and Bertoli, G. (1966). *Eur. J. Cancer* **2,** 211–220.
Bascom, K. F., and Osterud, H. L. (1925). *Anat. Rec.* **31,** 159–168.
Birmingham, M. K., Elliott, F. H., and Valero, H. L. P. (1953). *Endocrinology* **53,** 687–689.
Biskind, M. S., and Biskind, G. R. (1944). *Proc. Soc. Exp. Biol. Med.* **55,** 176–179.
Biskind, M. S., and Biskind, G. R. (1945). *Proc. Soc. Exp. Biol. Med.* **59,** 4–8.
Bloch, E., and Cohen, A. I. (1960). *J. Nat. Cancer Instr.* **24,** 97–107.
Bunker, M. C. (1966). *Can. J. Genet. Cytol.* **8,** 312–327.
Carlsson, S., Kullander, S., and Muller, E. R. (1972). *Acta Obstet. Gynecol. Scand.* **51,** 175–182.

Clark, J. L., Jones, K. L., Gospodorowicz, D., and Sato, G. H. (1972). *Nature (London), New Biol.* **236**, 180–181.

Cohen, A. I., Furth, J., and Buffett, R. F. (1957). *Amer. J. Pathol.* **33**, 631–651.

Dominquez, O. V., and Huseby, R. A. (1968). *Cancer Res.* **28**, 348–353.

Dominquez, O. V., and Huseby, R. A. (1969). *Endocrinology* **84**, 1039–1047.

Dunning, W. F., Curtis, M. R., and Segaloff, A. (1953). *Cancer Res.* **13**, 147–152.

Ely, C. A., Tuerche, R., and Chen, B. L. (1966). *Cancer Res.* **26**, 1441–1447.

Evgenjeva, T. P. (1970). *Eur. J. Cancer* **6**, 533–535.

Fawcett, D. W., Long, J. A., and Jones, A. L. (1969). *Recent Progr. Horm. Res.* **25**, 315–380.

Fiala, S., and Fiala, A. E. (1968). *Int. J. Cancer* **3**, 531–545.

Furth, J., and Furth, O. B. (1936). *Amer. J. Cancer* **28**, 54–65.

Gardner, D. A., Sato, G. H., and Kaplan, N. O (1972). *Develop. Biol.* **28**, 84–93.

Garren, L. D. (1968). *Vitam. Horm. (New York)* **26**, 119–145.

Garren, L. D., Gill, G. N., Masui, H., and Walton, G. M. (1971). *Recent Progr. Horm. Res.* **27**, 433–478.

Grower, M. F., and Bransome, E. D., Jr. (1970). *Science* **168**, 483–485.

Gunn, S. A., Gould, T. C., and Anderson, W. A. D. (1965). *J. Nat. Cancer Inst.* **35**, 329–337.

Huseby, R. A. (1958). *Ciba Found. Colloq. Endocrinol. [Proc.]* **12**, 216–230.

Huseby, R. A. (1960). *In* "Biological Activities of Steroids in Relation to Cancer" (G. Pincus and E. P. Vollmer, eds.), pp. 211–223. Academic Press, New York.

Inano, H., and Tamaoki, B. I. (1969). *Endocrinology* **84**, 123–131.

Inano, H., Machino, A., Tamaoki, B. I., and Tsubura, Y. (1968). *Endocrinology* **83**, 659–670.

Inano, H., Tamaoki, B. I., and Tsubura, Y. (1972). *Endocrinology* **90**, 307–310.

Jacobs, B. B., and Huseby, R. A. (1967). *J. Nat. Cancer Inst.* **39**, 303–309.

Jacobs, B. B., and Huseby, R. A. (1968). *J. Nat. Cancer Inst.* **41**, 1141–1153.

Jacobs, B. B., and Huseby, R. A. (1972). *J. Nat. Cancer Inst.* **49**, 1205–1212.

Jull, J. W. (1969). *J. Nat. Cancer Inst.* **42**, 961–966.

Kowal, J. (1969a). *Trans. N.Y. Acad. Sci.* [2] **31**, 359–378.

Kowal, J. (1969b). *Endocrinology* **85**, 270–279.

Kowal, J. (1969c). *Biochemistry* **8**, 1821–1831.

Kowal, J. (1970a). *Endocrinology* **87**, 951–965.

Kowal, J. (1970b). *Mt. Sinai J. Med., New York* **37**, 528–535.

Kowal, J. (1970c). *Recent Progr. Horm. Res.* **26**, 623–687.

Kowal, J. (1971). *In Vitro* **6**, 174–179.

Kowal, J. (1972). *J. Clin. Invest.* **51**, A51.

Kowal, J., and Fiedler, R. (1968). *Arch. Biochem. Biophys.* **128**, 406–421.

Kowal, J., and Fiedler, R. P. (1969). *Endocrinology* **84**, 1113–1117.

Kowal, J., Frenkel, R., and Angee, I. (1972). *Endocrinology* **91**, 1219–1226.

Krarup, T. (1970). *Brit. J. Cancer* **24**, 168–186.

Lacassagne, A. (1971). *Bull. Cancer* **58**, 235–275.

Lefkowitz, R. J., Roth, J., and Pastan, I. (1970a). *Nature (London)* **228**, 864–866.

Lefkowitz, R. J., Roth, J., Pricer, W., and Pastan, I. (1970b). *Proc. Nat. Acad. Sci. U.S.* **65**, 745–752.

Lefkowitz, R. J., Roth, J., and Pastan, I. (1971). *Ann. N.Y. Acad. Sci.* **185**, 195–209.

Lindsay, S., Nichols, C. W., Sheline, G. E., and Chaikoff, I. L. (1969). *Radiat. Res.* **40**, 366–378.

Lipschutz, A. (1968). *Perspect. Biol. Med.* **11**, 461–474.

Lucis, O. J., and Lucis, R. (1969). *Cancer Res.* **29**, 1647–1651.

Lucis, O. J., and Lucis, R. (1970). *Cancer Res.* **30**, 702–708.

McMillan, B. H., Ney, R. L., and Schorr, I. (1971). *Endocrinology* **89**, 281–283.

Marchant, J. (1961). *Brit. J. Cancer* **15**, 821-827.
Masui, H., and Garren, L. D. (1971). *Proc. Nat. Acad. Sci. U.S.* **68**, 3206-3210.
Maynard, P. V., and Cameron, E. H. (1972). *Biochem. J.* **126**, 99-106.
Mizejewski, G. J. (1972). *Experientia* **28**, 961-962.
Mizejewski, G. J., Beierwalter, W. H., and Quinones, J. (1972). *J. Nucl. Med.* **13**, 101-106.
Mobbs, B. G. (1970). *J. Endocrinol.* **48**, 545-552.
Mody, J. R. (1969). *Cancer Res.* **29**, 1254-1261.
Monsen, H. (1952). *Cancer Res.* **12**, 284-285.
Moudgal, N. R., Moyle, W. R., and Greep, R. O. (1971). *J. Biol. Chem.* **246**, 4983-4986.
Moyle, W. R., and Armstrong, D. T. (1970). *Steroids* **15**, 681-693.
Moyle, W. R., and Ramachandran, J. (1973d). *Endocrinology* **93**, 127-134.
Moyle, W. R., Moudgal, N. R., and Greep, R. O. (1971). *J. Biol. Chem.* **246**, 4978-4982.
Moyle, W. R., Jungas, R. L., and Greep, R. O. (1973a). *Biochem. J.* **132**, 407-413.
Moyle, W. R., Jungas, R. L., and Greep, R. O. (1973b). *Biochem. J.* **132**, 415-424.
Moyle, W. R., Kong, Y. C., and Ramachandran, J. (1973c). *J. Biol. Chem.* **248**, 2409-2417.
Mühlbock, O., van Nie, R., and Bosch, L. (1958). *Ciba Found. Colloq. Endocrinol. [Proc.]* **12**, 78-98.
Neaves, W. B. (1973). *J. Nat. Cancer Inst.* **50**, 1069-1073.
Neville, A. M., Anderson, J. M., McCormick, M. H., and Webb, J. L. (1968). *J. Endocrinol.* **41**, 547-554.
Ney, R. L., Hochella, N. J., Grahame-Smith, D. G., Dexter, R. N., and Butcher, R. W. (1969). *J. Clin. Invest.* **48**, 1733-1739.
Otten, J., Johnson, G. S., and Pastan, I. (1973). *J. Biol. Chem.* **247**, 7082-7087.
Pastan, I., Pricer, W., and Blanchette-Mackie, J. (1970). *Metab. Clin. Exp.* **19**, 809-817.
Pierson, R. W. (1967). *Endocrinology* **81**, 693-707.
Pokel, J. D., Moyle, W. R., and Greep, R. O. (1972). *Endocrinology* **91**, 323-325.
Rice, B. F., and Segaloff, A. (1967). *Acta Endocrinol. (Copenhagen)* **54**, 568-576.
Rivière, D., Vendrely, C., and Rivière, M. R. (1967). *C.R. Soc. Biol.* **161**, 1850-1854.
Roberts, D. C. (1964-Present). "Research Using Transplanted Tumors of Laboratory Animals: A Cross-Referenced Bibliography." Imperial Cancer Res. Fund.
Robison, G. A., Butcher, R. W., and Sutherland, E. W. (1971). "Cyclic AMP," pp.17-46 and 317-335. Academic Press, New York.
Rosner, J. M., Chaneau, E., Houssay, A. B., and Epper, C. (1966). *Endocrinology* **79**, 681-686.
Roth, L. M., Spurlock, B. O., Steinberg, W. H., and Rice, B. F. (1970). *Amer. J. Pathol.* **60**, 137-152.
Roth, L. M., Steinberg, W. H., Huseby, R. A., Macphee, A. A., Cole, F. E., and Rice, B. F. (1972). *Lab. Invest.* **27**, 115-122.
Rouiller, G., Schimmer, B., and Jones, A. L. (1969). *Anat. Rec.* **163**, 342.
Russfield, A. B. (1966). *U.S., Pub. Health Serv., Publ.* **1332**, 25-38 and 45-65.
Sato, G., Augusti-Tocco, G., Posner, M. (1970). *Recent Progr. Horm. Res.* **26**, 539-546.
Sato, G., Clark, J., Posner, M., Leffert, H., Paul, D., Morgan, M., and Colby, C. (1971). *Acta Endocrinol. (Copenhagen), Suppl.* **153**, 126-136.
Sato, G. H., and Yasumura, Y. (1966). *Trans. N.Y. Acad. Sci.* [2] **28**, 1063-1079.
Sato, G. H., Rossman, T., Edelstein, L., Holmes, S., and Buonassisi, V. (1965). *Science* **148**, 1733-1734.
Schimmer, B. P. (1969). *J. Cell. Physiol.* **74**, 115-122.
Schimmer, B. P. (1972). *J. Biol. Chem.* **247**, 3134-3138.
Schimmer, B. P., Ueda, K., and Sato, G. H. (1968). *Biochem. Biophys. Res. Commun.* **32**, 806-810.

Schorr, I., and Ney, R. L. (1971). *J. Clin. Invest.* **56**, 1295–1300.

Schorr, I., Rathnam, P., Saxena, B. B., and Ney, R. L. (1971). *J. Biol. Chem.* **246**, 5806–5811.

Sharma, R. K. (1972). *Cancer Res.* **32**, 1734–1736.

Sharma, R. K., and Hashimoto, K. (1972). *Cancer Res.* **32**, 666–674.

Shin, S. I. (1967). *Endocrinology* **81**, 440–448.

Shin, S. I., and Sato, G. H. (1971). *Biochem. Biophys. Res. Commun.* **45**, 501–507.

Shin, S. I., Yashumura, Y., and Sato, G. H. (1968).*Endocrinology* **82**, 614–616.

Snell, K. C., and Stewart, H. L. (1959). *J. Nat. Cancer Inst.* **22**, 1119–1155.

Stephens, R. J., Pourreau-Schneider, N., and Gardner, W. U. (1968). *J. Ultrastruct. Res.* **22**, 494–507.

Stollar, V., Buonassisi, V., and Sato, G. (1964). *Exp. Cell. Res.* **35**, 608–616.

Stone, D., and Hechter, O. (1954). *Arch. Biochem.* **51**, 457–469.

Taunton, O. D., Roth, J., and Paston, I. (1967). *Biochem. Biophys. Res. Commun.* **29**, 1–7.

Taunton, O. D., Roth, J., and Pastan, I. (1969). *J. Biol. Chem.* **244**, 247–253.

Temple, R., and Wolff, J. (1973). *J. Biol. Chem.* **248**, 2691–2698.

Temple, R., Williams, J. A., Wilber, J. F., and Wolff, J. (1972). *Biochem. Biophys. Res. Commun.* **46**, 1454–1461.

Trelford, J. D. (1970). *Cancer* **25**, 1122–1133.

Ueda, G., Coli, A., and Kunii, A. (1971). *Gann* **62**, 41–48.

Woolley, G. W. (1950). *Recent Progr. Horm. Res.* **5**, 383–405.

Yasumura, Y., Buonassisi, V., and Sato, G. (1966). *Cancer Res.* **26**, 529–535.

Zawirsha, B., and Medas, R. (1972). *Arch. Immunol. Ther. Exp.* **20**, 243–256.

CHAPTER XII

ENDOCRINE AND IMMUNOLOGICAL FACTORS IN TROPHOBLAST CANCERS

ROLAND A. PATTILLO

I. Introduction to the Model

The search for essential growth substances in malignant tumors has paralleled a similar quest for fundamental growth stimulants in normal tissues. The consideration of hormones in this role is supported by abundant biological data demonstrating the requirement for specific hormones in *differentiation*. It has not been determined, however, what role hormones play, if any, in the *growth* process prior to differentiated function. In malignant growth, on the other hand, it has been shown that antibody is produced against antigen within the malignant cell itself (uterine cancer). It was, therefore, suggested that "this capacity to produce self-directed antibody may be the basis of a locked in, self-stimulatory, mechanism involved in the continuous growth of cancer cells" (Charney, 1968). It may be alternatively suggested, however, that while antibody production is demonstrable in malignant cells derived from nonimmunocompetent epithelium (HeLa cells—cervix) (Holmgren, 1968), it may not be the basis of self-stimulation of growth but may rather be an autoimmune consequence of antigenic aberration associated with a transforming agent of malignancy induction, i.e., oncogenic virus, protovirus. Accordingly, recent immunochemical evidence has been presented suggesting that the carcinoembryonic antigen (CEA) found in colon, lung, breast, and prostate cancers may represent endogenously altered blood group substances of the ABO category (Alastair *et al.*, 1973). While it has been clearly established that the transformation of normal cells to the malignant state by polyoma virus is characterized by the appearance of new cellular antigens, more recent results have suggested that this tumor associated antigen may act as a specific activator of chromosome replication (Weil and Kara, 1970). These investigators studied the temporal relationship between the appearance of polyoma-specific "tumor antigen" and polyoma-induced activation of the cellular DNA synthesizing apparatus in mouse kidney cells. The experimental results were compatible with the hypothesis that virus-induced replication of the mouse cell chromosomes was triggered by the tumor antigen. The studies indicated that a few hours after adsorption of polyoma virus, but prior to the appearance of "T" antigen, trace amounts of "early, early" polyoma-specific RNA could be detected. It was suggested that this early, early RNA was the first transcription product of the intranuclear parental polyoma DNA. The appearance of polyoma-specific T-antigen, as detected by immunofluorescence, was found to precede the polyoma-induced activation of the cellular DNA-synthesizing apparatus. Thus, it may be speculated that self-stimulation of growth resulting from foreign antigens inducing chromosome replication may be a characteristic of autonomous malignant cells and may likewise form the basis of normal reproduction, as observed in normal pregnancy. In the latter instance, foreign paternal chromosomes inducing HL-A antigens foreign to the maternal germ cell may act as the signal for initiation of mitosis in the fertilized ovum.

On the basis of the preceding, it is proposed that an intrinsic mechanism for initiation of new growth from oncogenic agents in malignancy and from paternal and maternal genes in normal pregnancy may result from foreign genetic information inducing neoantigens which may provide the stimulus for mitotic self-replication. A parallel of this mechanism may exist in the instance of lymphocyte stimulation in mixed leukocyte cultures (MLC), wherein the stimulus for DNA synthesis and replication ensues from extrinsic histocompatibility antigen differences. Likewise, oncogenic virus incorporation into normal cellular genomes results in altered antigen expression which might constitute a similar basis for DNA synthesis, replication, and continuous growth. Another example of endogenous tumor growth stimulation was noted when stimulation of mouse mammary tumor growth was observed when small numbers of specifically immunized spleen cells were given to thymectomized, X-irradiated animals challenged with the mouse mammary tumor. These results are in direct variance with the concept of immunosurveillance which implies immunoinhibitory activity at the earliest stages of tumor induction (Prehn, 1972; Medina and Heppner, 1973).

A requirement for hormones as the *initiating* growth substances in the genesis of the human trophoblast in normal pregnancy or in trophoblastic cancers has not been demonstrated. Rather, the capacity for synthesis of the hormones necessary for *differentiation* follows the initiation of growth which occurs upon fusion of sperm and ovum. Human embryological studies (Hertig, 1968) indicate that the first cell division following ovum fertilization results in the two-cell stage which consists of one cell showing trophoblastic morphology, the other representing the forerunner of the embryo. This event occurs approximately 30 hours after fertilization. While the precise moment of initiation of endogenous trophoblast hormone production has not been established, maternal serum levels of human chorionic gonadotropin (HCG) can be demonstrated with present techniques by the ninth day following conception (Kosa *et al.*, 1973). However, since gonadotropin hormone production can be demonstrated from normal and malignant trophoblastic cells in culture, it is believed to be an intrinsic property of the trophoblastic cell from its inception at the two-cell stage (Pattillo *et al.*, 1971a). Thus, in the analogy of malignant growth induction and normal pregnancy, the initial stimulus for "growth" (mitosis) of the ovum, in addition to a possible male-specific antigen (Watchel *et al.*, 1973), might be the paternal–maternal genetic complex in fertilization expressing foreign histocompatibility antigens (HL-A haplotype) which may activate chromosomal replication and result in the first cell division. The appearance of the trophoblastic cell in the resulting two-cell stage may provide the first source of hormones to initiate the differentiation process in the accompanying embryonic cell.

The normal trophoblast shares many properties of cancer cells, as well as representing the source of the malignant tumor of the placenta–choriocarcinoma. Most prominent is the normal biological characteristic of invasiveness, a prerequisite for implantation of the fertilized ovum unto the uterine decidual bed. This maligant-like invasiveness anchors the trophoblastic and embryonic blastocyst into its maternal host. The essential requirement for survival and growth of the implanted blastocyst is a satisfactory nutrient source within the implantation bed. This is provided by the rich glycogen and glycoprotein matrix of the uterine decidual bed. Having achieved implantation, the derivation of an energy source depends on catalytic influences provided by multiple hormonal constituents of the trophoblast. Prominent in the acquisition of a nutrient and energy source is the abundance of simple and complex carbohydrates at the implantation site. In this connection, it is apparent that gonadotropin and steroid hormones interact to control carbohydrate utilization. The major source of ribose precursors for nucleotide synthesis in cell replication and function derives from ribose sugars synthesized in the pentose phosphate pathway. McKerns (1969) has suggested that the entry of metabolites into this pathway is controlled by the enzyme glucose-6-phosphate dehydrogenase (G6PD) under the control of pituitary hormones. In addition to serving as a source of ribose sugars for RNA and DNA, the pentose cycle also constitutes a major NADPH-generating system, which may serve as a rate-limiting step for steroid biosynthesis. The pleuripotential trophoblastic cell secretes glycoprotein, protein, and steroid hormones in ordered sequences for differentiation controls during the course of normal gestation. In addition to functioning in growth and differentiation as illustrated by HCG stimulation of nucleotide synthesis (McKerns, 1973), these hormones also have important immunosuppressant properties.

II.   Hormone Activity and Trophoblast Redifferentiation in Cancers of Diverse Somatic Tissues

The present recognition of trophoblastic redifferentiation in multiple forms of malignancies has been emphasized by recent reviews wherein trophoblastic elements and gonadotropin hormone production have been identified in cancers of virtually every organ of the body. This concept of trophoblastic reexpression in cancers of multiple organs includes: lung (Rosen *et al.,* 1968), esophagus (McKechnie and Fechner, 1971), kidney (Castlemen *et al.,* 1972), bladder (Ainsworth and Greshman, 1960), stomach (Regan and Cremin, 1960), pineal, pituitary gland (Edmonds and Cerrea, 1965), mediastinum (Bennington *et al.,* 1964), retroperitoneal space, and thymus (Jernstrom and McLaughlin, 1962). In breast cancer, adrenal carcinoma and melanoma, gonadotropin activity was found, however, tissue descriptions were not included (McArthur, 1963). Gonadotropin hormone production of chorionic and pituitary-like characteristics was reported in hepatoblastomas, although trophoblastic differentiation was not described histologically. Choriocarcinomas in ovary and testis (Rubin, 1970) are well known. Increasing numbers of lung carcinomas with gonadotropin activity have been reviewed by Rosen *et al.,* (1968). The patients have generally been men with histological patterns of undifferentiated carcinoma; however, squamos, mixed adeno and squamous oat cell, and bronchioalveolar carcinomas have also been reported. Other hormones, in addition to HCG have also been found in trophoblastic tumors.

III.   Multiple Hormone Secretions in Trophoblastic Cancers

A series of *in vitro* models of choriocarcinomas have been established which maintain hormonal function in continuous cultivation. The cell lines established in the author's laboratories (Pattillo *et al.*, 1971b) synthesize gonadotropic hormones, protein hormones, and steroids in similar fashion to the *in vivo* patterns in the normal placenta and in patients with choriocarcinoma. HCG, by far the most valuable clinical monitor of trophoblast activity, is secreted in these cultures in quantities of 1000 IU/gm of cells/24 hours. Human placental lactogen production is considerably less, amounting to $2/\mu g/gm$ cells. While chorionic gonadotropin is produced in large quantities and can be determined by bioassay or radioimmunoassay on several microliters of fluid in which the cells are incubating, human placental lactogen determinations require pooled media and chromatography for extraction and subsequent radioimmunoassay.

The enzymatic and metabolic capacity for synthesis of estriol in the trophoblastic tumor cells were documented using a schemata which paralleled normal placental pathways for synthesis of estriol from $1\dot{\text{o}}$-hydroxy-Δ ⁴-androstenedione, which is hydroxylated in the 16α-position in the fetal liver and is transported to the placenta where it serves as a precursor or estriol. Since the aromatizing enzymes for transformation of androgen into estrogens are abundant in trophoblastic cells, the 16α-hydroxylated androgen precursor was added to the incubation media of the trophoblastic tumor cells in culture. Approximately 1% conversion of this precursor to estriol was found in the BeWo cell line. Similar experiments using the radioactively labeled progesterone precursors, pregnenolone demonstrated conversion of this precursor to progesterone (Huang *et al.*, 1969). The synthesis of progesterone from pregnenolone was associated with dramatic depletion of cellular glycogen and a concomitant increase in glycogen phosphorylase (Pattillo *et al.*, 1970). Electron microscopic examination gave evidence of morphological differentiation of these tumor cells characterized by increased quantities of endoplasmic reticulum and electron dense lipid droplets characteristic of steroid secretion.

Trophoblastic tumors have been associated with increased thyroid function as demonstrated by the occurrence of hyperthyroidism in choriocarcinoma and in the benign form of this tumor associated with pregnancy, hydatidiform mole (Odell *et al.*, 1963). Extraction of such molar thyroid-stimulating hormone activity has been reported in cases of benign hydatiform molar tumors associated with toxemia of pregnancy and increased thyroid function (Pattillo *et al.*, 1972).

IV. Estrogen Synthesis in Postgestational Choriocarcinoma *in Vitro*

Steroid biosynthesis in the trophoblastic cell lines have been determined by radioimmunoassay on fluid in which the cells are incubated or by specific tritium-labeled steroid precursor incubations. These incubations are analyzed by celite column chromatography or more recently by thin-layer chromatography with radiochromatogram scanning. In order to document specific steroidogenic properties of these tumor cells, extensive investigations of biosynthetic pathways are being carried out. It has been found that as in the normal placenta, trophoblastic tumor cells convert tritiated Δ^4-androstenedione to estrone and 17β-estradiol. For these experiments, the standard format employs isotopically labeled Δ^4-androstendione, labeled in the 1 and 2 positions with tritium. This is incubated in 10 ml of culture medium in plastic Falcon flasks containing approximately 8×10^6 trophoblastic tumor cells (BeWo line in this example). Incubations are performed for 3–9 hours at 37°C under atmospheric conditions. The incubation is terminated by addition of equal volumes of 95% ethanol. The combined cell and solvent mixture is then extracted with acetone. The resultant supernatant solution is evaporated *in vacuo* and subsequently extracted with ether. This is repeated for a total of three extractions. The pooled ether extract is then subjected to alkali treatment for separation of phenolic from neutral fraction, using the procedure of Huang and Pearlman (1962). The phenolic fraction, containing estrogen, is analyzed by reverse phase column chromatography on siliconized celite. Approximately 80% of the applied radioactively was eluted in the areas of both estrone and estradiol (Fig. 1). The estrogen fraction was later pooled. Carrier estrone and estradiol were employed, and further purification by partition chromatography on a nonsiliconized celite column was carried out. In these experiments, both estrone and estradiol were clearly separated from one another, and the radioactivity and optical density profiles superimposed (Fig. 2). Approximately 15% of the radioactivity was associated with carrier estrone and 52% with 17β-estradiol. The estrone and estradiol peak were separately mixed with additional carrier, and isotope dilution studies were carried out.

For estrone, after three recrystallizations, the specific activities of both crystal and mother liquid became constant and equal. The estrone purity from partition chromatography was greater than 96%. In the case of estradiol, three crystallizations were also required to achieve constant and equal specific activities of both crystal and mother liquid. The purity of estradiol from partition chromatography was nearly 92%.

The analyses of two separate experiments indicated that 3 to 5% of the added precursor was converted to estrone in 10 hours, while approximately 9% of the tritiated androstenedione was converted to estradiol. Thus, the formation of estradiol from Δ^4-androstenedione was 2–3 times greater than that of estrone.

The estrone and estradiol areas from partition chromatography have further been acetylated with pyridine and acetic anhydride. The acetylated

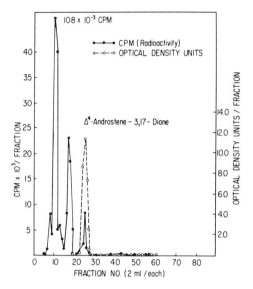

Fig. 1. Celite reverse phase column chromatography E_1 (estrone) and E_2 (estradiol) in initial peaks are pooled for partition reparation.

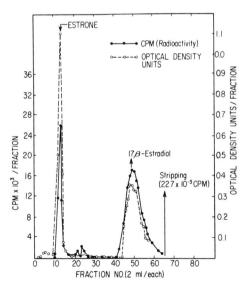

Fig. 2. Partition column chromatography on nonsiliconized celite column distinctly separates estrone (E_1) and estradiol (E_2).

products were resolved by partition column chromatography. The superimposition of both radioactivity and carrier steroid provided (Fig. 3) additional evidence that the two major peaks of radioactivity previously identified were indeed estrone and estradiol. The fact that these steroids as well as other placental hormones show immunosuppressive properties is of significance in this review (Waltman *et al.*, 1971).

V. "Spontaneous" Regression of Cancer

Of more than 1000 cases of "spontaneous" regression of cancer reported in the world literature (Everson, 1964), only 130 were accepted as having sufficient documentation to represent a probable example of true regression of cancer. Over 50% of the cases of spontaneous regression involved choriocarcinoma, hypernephroma, neuroblastoma, and malignant melanoma. More recent authors have investigated the effects of concomitant infections in spontaneous regression of cancers of the lung. It was found that abscess and empyema accompanying surgical therapy of lung cancers were associated with regression and ultimate resolution of persisting tumor. The overall 5-year survival rate for the associated empyema group of patients was 50% compared to an 18% survival rate for a

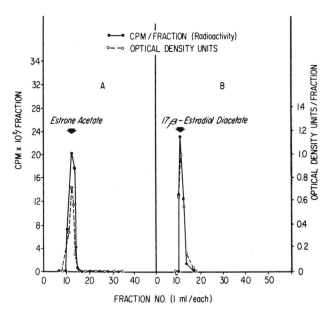

Fig. 3. Partition column chromatographic separation of acetylated estrone and estradiol derivatives indicated by complete superimposition of radioactivity and carrier steroid.

controlled group consisting of 34 random cases of lung cancer having surgical removal without associated empyemas (Ruckdeschel et al., 1972). It was postulated that this remarkable increase in survival was attributable to immunological defense mechanisms mediated by activation of regional immune cellular mechanisms. The reaction between immune lymphocytes and nonspecific bacterial antigens releases lymphokines and activates macrophages that may nonspecifically destroy residual tumor cells. The experiments of Coley (1906) using bacterial antigens in immune treatment of inoperable sarcomas have been largely ignored until the present time. The remarkable survival rate of these patients for more than 20 years following treatment with bacterial toxins of killed hemolytic streptoccocci and *Serratia marcescens* constituted the first successes with attempts to induce host reactions against autologous tumors.

Recent emphasis on stimulation of host defenses against neoplastic growth is based on many literature reports showing association between depressed immunological competence and the development of malignancies. Good (1972) has emphasized that the incidence of leukemia in Bruton type agammaglobulinemia shows that in patients with selective deficiencies of immunoglobulin synthesis and secretion, failure of antibody production, absence of plasma cells from the bone marrow and lymphoid tissues, and deficiencies of germinal centers is associated with a lack of B cells and plasma cells. This deficiency renders such patients unable to respond to intense antigenic stimulation. In contrast, their cellular immune mechanisms are completely intact as evidenced by the fact that these patients developed normal delayed type of sensitivity. Skin or graft rejection is not impaired. It can be concluded, therefore, that these patients, while not being able to form circulating antibodies, can handle cellular immune mechanisms quite normally. The incidence of leukemia in the Bruton type agammaglobulinemia is about 10% and is much increased over the normal expected incidence in this population.

In contrast to this depressed immune state, the association of tumor regression in the presence of lung abscesses depicts a heightened immune condition. These examples of spontaneous immune defense against neoplasia have stimulated investigators to attempt to actively immunize patients against their own tumor. Many such efforts have used specific tumor antigens, as well as nonspecific bacterial toxins, antigens, and adjuvants. Old et al., (1961) have utilized Bacillus Calmette-Guérium (BCG) strain of mycobacterium tuberculosis to protect animals from a series of experimental tumor challenges. In the human, Mathé et al., (1969) reported prolongation of chemotherapy induced remission of acute leukemia with the same immunogen, along with irradiated autologous leukemic cells. The success of treatment of malignant melanoma by direct injections of BCG organisms (Morton *et al.*, 1971) in localized skin lesions has given great impetus to this approach. Ruckdeschel *et al.*, (1972) have implicated specific macrophage reactions among the immune mechanisms responsible for the "spontaneous regression of residual tumor" in lung cancers. A possible mechanism involves tissue macrophage processing of antigenic information by the infecting organisms. The reactions to these organisms by immune lymphocytes generated by this macrophage lymphocyte interaction triggers a release of a group of soluble products or lymphokines that may destroy tumor cells. Prominent among these lymphokines is migration inhibitory factor (MIF), a soluble protein released by sensitized lymphocytes in the presence of antigen. It is capable of concentrating phagocytic macrophages at the site of the reaction. If macrophages destroy tumor cells (nonspecifically), the release of this factor would be of additional enhancement to tumor cell destruction by immune reactions against bacterial antigens. Other inhibitory factors include lymphotoxins (Granger *et al.*, 1969) and clonal inhibitory factor (CIF) (Lebowitz and Lawrence, 1969), which exhibit direct cytostatic or cytotoxic activity against human tumor cells in culture. Macrophage activating factor (MAF) (David, 1971), another product of lymphocyte antigen interaction, greatly enhances engulfing and killing capacity of macrophages. It has been emphasized (Mackaness, 1969) that specificity of antimicrobial cellular community exists only up to a certain degree in the efferent immune part. The production of immune lymphocytes, their accumulation at the site of inflammation, and their interaction with the synthesizing antigen, are all specific to the antigen in question. However, activated macrophages, the products of this reaction, are competent to destroy unrelated organisms. This may provide a mechanism of nonspecific tumor cell destruction. In addition to immune destruction of tumor cells by macrophages induced by bacterial products, the possibility of exposure of tumor-specific antigens on the surface of existing tumor cells by the activity of bacterial enzymes is also pertinent. This response of organisms elaborating various sialodases may permit tumors specific antigen exposure and with subsequent specific tumor cell response. It is likely that previously reported instances of "spontaneous regression" of cancer will likely be shown to have a host immunological basis.

VI. Malignancy and Immunosuppression

The success of kidney transplants in man has been to a large measure a result of the development of effective means for control of rejection phenomena. The employment of continuous immunosuppression, however, has been associated with a statistically significant increase in the incidence of malignancy arising in the immunosuppressed host. In several instances, the transplantation of malignancy has occurred in which inadvertent transfer of foci of malignant cells in the donor kidney occurred (Wilson *et al.,* 1968; Gatti and Good, 1971). In each instance, however, complete regression was achieved, even for widely metastatic tumors, by discontinuing the immunosuppression regimen. Both the allogenic organ transplant and the malignancy were rapidly rejected. In successful renal transplants, there is greater than 10-fold increase in the incidence of malignancy developing *de novo* in the immunosuppressed recipients (Gatti and Good, 1971).

The phenomena of aging or cellular senescence are associated with decreased immunological reactivity, particularly demonstrated in diminished cellular immunity shown in experimental mouse strains. In contrast, the capacity for immunoglobulin and autoantibody synthesis does not appear depressed with aging (Good, 1972). The imbalance of humoral and cell-mediated immune function may allow sufficient immunodeviation to permit an increased susceptibility to malignant proliferation with aging (Good, 1972).

Evidence has been presented that immunosuppressive procedures, including thymectomy (Defendi *et al.,* 1964), enhance chemical carcinogen induced malignancies. Other more recent analysis suggests that only malignancies induced by oncogenic viruses is influenced by immunosuppression (Allison and Law, 1968).

Some carcinogenic chemicals have immunosuppressive properties (Malmgren *et al.,* 1952), the duality of characteristics for immunosuppression and carcinogenic potential may provide increased carcinogenesis influence. The period of exposure and dose of the agents bear importantly on the potential of neoplastic induction.

Likewise, certain oncogenic viruses suppress cellular and humoral immune mechanisms (Dent *et al.,* 1965). Oncogenic viruses induce common surface antigens on transformed tumor cells which demonstrate tumor specific antigen properties (TSA). Virus-induced tumors produce specific antigens which are similar for all tumors induced by the particular virus in question. Accordingly, in experimental animals, a polyoma virus-induced malignancy, either hepethelia or stromal tissues, will display the same surface antigen. By contrast, a single chemical carcinogen inducing malignancy in different organs of the same animal will display different tumor specific antigen.

VII. Tissue Type Antigens

A. Histocompatibility

The major histocompatibility system in the human determining tissue types consists of a system of human leukocyte antigens (HL-A). A more extensively studied H-2 locus in the mouse has served as an accurate guide for transplantation experiments in the murine species (Bach *et al.,* 1972). Human graft rejection is in addition significantly affected by ABO blood group incompatibility. HL-A antigens are determined by genes on the single pair of autosomal chromosomes designated as the HL-A locus or region (McDonald *et al.,* 1970). They are complex loci divisible into two known (and possibly a "third") segments or subloci. The two subloci best defined are the first or "LA" and second or "Four" subloci. These loci contain four genes in every individual (two inherited from each parent) and are responsible for specifying a distinctive HL-A antigen on the surface of cells of that individual. There are at present 31 known HL-A antigens, each with its allele on the corresponding chromosome, i.e., HL-A 1, 2, 3, 9 located on LA locus; HL-A 5, 7, 8 located on "Four" locus (Fogerty Proceedings, 1972). The sublocus is used to designate the position on the chromosome wherein the genetic information for each segregant series of HL-A antigens is found. The corresponding alleles designates similar or alternate genetic determinants on the corresponding chromosome. Because there is very close linkage (0.5 recombinational units) between the two subloci, a given "LA" determinant will always travel together with the same "Four" determinants during fertilization, and thus haplotypes (the genetic information of the two series) on one chromosome of the offspring can be determined. The HL-A chromosomal region is inherited in block with the chromosomal combinations of one "LA" and one "Four" genetic determinant comprising the haplotype of that individual. These histocompatibility antigens are genetically controlled cell surface structures which differ between individuals. They are, in principle, defined by the fact that grafts exchanged between individuals which differ with respect to these antigens are rejected by the immune mechanisms of the recipient. At present, only some of these antigens are recognized by serological methods. This determination constitutes the current basis for tissue typing using the expression of these antigens on the formed elements of the blood. Most importantly, these cell surface gene products may play the critical role of control of the immune response in malignancy. Evidence has been presented suggesting that the H_2 locus in the mouse determines susceptibility to Gross leukemia virus in this species (Lilly, 1966). Methods for detecting HL-A antigens, include leuko-agglutination, cytotoxicity tests and mixed leukocyte cultures (MLC). Using cytotoxicity and agglutination tests for detection of tissue type surface antigens, various antisera will phenotypically identify these antigens controlled by the serologically definable loci (SD locus) in the human. In the mixed leukocyte test (MLC), responding lymphocytes of a recipient recognizes different antigens or foreignness on the stimulating lymphocytes of the donor. In the one way, MLC test the stimulator cells are blocked with mitomycin C, a DNA synthesis inhibitor, so that their antigens can be expressed but are inhibited from blast transformation and DNA synthesis, the measure of responsiveness.

B. HL-A in Choriocarcinoma, a Tumor Graft

It has been proposed (Mogensen and Kissmeyer-Nielsen, 1968) that survival of placental choriocarcinoma in the maternal host presupposes a high degree of histocompatibility between the fetus and mother as regards major transplantation antigens. This concept theorizes that choriocarcinoma, an allograft of fetal tissue in the maternal host, develops in an environment of homogeneity of maternal and fetal antigens. Accordingly, such tumors should receive one of the father's chromosomes carrying his histocompatibility antigens. Failure of tumor rejection may result if that chromosome fails to contain an antigenic determinant that can be recognized as foreign by the mother. Haplotype studies, obtained by serotyping the children of pregnancies in which choriocarcinoma developed showed that the children in 5 of these 6 families possessed no antigens not also present on their mother's cells (Mogensen et al., 1969). This finding provided the basis for their concept that the paternal chromosome inherited by these children and the associated choriocarcinoma contained no serologically detectable strong transplantation antigen not already present in the maternal genetic composition. However, evidence against this concept has recently been presented (Rudolph and Thomas, 1970) from histocompatibility studies in 3 patients with trophoblastic tumors and 14 of their children. Using one way mixed leukocyte cultures (MLC), cells from all 14 of the children stimulated the mother's lymphocytes, indicating the presence of antigenic differences. Significantly, leukocyte serotyping detected antigenic differences in only 6 children. It can be surmised, therefore, in contrast to (Mogensen and Kissmeyer-Nielsen, 1968) original findings, which employed only leukocyte serotyping with antisera, that all antigenic differences are not detectable by antisera alone.

Thus, the more sensitive MLC made it possible in this more recent study to detect antigenic differences. Thus, the results of these studies do not support the hypothesis that survival and dissemination of postgestational choriocarcinoma is dependent on a high degree of histocompatibility between the malignant graft deriving from the child's placenta and the maternal host. Similarly, mixed leukocyte cultures (Lewis, et al., 1966) from maternal and paternal pairs show that histocompatibility differences could be readily demonstrated by a responsive state between the paternal and maternal lymphocytes in the patients with trophoblastic tumors.

The above observations have been explained by Bach's findings (Bach et *al.,* 1972). He has differentiated these findings in the human HL-A and mouse H-2 systems by defining two regions of the respective chromosome, SD loci (serologically defined) and LD loci (lymphocyte defined). The former can be defined with antisera by serological means, whereas the latter can be defined only by lymphocyte interaction in mixed leukocyte cultures (MLC). These regions are the major histocompatibility loci, their allels controlling the respective tissue type antigens. In the mouse, genetic mapping of the H-2 locus (Bach *et al.,* 1972) has shown it to be composed of an SD region beginning proximal to the centromere, comprised of H-2K and H-2D loci. The LD region, on the other hand, contains the Ir locus (immune response) and an additional locus controlling serum protein levels. Though the presence of LD loci in man cannot yet be conclusively established, the striking similarities thus far identified make this a high probability. In the mouse, the Ir-1 gene product seems to be expressed in T lymphocytes and it has been suggested that it may control a T cell receptor site (Benacerraf and McDevitt, 1972). Bach *et al.,* (1972) has suggested that if the LD locus and the Ir locus are found to be the same, then the above noted receptors could act both as recognition molecules on responding cells and as foreign molecules on stimulating cells. Thus, any cell that has one or more Ir receptors which a second cell does not have might stimulate the second cell in MLC. If the LD locus product is different from the Ir product, the LD product might be recognized by T cells but may be incapable of stimulating B cells. An alternate possibility is that T lymphocytes may recognize differences in the spatial arrangement of antigens which may be controlled by the LD locus. At this point, it can only be stated that definition of immune response control mechanisms still pose a major challenge.

C. Histocompatibility in Pregnancy and Maternal Antibodies

In mixed leukocyte culture studies (Lewis *et al.,* 1966), lymphocyte transformation between normally pregnant women and their husbands have demonstrated that pregnant women exhibit a specific lack of responsiveness to their husband's leukocytes but do not show this in relation to the cells of unrelated males. This unresponsiveness appears to be specific for the paternal antigens of the existing gestation. However, no decrease in response to mitogenic stimuli could be detected in lymphocytes from pregnant females versus nonpregnant controls in studies with phytohemagglutinin (PHA) (Thiede *et al.,* 1968). Purtilo *et al.,* 1972) reported decreased responses to PHA. On the contrary, mixed husband–wife leukocyte cultures in 22 cases of aborted pregnancies (Halbrecht and Komlos, 1968) showed increased lymphocyte transformation and responsiveness suggesting a possible expression of failure to achieve "immunologic blocking necessary for allograft tolerance."

Since the fetus and its placenta are genetically distinct from its maternal host, a true biological example of an allograft is indeed present. Fundamental to the acceptance of such a concept is the demonstration of an immune response by the mother to the fetus and trophoblast. The entire placental organ derives from a single trophoblast precursor identifiable at the two-cell stage (Hertig, 1968). The primitive trophoblastic stem cell gives rise to the complete placental complex with its two epithelial cell types, the cellular or cytotrophoblast, and the plasmodial or syncytial trophoblast. The syncytial trophoblast is in direct contact with the maternal blood sinuses. Trophoblastic emboli can be found throughout the maternal blood stream and aggregate in the maternal lung, ultimately to be eliminated by the end of the postpartum period (Douglas et al., 1959). Antibodies to the placenta have been detected using fluorescent antibody methods (Hulka et al., 1961) on frozen tissue sections. The globulin factions of postpartum serum was obtained by precipitation with 20.4% sodium sulfate, tagged with fluorescein isothiocyanate and absorbed with mouse and rat liver powders. Specimens of the whole placenta obtained at delivery were frozen in the cryostat and submitted for immunofluorescence. Treatment of the sections with tagged postpartum globulin for 30 minutes resulted in localization of fluorescein in all cellular elements of the trophoblastic villus. When the section was first flooded with untagged postpartum globulin, sites of fixation on the tissue were blocked and subsequent treatment with tagged material failed to result in fluorescence.

It has been firmly established that leukocyte antibodies are present in the maternal host as a result of isoimmunization during normal pregnancy (Leventhal et al., 1970). Furthermore, the frequency of immunization significantly increases with parity, although leukocyte antibodies are also demonstrable in the primigravida (Ahrons, 1971). This can be shown by leukoaggluting and lymphocytoxic antibodies. These antibodies are likewise demonstrable in the umbilical cord circulation and were also directed against antigens from the father. Some leukocyte antibodies provoked by pregnancy disappeared shortly after delivery (Payne, 1962). Since placental trophoblastic emboli (Douglas et al., 1959) and blood cells carry antigens of the child, it may be suggested that immunization of the mother during gestation results from trophoblast and fetal cells in the maternal circulation. A third possibility is from HL-A antigens on the sperm (van Rood et al., 1964) since spermatozoa possess one of the 2 male HL-A haplotypes (Fellous and Dausset, 1970). Since no adverse effects of maternal leukocyte antibodies could be shown (Ahrons, 1971) and because of the enhancing effects of leukocyte antibodies in transplantation (Batchelor *et al.,* 1970), it has been suggested that leukocyte antibodies may be present in all normal pregnancies functioning as enhancing antibody which may represent a major mechanism of survival of the fetal allograft. A similar enhancing antibody may facilitate survival of malignant cells (Ahrons, 1971). Accordingly, maternal plasma has been shown (Leventhal *et al.,* 1970) by immunofluorescence to contain IgG antibodies which coat human lymphoid tissue culture cells of known HL-A specificity. In mixed leukocyte cultures, lymphocytes from five mothers were washed and tested against mitomycin treated cells from 13 of their children. This mixed leukocyte culture resulted in expected lymphocyte transformation *but* this could be abolished by addition of maternal plasma in 9 cases and diminished in 3. The decreased MLC activity could be shown to be a function of diminished stimulating capacity of cells bearing specific HL-A antigens. It was concluded that antibody present in maternal plasma can coat the cells to which the antibodies are directed as evidence by their decreased capacity to react immunologically in mixed lymphocyte cultures (Leventhal *et al.,* 1970). This effect may represent a "blocking" antibody mechanism which may protect the fetus from rejection by the maternal immune potential during gestation and may also protect malignant cells against host immune rejection. Indeed, it has been corroborated that autologous plasma factors (immunoglobulin or immune complexes) produce blocking of maternal cell mediated immune reactions to placental antigens (Youtananukorn and Matangkasombut, 1973).

VIII.   T and B Cells in the Immune Response

When grown in culture, the normal trophoblast undergoes cytolysis in the presence of allogenic or maternal lymphocytes (Currie and Bagshawe, 1967). Choriocarcinoma cells *in vitro* were likewise found to be lysed in the presence of host lymphocytes. Although the trophoblast expresses antigenicity *in vitro* (detectable by the maternal lymphocytes), there is no rejection of fetal trophoblast as would be expected of allogenic tissue. Currie and Bagshawe (1967) suggested that the sialomucin covering of the trophoblast when removed by trypsinization *in vitro* permitted expression of maternal lymphocyte cytotoxicity, an event which does not occur *in vivo* in normal pregnancy or in choriocarcinoma. These authors proposed that the negative electrical charge on the surface of the trophoblast, cancer cells, and host lymphocytes prevented effective cellular contact and cytolysis by immunologically competent lymphocytes. In addition to the net negative surface charge of choriocarcinoma cells in culture, it has been demonstrated in the author's laboratory that these cells also display a positive prepotential in common with other malignant cells in culture (Hause *et al.,* 1970).

Metcalf (1971) has emphasized that the initiation of an effective immune response against malignant cells requires processing of tumor antigens by macrophages which must be followed by contact with lymphoid cells which are specifically preprogrammed to bind the antigen. Such antigen-binding cells originate from multipotential hemopoietic stem cells which in the fetus arise in the yolk sac, migrate to the developing liver, and later populate in sequence the developing thymus, spleen, and bone marrow (Good, 1967). These stem cells during fetal and adult life continuously generate progenitor cells which are the precursors of the series of lymphoid, granulocytic, and erythroid lines. Antigen-binding cells develop in two organs, the thymus and bone marrow from which they migrate to lymph nodes and spleen. Although thymic and bone marrow lymphoid populations initially arise from a common source, there are specific properties acquired in the respective microenvironments which characterize the two populations as "T" (thymic derived/dependent) or "B" cells (Bursal-equivalent derived/dependent). The specialized function of these two populations involve production of cytotoxic or "killer" lymphocytes from "T" cell progenitors and antibody forming plasma cells and lymphocytes from "B" cell precursors (Miller and Mitchell, 1969). In the commonly used *in vitro* systems used to immunologically activate lymphocyte responses, the "T" lymphocytes respond to the mitogen, phytohemagglutinin (PHA) and "B" lymphocytes respond primarily to the pokeweed mitogen (PWM) (Janossy and Greaves, 1971). It has been suggested that the various mitogenic substances "bypass" the requirement for antigenic recognition and induce cells to undergo that pattern of response "normally" dependent on strict immunological activation (Coulson and Chalmers, 1964).

IX. Humoral Immunity and Blocking Antibodies (Antibody-Mediated Immunity—AMI)

Antibodies to the trophoblast in the postpartum period have been previously identified using the globulin fraction of postpartum serum and the fluorescent antibody method on tissue sections (Hulka *et al.,* 1961). Although the precise class of immunoglobulin to which these circulating antibodies belong was not identified, significant advances have been made in defining immunoglobulin classes as to structure and function. In general, immunoglobulins are glycoproteins synthesized by plasma cells and certain lymphocytes of the humoral immune system. All immunoglobulins consist of two pairs of light and heavy chains united by disulfide bridges. Light chains are designated by title kappa or lambda (not both), heavy chain by Greek letters denoting immunoglobulin class, i.e., IgA-α, IgG-λ, IgM-μ, IgD-8, and IgE$_E$). Protoeolytic digestion produces three fragments, two of which are identical (Fab) and contain a light chain and a portion of a heavy chain. Each Fab fragment contains a single antibody combining site, whereas the third fragment, the Fc fragment, containing the remaining portions of the heavy chain pair, is responsible for functional properties of the molecule. The various immunoglobulins, including IgA, G, M, D, and E all contain heavy chains by which their immunoglobulin class, and biological properties are identified.

Although immune reactivity to malignant tumors is mediated primarily by cellular toxicity, an initial humoral response precedes any such target cell destruction by immune lymphocytes. The presence of these two immunological responses in the host generally works in a complementary manner. However, in tumor immunology, there is a paradox in that there appears to be discordance between humoral- and cell-mediated immune responses. There is a substantial body of evidence demonstrating that antibodies actually protect tumors against otherwise effective sensitized lymphocytes (Hellström et al., 1971). The presence of such "blocking" or "enhancing" antibodies may result from the early development of humoral immunity preceding the appearance of cellular immunity with a resultant occurrence on noncytotoxic antibody. Recent evidence has indicated that this blocking activity may be mediated by an antibody–antigen complex (Sjögren et al., 1971). Similarly, "unblocking" serum activity has been identified in Moloney sarcoma regressor serum (Hellström and Hellström, 1970) and may correlate with antitumor effects of antiserum in vivo (Bansal and Sjögren, 1971). This noncytotoxic complex may prevent target cell destruction by "T" lymphocytes by covering surface antigenic sites without damaging or destroying the tumor cell. Similar mechanisms of immunological enhancement in tumor immunology may also exist in successful organ transplantation wherein blocking antibodies may prevent transplant rejection. Blocking antibodies were shown to play a significant role in immunological enhancement when hyperimmune serum from CBA tumor bearers was found to produce prolonged survival of tumor growth and to block target cell destruction by sensitized lymphoid cells (Takasugi and Klein, 1971). In addition, Acquired Tolerance has been suggested to be a result of the production of such blocking antibodies (Hellström et al., 1971). However, there is some evidence that the induction of antibody-mediated tolerance may depend critically on the ratio of antigen and antibody to which the cells were initially exposed (Feldman and Diener, 1971).

Immunoglobulin molecules on the membranes of lymphocytes were first discovered in the course of experiments wherein rabbit lymphocytes treated with anti-immunoglobulin allotype antisera induced transformation of these lymphocytes to blastogenesis (Sell and Gell, 1965). Subsequently, direct demonstration using immunofluorescence (Raff and Wortis, 1970), and "rosette formation" around lymphocytes with erythrocytes sensitized with immunoglobulins and bridged by antisera (Coombs *et al.,* 1970), permitted more direct demonstration of immunoglobulins on lymphocyte cell surfaces. Although "B" cells appear to carry far more immunoglobulins on their surfaces (Unanue *et al.,* 1971) than "T" cells; identification of theta antigens on "T" cells has provided a most accurate tool for exclusive differentiation of the latter cell type (Raff and Wortis, 1970).

Serum antibody levels have recently been the subject of intense investigation. Accordingly, there appears to be an equilibrium between circulating antibody and antigen in its free or antigen–antibody complex form. From the mass action principle, alterations in circulating antibody concentrations tend to induce a shift in the equilibrium towards free antigen or antigen–antibody complex with resulting increase or decrease in immunogenic stimulation of antibody synthesis (Bystryn *et al.,* 1970). Such antibody synthesis takes place within the immunogenic compartment of lymphoid organs rather than in the systematic circulation where the half-life of immune complexes is very short. Antigen is apparently fixed on macrophage cell surfaces which acquire contact with specific "T" and "B" lymphocytes. The resulting stimulated lymphocyte thus replicates and differentiates into an antibody-secreting cell (Nossal *et al.,* 1968).

The complement system represents an intricate biological complex interacting with immunoglobulins and cellular elements in the immune process. Characteristic multimolecular assemblages develop on cell surface membranes as a result of complement proteins activated by immune complexes. Complement and its associated enzymes thus cause marked alteration in cell surface properties eventuating ultimately in cell death. Many intermediate noncytolytic events take place however; these include release of histamine from most cells and platelets, directed migration of leukocytes and general properties leading to cell destruction, inflammation and promoting of coagulation (Müller-Eberhard, 1971).

"Blocking" or "enhancing" antibodies appear to play a major role in the survival of tumors as well as normal tissue allografts (Irvin *et al.,* 1967). Three major mechanisms have been proposed to explain these effects: (1) efferent inhibition of the immune response as a result of interference with the process, (2) central inhibition of the immune response by way of feedback inhibition, whereby circulating antibody inhibits the formation of sensitized lymphoid cells or more circulating antibody (Kaliss, 1966), and (3) efferent inhibition in which the enhancing antibody coats graft antigens so that they become inaccessible to sensitized lymphoid cells or to cytotoxic antibodies (Smith, 1968). Since cellular destruction occurs when antibodies react with target cells in the presence of complement, it would appear that efferent inhibition could only be mediated by noncytotoxic antibodies. In this regard, it has been shown that enzymatic digestion, which removes the

Fc portion of complement-fixing IgG antibodies, converts them from cytotoxic to enhancing antibodies (Chard, 1968). It must be noted, however, that both enhancing and cytotoxic activity against Sarcoma-I cells in mice were reported to reside in 7 S γ_2 fraction, whereas neither activity was present in the 7 S γ_1 fraction (Takasugi and Hildemann, 1969). Still further, it has been suggested that antigen density on cell surfaces may account for enhancing activity of cytotoxic antibody (Linscott, 1970).

X.   Cell-Mediated Immunity (CMI)

A lymphocyte dependent antibody (LDA) has been demonstrated in the serum of a patient with choriocarcinoma, which permits previously nonsensitized lymphocytes from the husband to destroy target tumor cells in the wife. The antibody in the patient's serum appeared to be directed against HL-A antigens of the father, presumably also present on the trophoblast tumor graft (Wunderlich et al., 1971). Several pathways of tumor cell destruction are believed to be operative in the course of immune reaction against malignant cells. Immune lymphocytes may destroy specific target cells as a result of direct interaction, with and without specific mediators. Most investigators agree that recognition of foreign tissue may be facilitated by a specific cell associated antibody (CAB) present on the surface of immune lymphoid cells. This antibody is believed to facilitate specific contact between immune lymphocytes and target cells. The actual process of cell destruction by the immune lymphocyte is believed to be brought about by interaction with the target cell membrane; release of nonspecific toxins and secretion of complement which combines with the humoral antibodies previously fixed on the target cell surface (Granger and Williams, 1971).

Since tumor associated antigens are generally localized on the plasma membrane and host cells are programmed to reject "foreign" tissue, the primary focus of tumor rejection phenomena is expressed through cytotoxic lymphocytes. After generation of sufficiently diverse antigen-binding cells in the bone marrow and thymus and their seeding in specific microenvironments in lymph nodes and spleen, the biological stage would appear to be set for necessary antigen processing by macrophages. This processing is thought to bring about antigen preparation suited for "T" and "B" cell interaction and for the generation of active progenies with killer cell and humoral antibody specificities.

Immunoglobulin surface antigen may act as antigen–antibody determinants on both "T" and "B" cells. Accordingly, cell surface antigen receptors on "B" cells have the general and specific properties of immunoglobulins of known classes (Makela and Cross, 1970). It is observed that anti immunoglobulin antisera bind to "B" lymphocyte receptors and that these immunoglobulins are similar, if not identical, to the antibody molecule eventually secreted by the same cell, that is, the particular cell surface receptors are believed to have similar specificity as the antibody to be secreted (Mäkelä and Cross, 1970). Likewise, antigen receptors on "T" lymphocytes have been alluded to as cell bound antibody or IgX where X is the unknown class of immunoglobulin. Using the "rosette" reaction in which lymphocytes bind foreign erythrocytes to their surface in a "rosette" arrangement, strong support for the presence of immunoglobulin on both "T" and "B" cells has been derived (Greaves and Hogg, 1971).

Mediators of cellular immunity constitute a large series of reactants in the cellular immune process. Cellular immunity clearly involves both immunologically specific and nonspecific components. While lymphocytes of thymus dependency comprise the major specific reactors, macrophages arising from a rapidly dividing pool of bone marrow promonocytes are also prominently involved. Critical in the cellular immune process is the large series of lymphocyte mediators which are released as a result of the interaction of sensitized lymphocytes with antigen or by the interaction with mitogens *in vitro*. These factors include those affecting macrophages directly, causing them to be attracted to the site, keeping them at the site and causing their activation. Significant among these factors are migration inhibitory factor (MIF), macrophage activating and macrophage aggregating factors, and chemotactic factors. Additionally significant in these reactions are the lymphocyte cytotoxic factors, i.e., lymphotoxins, growth inhibitory factors, such as clonal inhibitory factors. Other factors include skin reactive factors, blastogenic factors, interferon, immunoglobulins, and transfer factors. In addition to the important cellular factors in immunoresistance, there is also considerable evidence to suggest that specific genetic factors, (such as have been identified on the H-2 locus of the mouse chromosome, i.e., immune response gene, Ir), may be determinants of genetic susceptibility to neoplastic growth. There is also a suggestion of similar significance in the human HL-A system in some neoplasms.

XI.   Cell Surface Receptors in Choriocarcinoma and Prospects for Tumor Immunotherapy

Walborg *et al.* (1969) have shown that the agglutination of Novikoff ascites tumor cells by the plant lectins conconavalin A (Con A) and wheat germ agglutinin (WGA) is competitively inhibited by a crude sialoglycopeptide extract from the surface of these tumor cells. In collaboration with Walborg, we have studied similar receptor sites on the cell surface of choriocarcinoma cells in culture (BeWo Line) (Pattillo *et al.*,

1971b). With the Novikoff sialoglycopeptide, 5 μg per agglutination well resulted in 3-fold increases in the concentration of Con A necessary to yield half maximum agglutination of BeWo cells. The agglutination assays utilized 50,000 washed BeWo cells per well in plasmocrit floculation plates. The cell dispersion was mechanical in phosphate-citrate buffer and agglutinations were scored microscopically from 0 to 4+. The findings of cross-reacting binding sites on the surface of human trophoblastic and Novikoff tumor cells, demonstrated by sialoglycopeptide extracts and by the oligosaccharides methyl-α-D-mannopyranoside and 2-acetamido-2-deoxy-D-glucose, is a significant illustration of common cell surface changes in these unrelated mammalian tumor cells.

The recognition that human tumors are immunogenic to the host, and consequently, initiate an immune response, albeit insufficient to control tumor advancement, has given great encouragement to hopes for tumor immunotherapy. The observation that cancer patients exhibit depression of cell-mediated immunocompetence, in spite of continuously shed tumor antigens and circulating serum immunoglobulins, has focused significant attention on attempts to abrogate blocking factors. At the present time, the most helpful avenues for augmentation of tumor immunity appear in the area of (1) increasing the effectiveness of specific cell-mediated immunity, (2) general augmentation of immunity, (3) interfering with "blocking" or "enhancing" effects of antibody, and (4) contriving methods through which potentially cytotoxic lymphocytes and antibody may be concentrated against target tumor cells (Smith, 1972). In addition, encouraging results have recently indicated that significant inhibition of chemical carcinogen-induced tumors can be achieved by viral vaccines (Whitmire and Huebner, 1972). Of equal importance is the fact that these latter results add support to the concept that C-type RNA viruses may act as a major determinant in the development of cancers induced by chemical carcinogens. Because of the lack of knowledge of specific hormone effects on the immunology of neoplasia generally, this chapter has concentrated on a trophoblastic tumor model in which nearly all of the important endocrine parameters are maintained. This form of malignancy represents one of the most lethal tumors in biology, but at the same time may provide an ideal model in which major questions in clinical medicine may be posed and answered.

ACKNOWLEDGMENT

The author gratefully acknowledges the collaboration and stimulation of the Cancer Research and Reproductive Endocrinology Laboratory personnel in the preparation of this manuscript, particularly Robert O. Hussa, Ph.D., Michael T.Story, Ph.D., Eleanor Delfs, M.D., Richard F. Mattingly, M.D., Anna C. F. Ruckert, Martha Rinke, and to my secretary, Mary Konrad.

REFERENCES

Ahrons, S. (1971). *Tissue Antigens* **1**, 178–183.

Ainsworth, R. W., and Gresham, G. A. (1960). *J. Pathol. Bacteriol.* **79**, 185–192.

Alastair, D., Simmons, R., and Perlmann, P. (1973). *Cancer Res.* **33**, 313–322.

Allison, A. C., and Law, L. W. (1968). *Proc. Soc. Exp. Biol. Med.* **127**, 207–212.

Bach, F. H., Bach, M. L., and Klein, J. (1972). *Science* **176**, 1024–1027.

Bansal, S. C., and Sjögren, H. O. (1971). *Nature (London) New Biol.* **233**, 76–78.

Batchelor, J. R., French, M. E., Cameron, J. S., Ellis, F., Bewick, M., and Ogg, C. S. (1970). *Lancet* **2**, 1007–1010.

Benacerraf, B., and McDevitt, H. O. (1972). *Science* **175**, 273–279.

Bennington, J. L., Haber, S. L., and Schweid, A. (1964). *Dis. Chest* **46**, 623–626.

Bystryn, J. C., Graf, M. W., and Uhr, J. W. (1970). *J. Exp. Med.* **132**, 1279–1287.

Castleman, B., Scully, R. E., and McNeely, B. U. (1972). *N. Engl. J. Med.* **286**, 713–719.

Chard, T. (1968). *Immunology* **14**, 583–589.

Charney, J. (1968). *Nature (London)* **220**, 504–506.

Coley, W. B. (1906). *Amer. J. Med. Sci.* **131**, 375–430.

Coombs, R. R. A., Gurner, B. W., Janeway, C. A., Wilson, A. B., Gell, P. G. H., and Kelus, A. S. (1970). *Immunology* **18**, 417–429.

Coulson, A. S., and Chalmers, D. G. (1964). *Lancet* **2**, 819.

Currie, G. A., and Bagshawe, K. D. (1967). *Lancet,* **1**, 708–710.

David, J. R. (1971). *In* "Progress in Immunology" (B. Amos, ed.), pp. 399–412. Academic Press, New York.

Defendi, V., Roosa, R. A., and Koprowski, H. (1964). *In* "The Thymus in Immunobiology" (A. E. Gabrielsen and R. A. Good, eds.), pp. 504–520. Harper, (Hoeber), New York.

Dent, P. B., Peterson, R. D., and Good, R. A. (1965). *Proc. Soc. Exp. Biol. Med.* **119**, 869–871.

Douglas, G. W., Thomas, L., Car, M., Cullen, N. M., and Morris, R. (1959). *Amer. J. Obstet. Gynecol.* **78**, 960–969.

Edmonds, L. C., and Cerrera, G. M. (1965). *J. Pediat.* **67**, 94–98.

Everson, T. C. (1964). *Ann. N.Y. Acad. Sci.* **114**, 721–735.

Feldmann, M., and Diener, E. (1971). *Immunology* **21**, 387–404.

Fellous, M., and Dausset, J. (1970). *Nature (London)* **255**, 191–193.

Fogerty Proceedings. (1972). *Fogerty Int. Cent. Proc.* **31**, 1087–1104.

Gatti, R. A., and Good, R. A. (1971). *Cancer* **28**, 89–98.

Good, R. A. (1967). *In Birth Defects, Reprint Ser.* **PE RS-98**, 1–12 (reprinted from *Hosp. Pract.* **2**).

Good, R. A. (1972). *Proc. Nat. Acad. Sci. U.S.* **69**, 1026–1032.

Granger, G. A., and Williams, T. W. (1971). *In* "Progress in Immunology" (B. Amos, ed.), pp. 437–445. Academic Press, New York.

Granger, G. A., Shacks, S. J., Williams, T. W., and Kolb, W. P. (1969). *Nature (London)* **221**, 1155–1157.

Greaves, M. F., and Hogg, N. M. (1971). *In* "Progress in Immunology" (B. Amos, ed.), pp. 111–125. Academic Press, New York.

Halbrecht, I., and Komlos, L. (1968). *Obstet. Gynecol.* **100**, 173–177.

Hause, L. L., Pattillo, R. A., Sances, A., Jr., and Mattingly, R. F. (1970). *Science* **169**, 601–603.

Hellström, I., and Hellström, K. E. (1970). *Int. J. Cancer* **5**, 195–201.

Hellström, I., Hellström, K. E., and Allison, A. C. (1971). *Nature (London)* **230**, 49–50.

Hertig, A. (1968). *In* "The Human Trophoblast," pp. 24–27. Thomas, Springfield, Illinois.

Holmgren, N. B. (1968). *19th Annu. Meet. Tissue Cult. Ass.* Abstract No. 115, p. 53.

Huang, W. Y., and Pearlman, W. H. (1962). *J. Biol. Chem.* **237**, 1060–1065.

Huang, W. Y., Pattillo, R. A., Delfs, E., and Mattingly, R. F. (1969). *Steroids* **14**, 755–763.

Hulka, J. F., Hsu, K. C., and Beiser, S. M. (1961). *Nature (London)* **191**, 510–511.

Irvin, G. L., Eustace, J. C., and Fahey, J. L. (1967). *J. Immunol.* **99**, 1085–1091.

Janossy, G., and Greaves, M. F. (1971). *Clin. Exp. Immunol.* **9**, 483–498.

Jernstrom, P., and McLaughlin, H. (1962). *J. Amer. Med. Ass.* **182**, 147.

Kaliss, N. (1966). *Ann. N.Y. Acad. Sci.* **129**, 155–163.

Kosa, T., Levesque, L., Goldstein, D. P., and Taymor, M. L. (1973). *J. Clin. Endocrinol. Metab.* **36**, 622–624.

Lebowitz, A., and Lawrence, H. S. (1969). *Fed. Proc., Fed. Amer. Soc. Exp. Biol.* **28**, p. 630 (abstr.).

Leventhal, B. G., Buell, D. N., Yankee, R., Rogentine, C. N., Jr., and Terasaki, P. (1970). *In* "Proceedings of the Fifth Leukocyte Culture Conference" (J. Harris, ed.), pp. 473–486. Academic Press, New York.

Lewis, J., Jr., Whang, J., Nagel, B., Oppenheim, J. J., and Perry, S. (1966). *Amer. J. Obstet. Gynecol.* **96**, 287–290.

Lilly, F. (1966). *Nat. Cancer Inst., Monogr.* **22**, 631–641.

Linscott, W. D. (1970). *Nature (London)* **228**, 824–827.

McArthur, J. W. (1963). *Progr. Gynecol.* **4**, 146.

McDonald, J. C., Jacobbi, L., and Williams, R. W. (1970). *Transplantation* **10**, 499–504.

Mackaness, G. B. (1969). *J. Exp. Med.* **129**, 973–992.

McKechnie, C., Jr., and Fechner, R. (1971). *Cancer* **27**, 694–702.

McKerns, K. W. (1969). *In* "The Gonads" (K. W. McKerns, ed.), pp. 137–173. Appleton, New York.

McKerns, K. W. (1973). *Biochemistry* **12**, 5206–5210.

Mäkelä, O., and Cross, A. M. (1970). *Progr. Allergy* **14**, 145–207.

Malmgren, R. A., Bennison, B. E., and McKinley, T. W., Jr. (1952). *Proc. Soc. Exp. Biol. Med.* **79**, 484–488.

Mathé, G., Amiel, J. L., Schwarzenburg, L., Schneider, M., Cattan, A., Schlumberger, J. R., Hayat, M., and DeVassal, F. (1969). *Lancet* **1**, 697–699.

Medina, D., and Heppner, G. (1973). *Nature (London)* **242**, 329–330.

Metcalf, D. (1971). *Bull. Int. Union against Cancer* **9**, 308–310.

Miller, J. F. A. P., and Mitchell, G. F. (1969). Transplant. Rev. **1**, 3–42.

Mogensen, B., and Kissmeyer–Nielsen, F. (1968). *Lancet* **1**, 721–725.

Mogensen, B., Kissmeyer-Nielsen, F., and Hauge, M. (1969). *Transplant. Proc.* **1**, 76–79.

Morton, D. L., Holmes, E. C., Eilber, F. R., and Wood, W. C. (1971). *Ann. Intern. Med.* **74**, 587–604.

Müller-Eberhard, H. J. (1971). *In* "Progress in Immunology" (B. Amos, ed.), pp. 553–564. Academic Press, New York.

Nossal, G. J. V., Abbot, A., Mitchell, J., and Lummus, Z. (1968). *J. Exp. Med.* **127**, 277–289.

Odell, W. D., Bates, R. W., Rivlin, R. S., Lipsett, M. B., and Hertz, R. (1963). *J. Clin. Endocrinol.* **23**, 658–664.

Old, L. J., Benacerraf, B., and Clark, D. A. (1961). *Cancer Res.* **231**, 1281–1300.

Pattillo, R. A., Hussa, R. O., Delfs, E., Garancis, J., Bernstein, R., Ruckert, A. C. F., Huang, W. Y., Gey, G. O., and Mattingly, R. F. (1970). *In Vitro* **6**, 205–214.

Pattillo, R. A., Gey, G. O., Delfs, E., Huang, W. H., Hause, L., Garancis, J., Knoth, M., Amatruda, J., Bertino, J., Friesen, H. G., and Mattingly, R. F. (1971a). *Ann. N.Y. Acad. Sci.* **172**, Art. 10, 288–298.

Pattillo, R. A., Walborg, E. F., Jr., Hause, L. L., and Hussa, R. O. (1971b). *Proc. Conf.*

Workshops Embryonic Fetal Antigens Cancer, 1st, 1900 Vol. 1, pp. 313–329, CONF-710527.

Pattillo, R. A., Story, M. T., Hershman, J. M., Delfs, E. and Mattingly, R. F. (1972). *Proc. Conf. Workshops Embryonic Fetal Antigens Cancer, 2nd 1900* Vol. 1, pp. 45–52, CONF-720208.

Payne, R. (1962). *Blood* **19,** 411–424.

Prehn, R. T. (1972). *Science* **176,** 170–171.

Purtilo, D. T., Hallgren, H. M., and Yunis, E. J. (1972). *Lancet* **1,** 769–771.

Raff, M. C., and Wortis, H. H. (1970). *Immunology* **18,** 931–942.

Regan, J. F., and Cremin, J. H. (1960). *Amer. J. Surg.* **100,** 224–233.

Rosen, S. W., Becker, C. E., Schlaff, S., Easton, J., and Gluck, M. C. (1968). *N. Engl. J. Med.* **279,** 640.

Rubin, P. (1970). *J. Amer. Med. Ass.* **213,** 89.

Ruckdeschel, J. C., Codish, S. D., Stranahan, A., and McKneally, M. F. (1972). *N. Engl. J. Med.* **287;** 1013–1017.

Rudolph, R. H., and Thomas, E. D. (1970). *Amer. J. Obstet. Gynecol.* **108,** 1126–1129.

Sell, S., and Gell, P. G. H. (1965). *J. Exp. Med.* **122,** 423–439.

Sjögren, H. O., Hellström, I., Bansal, S. C., and Hellström, K. E. (1971). *Proc. Nat. Acad. Sci. U.S.* **68,** 1372–5.

Smith, R. T. (1968). *N. Engl. J. Med.* **278,** 1268–1275.

Smith, R. T. (1972). *N. Engl. J. Med.* **287,** 439–450.

Takasugi, M., and Hildemann, W. H. (1969). *Transplant. Proc., Part II* **1,** 530–534.

Takasugi, M., and Klein, E. (1971). *Immunology* **21,** 675–684.

Thiede, H. A., Choate, J. W., and Dyre, S. (1968). *Amer. J. Obstet. Gynecol.* **102,** 642–652.

Unanue, E. R., Grey, H. M., Rabellino, E., Campbell, P., and Schmidtke, J. (1971). *J. Exp. Med.* **133,** 1188–1197.

van Rood, J. J., van Leeuwen, A., Eernise, J. G., Fredericks, E., and Bosch, L. J. (1964). *Ann. N.Y. Acad. Sci.* **210,** 285–295.

Walborg, E. F., Jr., Lantz, R. S., and Wray, V. P. (1969). *Cancer Res.* **29,** 2034–2038.

Waltman, S. R., Burde, R. M., and Berrios, Jr. (1971). *Transplantation* **11,** 194–196.

Watchel, S. S., Gasser, D. L., and Silvers, W. K. (1973). *Science* **181,** 862–863.

Weil, R., and Kara, O. O. Jr., (1970). *Proc. Nat. Acad. Sci. U.S.* **67,** 1011–1017.

Whitmire, C. E., and Huebner, R. J. (1972). *Science* **177,** 60–61.

Wilson, R. E., Hager, E. B., Hampers, C. L., Corson, J. M., Merrill, J. P., and Murray, J. E. (1968). *N. Engl. J. Med.* **278,** 479–483.

Wunderlich, J. R., Rosenberg, E. B., and Connolly, J. M. (1971). *In* "Progress in Immunology" (B. Amos, ed.), pp. 473–482. Academic Press, New York.

Youtananukorn, V., and Matangkasombut, P. (1973). *Nature New Biol.* **242,** 110–111.

SUBJECT INDEX

A

ACTH
  adenylate cyclase activity, 311
  adrenal steroidogenesis, 309
  DNA synthesis, 347
  glycolysis stimulation, 347
  mitochondrial membrane influence, 294
  tumor action, 336
Acidic protein, transcription, 6
Adenine nucleotide, mitochondrial translocation, 184
Adenocarcinoma
  C3H Mouse, 12
  isoenzyme patterns, 35
Adenosine triphosphatase, tumor mitochondria, 141
Adenylate cyclase activity
  ACTH effect, 311
  hormone effect, 312
  rat adrenal, adrenocorticoid tumor, 310
Adenylate cyclase adrenocortical tumor, multiple hormone receptors, 321
Adenylate energy charge, 173
Adenylate kinase
  inductive response in liver, 188
  isozymes, 185
  kinetic comparison, 181
  mitochondrial function, 184
  neoplastic tissues, 178
Adenylate kinase molecular weight, 182
Adrenal steroidogenesis, calcium ion, 338
Adrenal tumor, 336
  ACTH binding, 336
  adenyl cyclase activation, 337
  adenylate cyclase activity, 312
  glycolysis, 347
  fine structure, 349
  metabolism of steroids, 351
Adrenocortical carcinoma, adenylate cyclase, 318
Adrenocortical cells, 11-β-hydroxylating enzymes, 294
Adrenocortical tumor
  adenylate cyclase, 324

cyclic AMP levels, 322
  hormonal control, 317
Aldosterone receptor, rat kidney chromatin, 11
Anti-estrogens, competition for receptor sites, 95
9-β-D-Arabinofuransyl adenine, DNA synthesis, 291
Aspartate reduction, tumor mitochondria, 150

B

Breast cancer cells, differences in acidic chromatin proteins, 23
Breast cancer remission, estrogen receptor correlation, 125
Breast cancer therapy, estrogen receptor assay, 96
Breast epithelial cell differentiation, estrogen and progestogen, 115
Breast tissue human
  biochemical characteristics, 108
  protein and nucleic acid content, 110

C

C3H adenocarcinomas
  glycolytic enzymes in, 37
  Krebs cycle enzymes, 41
C3H mammary adenocarcinoma, isoenzymes, 35
C3H mice
  breast cancer, 12
  phospholipid synthesis, 66
  preneoplastic mammary gland, 30
C3H mice mammary gland
  acidic chromatin protein, 18
  nucleic acid synthesis, 65
C3HBA adenocarcinoma, lactate utilization, 61
C3HBA mammary adenocarcinoma
  amino acid composition chromatin protein, 19
  chromatin protein separation, 17

389